Jean Meinke

303-791-1852

Praise for Best Herbs for Healing

"Both practitioners and patients will find this guide to popular herbal remedies useful. It is authoritative and readable."

—Andrew Weil, M.D., author of *Spontaneous Healing* and *8 Weeks to Optimum Health*

"Readers seeking detailed information on the most popular herbs ranging from aloe to vitex will find it all here. A unique state-of-knowledge rating system providing rapid evaluation of research, history, safety, and acceptance of each of the 40 herbs is invaluable."

—Varro E. Tyler, Ph.D., Sc.D., coauthor of *Tyler's Honest Herbal, Tyler's Herbs of Choice,* and *Herbal Medicine—Expanded Commission E Monographs*

"Of all the many recent books on herbal medicine, *Best Herbs for Healing* stands out as the one that is the best blend of evidence-based, rigorously researched herbal medicine, along with specific and practical guidelines for 21st century home health care."

—Christopher Hobbs, L.Ac., author of *Handmade Herbal Medicines*

"With their usual lucidity, McCaleb and associates assess 40 of the most important medicinal herbs."

—James A. Duke, Ph.D., author of *The Green Pharmacy*

". . . a magnificent reference to the appropriate and safe use of herbs. The authors are to be congratulated for pulling together so much information on how these botanical therapies work, from their traditional uses to clinical trials and contemporary applications in health care. This book belongs in the libraries of those who collect, utilize, or prescribe herbal medicines, as it is well-grounded in fact and scientific studies."

—Michael J. Balick, Ph.D., director and philecology curator of economic botany, The New York Botanical Garden

Best Herbs

FOR

Healing

The World's Most Potent
Herbal Remedies Scientifically
Ranked & Rated for Healing
Power & Safety

PRENTICE HALL

Robert s. McCaleb • Evelyn Leigh • Krista Morien

Illustrations by Wendy Smith

Prentice Hall edition reprinted with permission of Prima Publishing.

Originally published as *The Encyclopedia of Popular Herbs: Your Complete Guide to the Leading Medicinal Plants.*

1 2 3 4 5 6 7 8 9 10
Printed in the United States of America

ISBN 0-13-042553-2

ATTENTION: CORPORATIONS AND SCHOOLS

Prentice Hall books are available at quantity discounts with bulk purchase for educational, business, or sales promotional use. For information, please write to: Prentice Hall Special Sales, 240 Frisch Court, Paramus, New Jersey 07652. Please supply: title of book, ISBN, quantity, how the book will be used, date needed.

PRENTICE HALL
Paramus, NJ 07652

http://www.phdirect.com

Contents

PART III

Appendixes 399

Acknowledgments

The authors would like to express their gratitude to the dedicated team who helped make this book a reality. Special thanks to Margaret Blank, Mady Borofsky, Sandy Cottriel, Mindy Green, Aler Grubbs, Kathleen McKeon, Christine Meadows, Brenda Mehos, Timothy Minger, Lisa Podmajersky, Leslie Stevens, and the rest of the HRF staff and volunteers. Special acknowledgment also goes to Richard Scharffenberg, who has worked with us for the past 15 years to help build the HRF library of international journal literature. Thank you to Prima editors Marjorie Lery and Jennifer Risden for their skill and dedication as the manuscript assumed its final form.

The writers would also like to acknowledge the contributions of authors Paul Bergner, Kerry Bone, Steven Foster, David Hoffmann, Christopher Hobbs, Michael Murray, and Roy Upton, whose work was consulted in the preparation of the manuscript.

A PERSONAL NOTE

From Krista: I would like to thank Xavier for rubbing my temples after long hours of work. I am also grateful to Steve Luiting, Theo, and to the plants—especially violets and mullein.

From Evelyn: I would like to thank Rich Fifield for making me laugh, and my garden, for waiting for me.

From Rob: I would like to thank Susan Satter for helping both my life and my garden to blossom, and the mountains and the sky for inspiration and perspective.

How to Use This Book

In preparing this book, we have tried to keep in mind the information needs of our readers. First and foremost, the book is intended to be *practical*. In order to make the book both useful and complete, we wanted to present information in terms that everyone could understand as well as to include important details about the research on the use of each herb. The result is a book that presents herb uses, dosages, and other practical information that allows consumers to use herbs wisely, all presented in what we hope is an accessible and interesting format.

This book also includes detailed descriptions of some of the best research on each herb, which can help health-care professionals (including physicians, pharmacists, herbalists, and others) to evaluate the strength of the research support for each herb we discuss. In a sense, it is an herb book for you *and* your doctor, or if you *are* a doctor, for you and your patients. The general reader does not need to understand all of the specifics presented in the sections Scientific Support, Specific Studies, and How It Works, which tend to be a bit more technical than the other sections.

Here is a guide to the format used in the herb entries:

- **Names:** The common and scientific names as well as the plant family.
- **Part Used:** The part or parts of the plant most often used.
- **Primary Uses:** The most common uses for the plant. When the uses are not supported by strong clinical evidence, we list them as *traditional* or *experimental*.
- **State of Knowledge (Five-Star Rating System):** This chart offers a subjective judgment about the amount of research, the traditional use, the safety, and the international acceptance of each plant. The quantity and quality of evidence available for each plant is indicated by the number of stars, as shown:

Excellent	★★★★★
Very Good	★★★★
Good	★★★
Fair	★★
Poor	★

It is important to note that everything is relative. We have credited few herbs with 5 stars in any category, and a 4-star clinical rating does not necessarily indicate that the herb has undergone what might be considered contemporary state-of-art pharmaceutical efficacy and safety testing. Remember that any substance that has been the subject of the hundreds of millions of dollars worth of research typically expended on synthetic pharmaceutical drugs is probably a patented prescription drug, not a dietary supplement.

On the other hand, all herbs with four-star research and most with three-star research enjoy government approval *as drugs* in dozens of countries throughout the world. Our goal in providing this information is to show, at a glance, how strong the support is for each plant. We have separated the different kinds of evidence, as follows:

Clinical (human) research: Evidence resulting from direct clinical trials, which we consider the strongest evidence. However, not everyone believes the randomized clinical trial is the best way to research herbs.

Laboratory research: This category combines laboratory experiments conducted in glassware *(in vitro)* as well as animal-based *(in vivo)* pharmacological research. These types of research can be especially useful in determining mechanisms of action, or how an herb works, and are almost always used for initial research studies. We are well aware that there are serious ethical considerations pertaining to *in vivo* research, which we will not address in this book. There are, however, some cases in which clinical research would be impossible. For example, the research proving that milk thistle protects the liver from dangerous liver toxins obviously could not be conducted in humans. Our goal is to present the evidence, and we have not excluded evidence based on value judgments.

History of use/traditional use: The extent of historical, traditional use of herbs is a strong form of evidence. In most cases, we would not have *any* scientific research on an herb if it had not acquired a reputation through traditional use. Different people weigh this type of evidence in different ways. Some trust it more than laboratory research. Others tend to discount it as anecdotal and unreliable.

Safety record: The safety of an herb is evaluated in a number of ways (see Herb Safety in chapter 4). This rating is a subjective combination of traditional knowledge, pharmacology, clinical research, clinical use, and chemistry. We do not intend to imply that we have conducted comprehensive safety reviews for all of the herbs in this book, but we do believe this rating is a fair and accurate representation of the state of safety knowledge on each herb.

International acceptance: Many countries have developed ways to assess the safety and effectiveness of herbs used by their citizens. We list a general rating indicating the degree of acceptance for each herb, based on whether it appears in pharmacopoeias, is widely used, or has a strong reputation among scientists and practitioners.

After the rating system, we provide some general information about the herb, including interesting facts about the herb, its most common uses, and a summary of the sections that follow. These sections include:

• **History:** The history of an herb is often fascinating and relevant to modern use. This section describes how each herb came to humanity's attention and how it has been used in traditional medicine systems.

• **International Status:** This part gives some indication of the level of official acceptance and approved uses of the herb in various countries. It can help provide clues to how much human experience there has been with the herb and how much respect it is afforded by governments worldwide. This section is not intended to be comprehensive. There are many pharmacopoeias to which we did not have access in preparing this book. Their omission was not intentional.

• **Botany:** This section provides botanical details about the plant, but also often includes information about sources of supply, manufacturing processes, and other data about the herbal raw material.

• **Benefits:** A list of the health benefits provided by each plant. Please note that we have included some information that is not conclusive, using the term *may* to indicate the uncertainty.

• **Scientific Support:** This key section describes the scientific research on each herb, including studies that support the use of the herb and those that do not.

• **Specific Studies:** Under this heading, we include detailed descriptions of some of the best studies. This part may be more technical than some readers are comfortable with. It is not necessary to understand all of the information presented to gain an appreciation for the depth of scientific inquiry represented by each study. Things to watch for in evaluating the quality of individual studies include the number of partici-

pants, the duration of the study, and the statistical significance of the results. Also note the specific measurements used to evaluate the results and their relevance to the effect(s) being investigated.

• **How It Works:** Many scientists consider an understanding of the mechanism of action a critical part of the evidence for the use of drugs. However, often we know *what* something does long before we understand *how* it works. We have attempted to thoroughly describe the known or proposed actions of each herb, at the same time demystifying the subject as much as possible by explaining some details of physiology and the significance of specific actions.

• **Major Constituents:** A list of some of the chemical compounds found in the herb. Wherever possible, we have included those that are considered most important to the herb's benefits. However, in many cases, we simply do not know which compounds contribute most significantly to an herb's effects.

• **Safety:** This section includes information about the overall safety of each herb, plus side effects, contraindications, and drug interactions, if any are known.

• **Dosage:** Research on many herbs has included a variety of forms (powdered herb, standardized extracts) and dosages, plus laboratory studies in which doses must be calculated to account for human body weight. Our first choice is to list dosages shown to be effective in clinical trials, followed by those from official sources, and finally, those based on traditional use. To avoid confusion, we have not presented all available dosage information, only that which we consider to be the most reliable.

• **Standardization:** In most modern nations, standardized herb extracts are the most popular herbal products in use today, as well as the most extensively researched and the most accepted by researchers, physicians, and regulators. Whenever possible, we include details about the compounds and levels to which each herb is typically standardized.

• **References:** All studies cited in the book are referenced. Keep in mind, though, that there are often many more studies that we could not include. We have tried to select and present the best research available on each herb. As one of its primary activities, the Herb Research Foundation maintains a specialty library of the latest medicinal herb information. This book has been made possible by more than 15 years of determined collection of scientific information on the health benefits of plants.

PART I

The Modern Herbal Renaissance

CHAPTER 1

What Are Herbs?

When we talk about herbal medicine, many images come to mind: the medicine man or shaman in the rainforest, the wise Chinese sage, the Greek philosopher/physician, and the modern scientist searching the jungle for the next new medicine. The plants we call herbs include all types: grasses and flowers, trees, vines and shrubs, even mosses and mushrooms. There are thousands of them—probably more than 10,000 different species worldwide. When talking about medicinal plants, the botanical definition of "herb"—that is, a nonwoody plant that dies back in winter—doesn't really apply. After all, herbal medicine includes both herbs, such as ginseng and garlic, and woody plants, such as ginkgo and Siberian ginseng. In the botanicals business, herbs are defined as "plants or plant parts that are used for savory, aromatic, or other uses." In this context, "other uses" might mean nutritional, medicinal, or even religious uses, like the burning of sagebrush in Native American spiritual rituals.

In the modern world, the primary uses of herbs have settled into three categories, more or less: cooking, health care, and fragrance. The uses, properties, and varieties of plants commonly called herbs are so vast that it is virtually impossible to come up with an all-inclusive definition. This book is about some of the most popular medicinal plants used in health care, so here, for our purposes, is a working definition of "herbs":

> Herbs are plants or plant parts that are used in fresh, dried, or extracted form for promoting, maintaining, or restoring health.

HISTORY OF HERBS IN MEDICINE AND PHARMACY

Herbs were our first source of medicine, and their use far predates history. No one knows exactly when humans first began using plants for medicine, but evidence of at least six medicinal plants was found in a

3

Neanderthal burial site estimated to be at least 60,000 years old.[1] The early history of medicine is also the history of herbal medicine. The first books written about medicine were also the first books written about herbs, including Chinese texts from 5,000 years ago, such as the famous herbal of the Yellow Emperor, and the Ebers papyrus, an Egyptian text written 3,500 years ago. In Western medicine, the father of modern medicine is Theophrastus, also the father of modern botany. In 320 B.C., Theophrastus published the first book describing plants in detail, which was also the first Western book (Greek, in this case) about their medicinal uses.

Simply stated, herbal medicine has been at the heart of medicine in every culture in the world at every time throughout history. Even today, according to the World Health Organization, more than 80 percent of the world's population rely on herbal medicines as their main source of health care.[2] This figure includes not only the large populations of China and India and all of the less-developed countries of the world, but also many modern nations. In fact, even in the United States, about 25 percent of our prescription medicines are still extracted from plants or are synthetic copies of plant chemicals,[3] and at least 57 percent of our top prescription medicines are derived in some way from plants. That is, they are *semisynthetic,* meaning that plant chemicals are used as building blocks for synthetic drugs.[4] For example, vitamin C can be made from corn-starch. A drug made from a plant chemical doesn't necessarily resemble anything naturally found in the plant, but it could not be made without the plant chemical as a starting point.

Herbs Versus Drugs

The concept of making drugs in the laboratory is newer than most people realize. The first synthetic chemical was produced in the mid-nineteenth century, and the widespread use of synthetic drugs began during the last 70 years. In the United States, more than in any other nation, natural remedies were replaced by powerful synthetic or highly purified "wonder drugs." The advances of modern medicine in the twentieth century have truly been wondrous. New medicines, especially antibiotics, provided cures for previously incurable diseases, and vaccines brought under control fatal or crippling diseases, including smallpox and polio. On the other hand, in our haste to embrace "scientific" medicine, we quickly forgot the contributions nature made and still makes to medicine. Indeed, neither antibiotics nor vaccines are synthetic. And most synthetic drugs are just duplicates or modifications of the same plant chemicals that make herbs work.

For example, one of the world's oldest known cultivated medicinal plants is the Chinese herb ma huang, or ephedra, which has been grown for over 5,000 years in China for treating respiratory disease, including asthma. Ephedra is the source of the modern drugs ephedrine, still used today to treat asthma, and pseudoephedrine (what we know as Sudafed), which is used as a nasal decongestant. These chemical compounds can be made synthetically in a laboratory, but they are no more effective than the plant itself; they are merely more concentrated.

During the last two centuries, scientists began conducting laboratory experiments to learn more about medicinal plants, how they work at the cellular level in the body, what chemicals are the most powerful, and in some cases, how herbs can be risky if overused or if used in improper combinations. However, the focus of research in the twentieth century shifted away from the study of whole plants toward single "active principles" and synthetic chemicals. Plant medicine research in the United States came to a virtual standstill as doctors and scientists turned increasingly to potent medicines fabricated in the laboratory. The medicinal use of plant drugs declined, although single pure plant chemicals were still in use.

Soon, pharmacists and doctors no longer needed to know about the plants themselves, and courses on plant medicines disappeared from medical and pharmacy schools. At the same time, public funding for medical research became focused primarily on cancer and later on AIDS, leaving little support for research on innovations in natural medicines. Drug companies focused their research efforts on developing synthetic drugs they could own through patent protection (see Government Regulation of Herbal Products).

The scientific study of medicinal plants continued, but mostly in places where they were still considered an important part of health care, such as Europe and Asia. In the United States and western Europe, researchers who concerned themselves with plant drugs concentrated on isolated plant constituents rather than whole herbs or crude extracts. For example, until recently, there was hardly any research on the health effects of green tea, whereas thousands of studies were conducted on caffeine. There is much more research on the alkaloid berberine derived from goldenseal than on goldenseal itself, and although numerous studies exist for ephedrine and pseudoephedrine, few have examined the plant ephedra (ma huang) or its extracts.

The pace of medicinal herb research done by European scientists accelerated rapidly from the 1960s to the present. Today, most of the best herb research is performed in Europe, primarily because European modern medicine never abandoned the use of complex or "crude" plant drugs and their extracts. In fact, with favorable treatment from European governments, *phytomedicine* (plant medicine) flourished, and companies developed sophisticated herb extracts, sponsored research, and built the European phytomedicine empire that today is revolutionizing medicine worldwide. While American doctors, scientists, and regulators decried the lack of sound evidence for medicinal herbs, European scientists conducted the studies that made phytomedicine a dominant form of therapy there.

CURRENT WORLDWIDE USE OF HERBS

Today in many modern nations, herbal phytomedicines (sometimes called *phytopharmaceuticals*) are among the most popular and widely used medicines. Germany is probably the most advanced in the use of these high-tech plant medicines. Herbal medicines are government approved and sold with medicinal claims throughout Europe and most of Asia, as well as in Australia, Mexico, and Canada. In other countries, limited health claims are allowed, based on traditional uses. In fact, in an informal review by the U.S. Commission on Dietary Supplement Labels, 11 of the 14 countries reviewed had an abbreviated method for allowing informative medicinal label claims on herbal products.

In many parts of the developing world, herbal medicine is practiced virtually the same way it was centuries ago. Traditional healers diagnose conditions and prescribe often-complex mixtures of dried roots, barks, leaves, flowers, and fruits, which are taken in a variety of ways. Technologically advanced nations attempt to control and regulate herbal medicines like other drugs, sometimes improving the reliability of these time-honored treatments, but sometimes creating unforeseen problems.

The most widely practiced form of herbal medicine in the world is probably traditional Chinese medicine (TCM), in use not only in China but also throughout Asia and, as a form of alternative medicine, in the United States and Europe. TCM, which frequently combines 10 or more herbs in each formula, is probably used to some extent by more than one-third of the world's population. However, by far the most officially accepted forms of herbal therapies today are those supported by modern clinical research, usually involving semipurified, standardized extracts of single herbs or simple combinations of less than six herbs. The highest-quality research is on single-herb extracts such as ginkgo, St. John's wort, and saw palmetto.

GOVERNMENT REGULATION OF HERBAL PRODUCTS

Many people believe that the decline of herbal medicine was the result of the discovery or invention of safer or more effective medicines than the herbal remedies used by our ancestors. The truth is that synthetics overtook natural medicines in the pharmacy because of money and laws, not science and medicine. In the early twentieth century, the U.S. Congress became alarmed by questionable "patent medicines" sold by unscrupulous medicine men. Some of these medicines were quite dangerous and some were useless. Congress passed laws that established the Food and Drug Administration

(FDA) and required foods and drugs to be proven safe before they could be sold. In the decades that followed, as more sophisticated and expensive testing methods were devised, it became increasingly expensive to establish the safety of drugs.

In 1962, Congress passed the additional requirement that drugs be proven effective, further increasing the cost of drug approval. According to the drug industry, it now costs an average of $350 million to prove that a drug is safe and effective, and it can take 5 to 12 years, or even more, to gain approval to sell the drug. Once a drug is on the market, a drug company can recover its losses through the sale of the drug, but only if the company has the exclusive right to sell it. The problem with herbal medicines is that herbs are not patentable, so no one can gain the exclusive right to sell an herb. Patent law is designed to protect inventors, but it also prevents people from claiming they invented common things that were already known. Common substances such as ice— or ginseng—have been known for too long to be patentable. So if a company chose to spend $350 million to prove that ginseng is safe and effective, anyone could sell it as a safe and effective drug. Patent law prevents them from "owning" ginseng, and rightly so. No one owns folk medicines. They belong to everyone.

Still, the effect of regulation and economics on herbal medicine and plant-based pharmaceuticals has been chilling. Since 1962, not a single new complex plant drug has been approved in the United States. Since herbs could not be sold and promoted as medicines, they were regulated as foods, or sometimes as food chemicals (additives). Today, herbs, as well as vitamins and minerals, are classified as dietary supplements in the United States.

The Introduction of DSHEA

The FDA and the U.S. herb industry have locked horns repeatedly during the past 30 years. In 1994, the U.S. Congress unanimously passed a bill called the Dietary Supplement Health and Education Act (DSHEA), which defined dietary supplements and forbade the FDA from treating them as food chemicals or drugs unless manufacturers made drug claims for their products. Most important, DSHEA allows dietary supplements to bear health benefit claims called "statements of nutritional support," which are commonly referred to as *structure/function claims* because they may describe the effect of the supplement on the structure or function of the body. These statements cannot be drug claims, however, and must be truthful and not misleading. They must be supported by scientific evidence, and must be accompanied by a disclaimer that the product is not intended for treating or preventing disease. With the passage of DSHEA, the United States changed virtually overnight from one of the most hostile regulatory environments in the world for herbs to one of the most progressive.

Although details must still be worked out, DSHEA allows fairly informative labeling of products without prior government approval, yet requires a scientific basis and truth in labeling, which the FDA is empowered to enforce. There have been some abuses of the new law, however, both because of opportunists making exaggerated claims and because of inadequate scrutiny by the FDA.

There is no doubt that DSHEA played a major role in influencing the growth of herb sales in the United States. Shortly after its passage, major drug companies that had always opposed the use of alternative medicines (for obvious financial reasons) suddenly began to develop herbal product lines, which are sold today in virtually every pharmacy, discount store, and grocery in America. However, DSHEA is clearly a compromise solution to the regulation of herbs for health care. Better models allowing more frank and informative labeling of herbal products will surely arise. Ways to incorporate traditional medicines such as TCM and Ayurvedic medicine into regulatory models are also needed, as these systems do not fit well within the framework of DSHEA. The German regulatory system also lacks an appropriate mechanism for those remedies, whereas the system used in France and Canada may work somewhat better. The latter type of system focuses on informing the public about traditional uses, rather than expecting strong scientific backing of all remedies.

The Future of Herb Regulation

As herb use continues to increase worldwide, wise and appropriate regulation of herbs in health care will continue to be developed and refined. As health-care consumers, we all have the same goals. For our families and ourselves we want the best, safest, most appropriate, and cost-effective remedies available, whether natural or synthetic. We want safety, effectiveness, and quality. We want to know what our options are, and we want full, frank, and honest disclosures of everything known about the substances we use in health care. Government regulation should be designed to deliver just that.

As the U.S. Congress affirmed with the passage of DSHEA, people want to assume a more active role in their own health decisions. Although the government has a legitimate role to play in protecting the public from fraud, it should go no further than necessary in controlling information. Information is the key to informed self-care and individual choice. The best solutions in regulation are those that create incentives for research and the development of innovative, high-quality health products.

In the area of herbs, it is crystal clear that the European regulatory model has provided greater research incentives for herbs than the FDA model, which crippled American medicinal plant research. European regulations made European drug companies the leaders in natural products medicine. The changes in U.S. supplement regulation have finally opened the doors in a way that brings better funding and a greater diversity of companies into the health-care marketplace. The resulting competition will quickly punish those who are shown to have inferior products, whereas high quality will be rewarded with increased consumer trust.

REFERENCES

1. Soleck RS, Shanidar IV. A Neanderthal flower burial in Northern Iraq. *Science* 1975; 190: 880.

2. Farnsworth NR, Akerele O, Bingel AS, et al. Medicinal plants in therapy. *Bulletin of the World Health Organization* 1985; 63(6): 965–981.

3. Farnsworth NR. The role of medicinal plants in drug development. In: Krogsgaard-Larsen P, Christensen SB, Kofod H, eds. *Natural Products and Drug Development.* Copenhagen: Munksgaard, 1984: 17–30.

4. Grifo F, Newman D, Fairfield AS, et al. The origins of prescription drugs. In: Grifo F, Rosenthal J, eds. *Biodiversity and Human Health.* Washington, DC: Island Press, 1997: 131–163.

CHAPTER 2

Herbs in Modern Health Care

There is a major trend today toward greater personal responsibility and choice in health care. People are taking the initiative to learn more about their health and different treatment options for health conditions. They are less willing simply to follow "doctor's orders" without better understanding what alternatives may exist. People are becoming more involved in the decision-making process on issues affecting their own treatment. This trend toward self-care is a positive one, and one that has the potential to dramatically reduce health-care costs. As U.S. Congressman Henry Waxman said, "Pennies spent on self-care save dollars on health care." Currently, Americans pay twice as much as Europeans and three times as much as Japanese for health-care costs as a percentage of the gross national product, yet fare worse than both groups in health statistics such as longevity, infant mortality, cancer, and heart disease rates.[1]

THE IMPORTANCE OF PREVENTIVE MEDICINE

The American culture is liberally steeped in the value of preventive medicine. From an early age, we learn that "an ounce of prevention is worth a pound of cure," "an apple a day keeps the doctor away," and "a stitch in time saves nine." Physicians have long advocated changes in diet and lifestyle to reduce risk factors for serious diseases. In the past decade, doctors and pharmacists have become more aware of using herbs and nutrients as preventive medicines, and many are now recommending them. Partly this is due to increased research and publicity, and partly to increased education about health-care alternatives. The past few years have seen a steady increase in the number of physicians attending continuing education courses in alternative medicine, including seminars taught by the Herb Research Foundation through programs at Harvard and

Columbia Medical Schools, among many others.

Although preventive medicine is not a new concept, it does not seem to fit easily into our current health-care system. Joseph Jacobs, M.D., former director of the National Institutes of Health, Office of Alternative Medicine, described the American medical system as "a sick-care system, not a health-care system." In other words, the term "preventive medicine" is typically used to describe early disease detection (for example, mammograms, regular physical exams, and blood testing)[2] and not the concepts of wellness and preventive medicine.

In more than 50 years of regulation by the U.S. Food and Drug Administration (FDA), not a single over-the-counter (OTC) medication was approved for internal use in the prevention of any major disease. Ironically, aspirin was approved not long ago for stroke prevention, although it may be the most toxic blood thinner available. Prior to this, the only FDA-approved OTC preventive medicines were fluoride toothpaste, sunscreens, motion sickness pills, and, recently, indigestion preventives.

Clearly, something has been missing in American health care. Today, growing numbers of people recognize that preventive medicine and self-care are the keys to lowering health-care costs while improving overall health. And more and more people realize that herbs—in combination with positive lifestyle changes—can play a vital role in helping them lead longer, healthier lives.

Safe, low-cost herbal remedies are becoming the first choice of thousands for the treatment of simple, everyday health problems. But perhaps most promising of all, herbs have value as preventive medicines. Clinical research continues to shed light on the potential health-protective properties of a wide variety of medicinal plants.

Examples of Preventive Herbal Medicines

Among the best-researched European phytomedicines, all of which are available in the United States, are agents that can reduce the risk of all four of the leading natural causes of death in the United States: heart disease, cancer, respiratory disease, and liver disease.

Heart Protectants

Since heart disease is America's most serious health risk, any program designed to maintain and optimize health must start with protecting the cardiovascular system. This means reducing artery-clogging cholesterol, preventing the oxidation of blood fats, and maintaining a strong, steady heart beat. The best-researched herbal remedies for reducing blood fat levels (cholesterol) and for obtaining other cardiovascular benefits include garlic, hawthorn, ginger, horse chestnut, bilberry, reishi mushroom, and the Ayurvedic herb guggul.[3–9] (See specific herb entries for more information.)

ANTICANCER HERBS

Cancer is perhaps the most feared disease because of its relentless progression and often poor prognosis. Population studies have shown that garlic protects against stomach cancer, one of the most common and least treatable cancers.[10] Reishi mushroom has impressive antioxidant and anticancer benefits, as do shiitake and maitake mushrooms. Siberian ginseng is a powerful immune system stimulant, and green tea extract can inhibit the production of cancer-causing chemicals in the intestines. Astragalus has been shown in the laboratory to stimulate the white blood cells of people with cancer, an action that strengthens the body's natural defenses. (See specific herb entries for more information.) In addition, the group of compounds called *flavonoids*, found in many of the most popular and healthful herbs, fruits, and vegetables, offers strong antioxidant properties that can protect DNA and strengthen immune function. Population studies clearly show less cancer in people who consume more flavonoid-rich foods and herbs.

Flavonoids and other antioxidants are important protection for the human body against the damaging effects of oxygen "free radicals." These free radicals (now more properly called *reactive oxygen species*) are produced each day as our cells burn fuel for energy, and can damage cell walls, lipids, DNA, and proteins, including enzymes.

The effect of free radicals in the human body has been compared to the damage caused by oxygen in a home furnace. The damage occurs so slowly that it is invisible until the day the furnace breaks down. Scientists consider oxidative damage to be one of the main mechanisms of aging, and antioxidants are considered anti-aging compounds. They work by capturing or "quenching" oxidants (free radicals), preventing them from producing damage.

PREVENTION OF LIVER DISEASE

The liver is one of the most vital organs in the body, equal in importance to the brain and the heart. Because the liver is responsible for metabolizing and eliminating toxins, and because all the blood in the body flows through it daily, it is subject to damage from a variety of toxic substances. Milk thistle protects the liver through powerful antioxidant effects and other mechanisms of action, and its extract is used in clinics and emergency rooms in Europe to combat serious cases of liver poisoning, to treat cirrhosis and hepatitis, and to aid in detoxification from alcohol or drug abuse. Scientific evidence suggests that artichoke leaf, medicinal mushrooms, turmeric, and other herbs also have liver-protective promise.

RESPIRATORY PROTECTION

Most people are surprised to learn that respiratory disease is the third major cause of death in America. In the elderly, as immune function declines, simple colds and flu often progress to life-threatening pneumonia. Especially for highly susceptible people, it is important to use every defense available to keep these "nuisance" diseases from raging out of control. Clinical research shows that echinacea stimulates the immune system and is effective in lessening the severity and shortening the duration of colds and flu. Astragalus also decreases the duration and frequency of colds.

Migraine Prevention

Although migraines are rarely life-threatening, they can seem that way to those who suffer from them. Feverfew leaf is a safe, inexpensive migraine preventive that has been shown to work even for some individuals who do not benefit from conventional treatments for migraine. It is thus one of the best examples of effective preventive medicine for a specific health condition.

Men's and Women's Health

Saw palmetto, nettle root, and pygeum have been proven effective in preventing the progression of benign prostate disease in men, while black cohosh and vitex (chasteberry) have a long history of use and a strong reputation for helping to maintain normal hormonal balance in women. The latest popular botanicals for easing menopause symptoms—and possibly preventing cancer—are plants high in compounds called isoflavones, such as soy and red clover.

Vision Problems

Bilberry, a stimulant of microcirculation in tiny blood vessels known as capillaries, appears to have unique benefits for the eyes, protecting against night blindness, cataracts, and possibly glaucoma. It also has cardiovascular benefits, tones and strengthens the capillaries, and helps protect against ulcers. Grape seed extract also has been shown to improve symptoms of some vision problems and to support the health and structure of the eye.

Overall Well-Being

Ginseng, Siberian ginseng, and astragalus show intriguing benefits in improving both mental and physical performance. Ginkgo increases the circulation of blood and oxygen to the brain to help improve and maintain memory and mental function. The medicinal mushrooms, revered as longevity tonics in the Orient, have protective effects against cancer, heart disease, and liver disease, and also stimulate the immune system. Although people have long scoffed at the idea of a longevity pill, today it is less and less far-fetched to think that we may live better and longer lives through the use of natural remedies that protect against so many of our greatest health risks.

Treating Illnesses with Medicinal Herbs

In addition to preventive actions, natural remedies from plants can serve as safe and effective direct replacements for proprietary prescription and over-the-counter drugs. One of the strongest benefits of herbs is that they work with the body, often bringing equal or superior results with less risk than strong synthetic drugs. Echinacea and other immune stimulants can boost our natural resistance to simple infections by making our white blood cells work harder. Antibiotics, on the other hand, are lethal to bacteria, but can promote the emergence of dangerous, antibiotic-resistant microbes.

The common cold provides a well-documented example of how effective herbs can be in providing symptomatic relief. Herbal immune stimulants can not only help prevent colds, but can also shorten the duration and lessen the severity of colds once symptoms have set in. The best-known herbal immunostimulant is echinacea, which heightens the overall activity of the immune system.[11] The Chinese immune stimulant herb astragalus has also demonstrated clinical effectiveness against colds.[12] Eucalyptus leaves, peppermint, chamomile and lavender flowers, cardamom, wintergreen, and many other botanicals are well known for containing beneficial aromatic compounds that help alleviate nasal congestion.

The Chinese herb ma huang, or ephedra (*Ephedra sinica*), contains pseudoephedrine, the same powerful decongestant compound used to make over-the-counter decongestants such as Sudafed, as well as ephedrine, used in asthma medications such as Primatene.[13] In China, ephedra has been used in combination formulas for the treatment of respiratory disease, including asthma, for more than 5,000 years. (Some safety precautions apply when using ephedrine and pseudoephedrine, but the same cautions apply to both the natural herb and the chemical versions.)

In many cases, herbs can produce results comparable to the best conventional treatments at substantially lower cost. For example, compare the costs of treating stomach ulcers with surgery, the prescription drug Tagamet (cimetidine), and licorice extract (*Glycyrrhiza glabra*) or deglycyrrhizinated licorice (DGL) (see table 1).[14] Although licorice extract has the potential to cause certain side effects that could limit its long-term use, it is safe enough to have been ap-

Table 1
Comparison of Treatment Costs for Stomach Ulcers

Treatment	Cost ($)
Surgery	25,000
Tagamet (per year)	1,000
DGL (per year)	300
Licorice extract (per year)	20

proved by FDA as a food ingredient: Concentrated extracts of up to 24 percent may be used in licorice candy. DGL appears to cause no side effects and can be safely used for longer periods.

Another good example is treatment of benign prostatic hyperplasia (BPH). Benign enlargement of the prostate gland affects nearly half of all men over age 40, and 75 percent of those over 60.[15] Table 2 compares the FDA-approved prescription drug Proscar (finasteride) with a European over-the-counter remedy made from a standardized extract of saw palmetto (Serenoa repens).

Table 2
Comparison of Treatment Costs for BPH

TREATMENT	COST ($)	RISKS
Surgery	5,000	All surgery carries with it the potential for serious or fatal complications. Complications specific to prostate surgery include incontinence, impotence, bleeding and infection.
Proscar (per year)	657	Impotence (3.7% risk), decreased libido, ejaculatory dysfunction, decreased sexual function; dangerous when used in men with liver problems.
Serenoa standardized extract (per year)	255	None known. Saw palmetto berries were used as a staple food by Native Americans, and have shown no toxicity in European use.[16]

These are just a few examples of the many botanical remedies that offer safe, effective, and inexpensive ways to maintain wellness and to help prevent and treat a variety of common health conditions. Supported by a combination of ancient history and modern scientific research, herbs are winning over an entire generation of physicians, pharmacists, and health-conscious individuals. Their history includes well-established use in treating both simple and serious diseases in Western medicine and an ancient history of use as general health tonics in the East. Today, both the therapeutic and preventive uses of herbs have received new respect and acclaim, as science, clinical practice, and the experience of millions of people worldwide combine to affirm their power and potential.

REFERENCES

1. Farnsworth NR. The role of medicinal plants in drug development. In: Krogsgaard-Larsen P, Christensen SB, Kofod H, eds. *Natural Products and Drug Development.* Copenhagen: Munksgaard, 1984: 17–30.

2. Jacobs J. Regulatory issues and medicinal plants. Presentation at the WHO/Morris Arboretum of the University of Pennsylvania Utilization of Medicinal Plants Symposium; April 19–21, 1993; Philadelphia, PA.

3. Barrie SA, Wright JV, Pizzorno JE. Effect of garlic oil on platelet aggregation, serum

lipids and blood pressure in humans. *Journal of Orthomolecular Medicine* 1987; 2(1): 15–21.

4. Silagy CA, Neil HAW. Garlic as a lipid-lowering agent—a meta-analysis. *The Journal of the Royal College of Physicians* 1994; 28(1): 39–45.

5. Yokozawa T, Seno J, Oura H. Effect of ginseng extract on lipid and sugar metabolism. I. Metabolic correlation between liver and adipose tissue. *Chemical Pharmaceutical Bulletin* 1975; 23(12): 3095–4000.

6. Shi L, Fan P-S, Wu L, et al. Effects of total saponins of *Panax notoginseng* on increasing PGI_2 in carotid artery and decreasing TXA_2 in blood platelets [in Chinese with English abstract]. *Acta Pharmacologica Sinica* 1990; 11(1): 29–32.

7. Li X, Chen J-X, Sun J-J, et al. Protective effects of *Panax notoginseng* saponins on experimental myocardial injury induced by ischemia and reperfusion in rat [in Chinese with English abstract]. *Acta Pharmacologica Sinica* 1990; 11(1): 26–29.

8. Farnsworth NR, Kinghorn AD, Soejarto DD, et al. Siberian ginseng *(Eleutherococcus senticosus):* current status as an adaptogen. In: Wagner H, Hikino H, Farnsworth NR, eds. *Economic and Medicinal Plant Research.*

Vol. 1. New York: Academic Press, 1985: 155–215.

9. Komoda Y, Shimizu M, Sonoda Y, et al. Ganoderic acid and its derivatives as cholesterol synthesis inhibitors. *Chemical Pharmaceutical Bulletin* 1989; 37(2): 531–533.

10. You WC, Blot WJ, Chang Y-S, et al. Allium vegetables and reduced risk of stomach cancer. *Journal of the National Cancer Institute* 1989; 81: 162–164.

11. Wagner H, Proksch A. Immunostimulatory drugs of fungi and higher plants. In: Wagner H, Hikino H, Farnsworth NR, eds. *Economic and Medicinal Plant Research.* Vol. 1. New York: Academic Press, 1985: 113–153.

12. Hou YD, Ma GL, Wu SH, et al. Effect of radix astragali seu hedysari on the interferon system. *Chinese Medical Journal* 1981; 94(1): 35–40.

13. Weil A. *Natural Health, Natural Medicine.* Boston: Houghton Mifflin, 1990: 239.

14. Rountree R, MD. Personal communication. Boulder, CO; 1992.

15. Denis LJ. Quantification and incidence of benign prostatic hyperplasia. *Drugs of Today* 1993; 29: 328–333.

16. Saw palmetto extract vs. Proscar. *American Journal of Natural Medicine* 1994; 1(1): 8–9.

CHAPTER 3

Choosing Herbal Products

Today's herbal products span a vast range, from jars of dried leaves and flowers and roots to slick, full-color boxes of blister-packed, coated tablets that look much like conventional over-the-counter drugs. By far the most popular forms of herbal products today are capsules and tablets, which are convenient and easy to use. They are also the easiest transition for Americans who are accustomed to taking medicines and dietary supplements in these forms, as are people in most industrialized countries. Most of these products contain standardized extracts of herbs, which will be explained in the next section.

The concept of making pills out of herbs is hardly new. The earliest pills were probably those made thousands of years ago in China by mixing powdered herbs with honey and rolling them into small balls, which were swallowed with water. The Chinese still make these simple herb powder tablets, and some can be found in Chinese herb shops.

Other ancient types of herbal products are also still available. Many health-food stores continue to carry hundreds of herbs in the original bulk form, that is, dried herbs, either whole or powdered, usually sold out of big glass jars and weighed out by the ounce. Herbal teas, also called *infusions,* are so popular they can be found in nearly every restaurant and hotel throughout the world. Herbal teas are usually just flavorful hot or cold beverages but sometimes have a medicinal effect, too. European herbal teas are especially popular for their effects on digestion and appetite. Aromatic teas, including those with mint or ginger, can help soothe the stomach after a heavy meal; others, like chamomile and linden flowers, can calm the nerves at the end of a busy day. Boiled herb teas called *decoctions* are still a major form of medicine in China and throughout Asia. After diagnosing a condition or "imbalance" in a patient, Asian physicians will prescribe a mixture of up to a dozen or more herbs, which are simmered, sometimes for hours, to produce a potent brew that is sipped throughout the day.

Herbal products also include liquid extracts, cough syrups, and lozenges. More recently, manufacturers have begun incorporating herbal extracts into selected food products, such as food bars, cereals, and even snacks. These are sometimes called *functional foods.* In general, it is difficult to add enough of an herbal extract to food to make a product that is truly effective yet still good tasting. Remember, the effectiveness of any herb, or for that matter anything used for health care, is dependent on how much of it we consume. An inadequate dose is useless, whereas an excessive dose may be hazardous in some cases.

ABOUT EXTRACTS

The hottest products on the market today are *standardized extracts,* a term that means that every dose of the extract contains the same level of important compounds. These are usually sold in tablet or capsule form, and are the major herbal products found in pharmacy, grocery, and discount stores. They are the favorite products of doctors and pharmacists because they add a level of consistency that appeals to professionals. It also helps that nearly all of the best clinical research on European phytomedicines is on standardized extracts. At the same time, standardized extracts are somewhat controversial to some herbalists precisely because they are high-

tech and highly processed. Some people worry that extremely sophisticated or refined herbal products are once again taking us away from nature in the same direction that synthetic medicines have led us. Before we plunge into a debate on the subject, here are some basics about extraction.

Plants contain a complex mixture of thousands of chemical compounds, including water and fiber, chlorophyll, starches, fats and proteins, plus unique compounds that give each herb certain effects. To make an extract, manufacturers grind the herb and use a solvent such as alcohol to dissolve beneficial compounds from the herb. The used herb is then discarded, just like coffee grounds. Why not just use the whole herb and get everything nature put in the plant? In some cases we can do just that. Not all herbs need to be extracted. But for several reasons, some are best used in extract form.

• **Concentration:** Some herbs are so mild that it is unrealistic to use them without concentrating them. Bilberry is a good example. The dark blue pigments in bilberry fruit are responsible for its benefits to the eyes. But to get enough of these compounds into a few easy-to-take capsules, we need to concentrate them by 100. In other words, to get an effective dose of simple dried bilberry fruit in a capsule, we would need to take up to 100 capsules a day. Instead, we take a concentrate. This concentrate, called a 100 to 1 concentrate, is usually written this way: 100:1.

• **Selection:** When we concentrate an herb, we leave something out of the extract. The largest part of what is not present in an extract is the insoluble fiber. In making the extract, we are deciding to select some parts of the plant and not others—in this case, not the fiber. That's all right: We are rarely taking an herb as a source of fiber. The herb contains more important things that we want to add to our diets.

Standardized Extracts

To standardize an extract, scientists test for key compounds in the plant and adjust the extract to ensure that the level of these compounds remains consistent. For instance, if a company processes a batch of a weaker-than-usual ginseng, the extract produced will be lower in the ginseng compounds called ginsenosides. To ensure that the extract is just as strong each and every time it is made, the company can either concentrate the extract or simply use more ginseng, just as you might if your morning coffee were too weak. Nature is variable, so we can't assume that every batch of any herb is the same as the last.

One problem with standardizing extracts is that we usually don't know exactly which chemicals in an herb are responsible for its health benefits. Of the hundreds of herbs on the market, only a half dozen or so are standardized to known active principles. Examples include kava, senna, ginseng, ephedra, and caffeine sources, such as cola and maté.

Other extracts are standardized to marker compounds. These constituents may not be the key to the plant's effectiveness, but there is usually evidence that if the extract contains enough of the marker compound, it will be effective. St. John's wort provides an excellent example. Extracts of this herb have well-researched antidepressant effects. Most St. John's wort extract is standardized to contain 0.3 percent hypericin. Research has shown that hypericin alone is not an active antidepressant; hence, it is not a known active principle. However, the clinical trials prove that an extract that has enough hypericin is effective against depression. Whatever chemical, or, more likely, combination of chemicals, that is responsible for this effect is extracted along with the hypericin, so the hypericin serves as a good marker.

One of the risks of standardizing extracts to a single chemical compound is the possibility that an unscrupulous manufacturer or ingredient supplier could boost the level of that compound with a cheap, synthetic chemical. This is called *spiking* and is believed to be very uncommon, partly because cheap synthetic sources of most marker compounds are not available. There have been reports of spiking in ephedra products—inexpensive ephedrine is available—but this is a dangerous practice for manufacturers. Not only is it the kind of unethical practice that could ruin a company's reputation, but it is also illegal.

A larger problem is that in independent tests, some products have been found to contain a far lower amount of marker compounds than is stated on the label. This could be the result of either poor quality control or intentional fraud. The pressure of intense competition in the herb industry will likely bring an end to such practices, but for now it is important to buy from quality-oriented companies with strong reputations.

Hydroalcoholic Extracts (Tinctures)

The simplest extracts on the market are the *hydroalcoholic extracts,* sometimes called *tinctures,* which are sold in dropper bottles. These should be labeled with a ratio that tells you how much of the herb is present in a given quantity of extract. In other words, the ratio is a measure of the weight of herb (the first number) used to make a certain amount of extract (the second number). If 1 kilogram of herb is extracted to produce 1 kilogram of extract, the extract is a "one to one," or 1:1, extract.

For dosage purposes, an extract labeled 1:1 is roughly equivalent to an equal weight of the herb. One dropperful usually contains about 1 milliliter (abbreviated as ml) of extract, which weighs around 1 gram, so a dropperful of a 1:1 extract is approximately equal to 1 gram of the herb. In a 1:5 extract, 1 gram of herb is present in 5 grams (5 ml) of extract. It takes 5 dropperfuls of a 1:5 extract to equal 1 gram of the herb, and a dropperful of a 2:1 extract is equal to 2 grams of herb.

A Basic Tincture Recipe

It's fairly easy to make your own tinctures. Vodka is a good solvent because it contains 40 percent alcohol and no flavorings. Thus it should extract a good range of water-soluble and oil-soluble compounds, both of which are usually soluble in alcohol. Place the herb to be extracted in a wide-mouth glass jar. (1-quart canning jars work well.) The herb should be powdered or at least cut fairly fine. Fill the jar no more than two-thirds full of herb, because the herb will expand when it gets wet. Fill the jar with vodka, cap tightly, and let it extract for several weeks, shaking it daily. Strain through cheese cloth, muslin, or a coffee filter, squeezing as much of the liquid as possible out of the herb. To get a rough idea of the strength of the extract, weigh the dry herb used in each jar before adding the alcohol, and later measure the amount of finished extract to figure out the ratio of extract to herb. See appendix A for books that provide more details on making your own tinctures and other herbal preparations.

To extract an herb with high levels of compounds that are not water soluble, manufacturers use more alcohol, up to 80 percent (160 proof!). About 25 percent alcohol is necessary to prevent an extract from spoiling, but the alcohol content in extracts varies from 25 percent up to 80 percent alcohol, depending on the requirements of the herb being extracted. For example, the flavor components and pungent principles in ginger are all soluble in alcohol, and ginger extracts may contain 80 percent alcohol. In other cases, such as with green tea extract, the beneficial components are soluble in water, and only enough alcohol to preserve the extract is needed. Sometimes extract makers use other solvents, including acetone and hexane. When toxic solvents are used, it is important for the manufacturer to test for solvent residues.

GUIDELINES FOR CHOOSING PRODUCTS

One of the most common questions today is how to choose herbal products. Dozens of brands are available, each claiming to be the best. Frequent stories in the media proclaim that the herb industry is "unregulated" and warn that products may not contain the ingredients they claim. The result is confusion that leaves the pharmacist, the physician, and the general public wondering how to select the highest quality product. As with all industries, the herb business includes companies committed to quality with the highest ethical standards, but also opportunists with only profit in mind.

The Importance of Quality, Testing, and Good Manufacturing Practices

When we choose something for health purposes, whether it is a drug, a vitamin, or an herbal product, we want three things: safety, effectiveness, and quality. These are like a three-legged stool that supports the value and validity of any product. Quality is the key to ensuring safety and effectiveness, and it is quality that will separate the successful companies from the failures in this competitive market. Marketing and advertising are important to building a strong business, but ultimately, a manufacturer cannot succeed without providing high-quality products.

Good manufacturing practices (GMPs) refers to the steps a company takes to ensure quality in their products. These include proper sanitation, good record keeping, laboratory testing, and the use of appropriate raw materials and processing equipment. Testing doesn't always detect poor manufacturing practices, but following GMPs dramatically reduces the risk of a critical failure in quality, safety, or effectiveness.

Laboratory testing is an important part of the manufacture of any health product, especially the more sophisticated extracts. An overwhelming failure of GMPs and lab testing occurred only a few years ago, when at least seven companies sold products that supposedly contained mild, harmless plantain leaves (*Plantago major*) but actually contained the powerful heart drug *Digitalis lanata*. Testing should have uncovered the problem long before it reached the retail shelf. The type of testing needed to ensure quality depends on the product itself. Here are some of the things companies test—or should test.

- **Identity:** The first question to be answered before starting to make an herbal product is "Do we have the right herbs?" Identity can be verified in whole herbs by botanical features (leaf shape, types of flowers, fruits, etc.), by microscopic inspection, and by chemical profiling or "fingerprinting." However, the more processed the product, the fewer ways there are to test it. For example, a powdered herb can be tested microscopically or chemically, but an extract can only be examined chemically.

- **Purity:** Even if it is the right plant, is it all the right plant? The batch may contain some weed leaves, a completely different herb, or perhaps the wrong part of the herb being purchased, such as ginseng leaves mixed in with the ginseng root. Purity also means freedom from contaminants, which may include pesticides, heavy metals, dirt, disease-causing bacteria, mold, or animal or insect contamination, to name a few.

- **Potency:** If it's the right plant and free from any serious contaminants (also called *adulterants*), is it strong enough to be effective? This is a much more difficult question to answer. For the very few herbs whose most active constituents are known, those are the compounds for which to test. But for the many herbs whose active principles are not known, we can only test for markers or assess potency in some other way.

Sometimes we overlook the obvious in seeking ways to assess herbs: our senses. For centuries, spice buyers have judged the quality of ginger, red pepper, cinnamon, and dozens of other spices by taste, smell, and color. Now scientists have identified important compounds in many of the spices and can test for them chemically, but usually such tests are no better than taste testing. I would trust a good spice buyer to judge the quality of a sample of ginger as much as any chemical analysis. I would trust a good wine, coffee, or tea taster far more than any lab equipment. Unfortunately, we cannot simply use our senses—called *organoleptic analysis*—for quality control of most herbal products today. The sophistication of the market demands a more precise and numerical method, hence the popularity of standardized extracts.

Benefits of Organic, Sustainable Herb Sources

Today, many herbs are cultivated, but a surprising amount are still picked from the wild, or *wildcrafted*. As herbs have become more popular, wildcrafting has become controversial. Many North American wild plants are now threatened with over collection. Some, including wild American ginseng, goldenseal, and ladyslipper, are considered threatened or endangered, and with the demand for herbs increasing, others could soon follow. In most cases, the solution is cultivation. One of the advantages of growing medicinal plants instead of making medicines in pharmaceutical factories is that herbs support farmers and keep agricultural land in productive use. The other main advantage is that it spares threatened plants in the wild.

To avoid pesticide and other residues not only in the herbs but in the soil, it is essential to grow plants organically, without synthetic fertilizers, herbicides, and pesticides. Good organic farming methods build the soil rather than deplete it and yield healthier, higher-quality herbs. Organic crops are better for the farmer, too, because they bring a higher price, rewarding the farmer for the extra care and work it takes to grow organically.

Not everything can be cultivated. Saw palmetto is a good example. No one knows how long it takes for a saw palmetto plant to bear fruit, but at least one farmer has had some in the ground for 10 years with nothing to show for the effort. It may take 12 years, or 20. Tree barks are another challenge. Elm, yohimbe, and pygeum barks are three examples of herbal raw materials taken from trees that are many years old, perhaps 20 to 30 years or more. Barks can be harvested sustainably, but the temptation to remove all the bark from the tree, killing it, is hard for harvesters to resist when the bark is valuable. For plants that realistically cannot be grown, we must learn to harvest them sustainably from the wild, without substantially reducing their numbers. Otherwise, we will need to find substitutes as the plants become scarce and expensive.

Several organizations, including the Herb Research Foundation (HRF), the U.S. Department of Agriculture (USDA), and the U.S. Agency for International Development (USAID), are working to foster sustainable herb production worldwide. This effort helps to increase income to disadvantaged farmers, improve the quality of herbs available to American, European, and Asian manufacturers, and ensure a long-term supply of sustainably produced herbs.

Reputation and Trust

Buying herbal products requires us to trust the manufacturer. Unfortunately, there have been cases in which product marketers have been caught selling inferior products. Whether by accident or intentional fraud, such events erode public trust in all herbs. It is difficult to make hard-and-fast statements about issues of reputation and trust, because there are ethical and unethical herb companies of all sizes.

In general, large companies that are household names have the most to lose from lapses in quality. Their continued success relies on a good reputation, and they are not likely to risk their reputations to save a few pennies a pound on ingredients. This is not to say small companies cannot also make good products. Indeed, many small companies use the same ingredient suppliers as their better-established competitors, and some large companies have faltered on quality.

In addition to asking about a company and its reputation, it is a good idea to ask lots of questions about quality, testing, and expertise. Lists of such questions can be found in the following section.

Questions to Ask

Just as we should ask our doctors for complete information about any medications, procedures, or other health-care options, it is important to be curious about self-care products. If a store or a company wants to sell a product, they should be able to answer some basic questions. Here are some issues to consider when choosing herbal products.

Before going shopping

- Consult a few herb reference books. Get a consensus of opinion from several authors about the herb's use and dosage, as well as what plant part should be used.
- Learn to read dietary supplement labels (see Interpreting Supplement Labels, later in this chapter).
- Ask friends which retailer in your area has the best herb department and why they think so.
- Ask friends which herbal products manufacturer they most trust and why.

When choosing a brand, ask your retailer:

- Would he or she take this brand? Why or why not?

- Does the manufacturer of the brand have a good reputation in the industry?
- How long has the retailer been doing business with this company?

Ask the manufacturer

- How long have they been selling herbal products?
- Do they test their herbal products for active constituents?
- How do they evaluate the quality of their herbs?
- What quality-control tests have been performed on the ingredients?
- Do they check their fresh herbs for foreign matter or adulteration?
- Are batch numbers written on the product label?
- Who is their on-staff herbal expert?
- What exactly is this product for?
- What evidence is there that it works?
- Has this specific product been clinically researched?
- If not, have the ingredients been well researched?
- Has this specific extract or herb been proven to work at the recommended dosage?
- Does the company have its own laboratories or does it use independent labs?
- Will the company send copies of test results?
- Are the ingredients of the product grown or collected in an earth-friendly way?

- Does the company support research and education organizations or initiatives?
- Does it offer free customer support?
- What kinds of questions will customer support answer?

Interpreting Supplement Labels

Government regulations in many countries prevent companies from making forthright claims about medicinal uses of herbal products. In the United States, companies can make "statements of nutritional support," often called *structure/function claims* because they relate to the way an herb affects the structure or function of the body. Claims about supporting wellness and maintaining healthy body functions are acceptable if there is evidence to support such claims. Consider, for example, possible label claims for garlic, which lowers cholesterol. A garlic label might claim that the product "helps maintain healthy cholesterol levels" or "helps maintain heart health." However, if a garlic label claimed that the herb "helps prevent heart disease," the product would be considered an illegal drug. This creates an unfortunate level of vagueness in the labeling of many herbs. Here are some more examples:

- Saw palmetto has been proven effective against prostate enlargement. Illegal drug claim: "Relieves symptoms of prostate enlargement." Legal statement of nutritional support: "Helps maintain prostate health."

- Echinacea stimulates the immune system and reduces the frequency and duration of colds. Illegal drug claim: "For colds and flu." Legal statement: "Boosts natural resistance."

Other countries have adopted similar compromises. In England, products may say "a traditional herbal remedy for [insert condition: sleep, menstrual disorders, etc.]." In France, herbs may be labeled "traditionally used for [condition]."

These approaches, while not ideal, have not caused serious problems. People are capable of understanding that there is a difference between "take two for headache" and "a traditional herbal remedy for headache." The situation in the United States is a bit more complex, but people understand that herbal dietary supplements are not the same as conventional medicines, although they have particular uses in health care.

One unfortunate result of the fact that companies can make only indirect claims is that there is currently no standard for what types of evidence are necessary before a product can make a health benefit claim. The law in the United States requires that statements be truthful and not misleading, and that they be supported by scientific evidence. However, the exact wording of claims and the amount of evidence required is not detailed. In some cases, health benefit claims are exaggerated or carry implications that are not supported by sound evidence. A little bit of common sense goes a long way in evaluating claims. As with any products sold through clever marketing, remember that any claim that sounds too good to be true probably *is* too good to be true. Be especially wary of products offering easy weight loss, enhanced virility, and other nice but unlikely dreams.

In the United States, dietary supplements that make structure/function claims must carry the following disclaimer:

> This statement has not been evaluated by the Food and Drug Administration. This product is not intended to diagnose, treat, cure or prevent any disease.

The FDA's purpose in requiring the statement is to alert the buyer that the FDA has not reviewed or approved the claim and that the product should not be considered an approved drug. The law requires that claims be truthful, not misleading, and be supported by scientific evidence; the disclaimer is a reminder that the FDA has not reviewed the evidence.

Supplement laws in the United States now require full disclosure of ingredients, including binders, fillers, and other inert ingredients that are used to make tablets and other herbal products. Some companies explain what each compound is for; others do not. The key ingredients in a supplement— the herbs or nutrients included—are listed in a special place on the package called the "Supplement Facts" panel. This panel lists required information about the ingredients,

including what part of the plant is used, the genus and species, and the content of key ingredients. For reasons of confidentiality, companies are allowed to use mixtures in which the exact quantity of each ingredient is not disclosed. Such a product might be labeled "a blend of . . ."

Potency claims are sometimes difficult to interpret. Careful reading is necessary to ensure that you are not being misled about the strength of the product. For example, one product may contain a concentrated and standardized extract of an herb, whereas another might contain just powdered herb, which, although seeming to provide more of the herb, actually delivers less. There are even some confusing but clever labeling tricks that may be designed to intentionally mislead the buyer. Consider the following example.

Ginkgo biloba standardized extract is well researched. The dose is 120 mg per day of an extract standardized to 24 percent ginkgo flavone glycosides. This extract is approximately a 50:1 concentrate. But a product may be labeled "Contains all the ginkgo flavone glycosides present in a 24 percent extract." Although it may in fact contain a true 24 percent extract (that is, less than one-fourth of the potency of ginkgo leaves), this extract contains far less than the 24 percent glycosides contained in a standardized extract. A ginkgo extract standardized to 24 percent glycosides is around 50:1, while a "24 percent extract" is 1:4. The latter probably contains 1/200th of the glycoside content of the former. This is a clever deception and somewhat difficult to explain simply. This kind of labeling exploits the public's understandable confusion. Use great care in reading labels, and seek out companies that do not play games with the wording of their ingredient statements.

With hundreds of herbal products available, it is easy to become confused about how to choose herbal products wisely. The key is to arm ourselves with a basic understanding of the types of products and differences between them, to ask lots of focused and probing questions, and to determine to buy based on top quality, not low price. Avoid companies that make extravagant claims and those who use tricky wording to describe the strength or potency of the product. The best attitude with which to approach the herbal marketplace is open-minded skepticism.

CHAPTER 4

Safety Guidelines for Using Herbs

We know that different levels of training and education are required for physicians, pharmacists, nurses, and health-food store clerks. There are also major differences between emergency medical treatments and taking an aspirin for a headache. In the world of pharmaceuticals, there are different standards for prescription drugs and those sold over the counter (OTC). OTC drugs are restricted to the treatment of *self-limiting* conditions, that is, ones that will go away in time by themselves, such as colds and headaches. There are no OTC drugs for life-threatening diseases. Likewise, dietary supplements and herbal remedies are sold over the counter and should not be considered life-saving medical interventions. Instead, herbs and nutrients are often most effectively used to support and maintain health, to improve health and protect the body.

We must use common sense in decisions about conventional self-care with OTC drugs versus seeing a doctor. We know when we have a cold or a headache or motion sick-

ness, and it is usually appropriate to self-medicate for such simple ailments. These conditions will go away anyway, with or without treatment. The same holds true for self-care with herbs. Many conditions are serious and not appropriate for self-care. We don't expect to walk into a pharmacy and pick up a cure for cancer off the shelf. We certainly shouldn't expect dietary supplements to substitute for qualified medical care, either. If you have any symptoms that could indicate serious illness, by all means seek professional help.

Too often people look to herbs as miracle cures when nothing else has worked. In some cases, herbs have provided striking results in conditions that seemed to be beyond conventional treatment, but this is rare. If we build up the expectation that herbs are miraculous, we may easily overlook the major role they can play in modern health care. Herbs can enhance the function of our organs and body processes to help us stay healthy and maintain our performance.

WORKING WITH A PRACTITIONER

Herbs are used mostly for self-care, but they are also finding their way into practitioner-mediated care. Physicians, naturopaths (practitioners who use natural agents and means to treat diseases), chiropractors, and other health-care providers are including herbs in their practice, both as alternatives to conventional drugs and as combination therapies. The greatest challenge is finding qualified practitioners who are knowledgeable about herbs. For the past few decades, medical doctors as a rule have scorned the use of herbs or other "unorthodox" remedies, so the chances of happening upon a physician who can advise you about choosing and using herbs for medical purposes are not good. American medical and pharmacy schools long ago stopped teaching about herbal remedies, and, for the most part, high-quality education for herbalists or other herbal practitioners failed to materialize. There are herbalists who have considerable knowledge about herbs, and some who are adept at diagnosing health conditions. Unfortunately, in the United States there is no official certification program for "herbalists," and technically, anyone can claim that title without any training or experience at all. Naturopathic education has filled in the gaps to some extent, as there are several accredited schools with rigorous and scientifically based programs. The Naturopathic Degree (N.D.) though, is unfortunately also an uncertain guide since there are poor-quality programs and correspondence courses that grant the same degree without the same standard of training as the accredited schools.

In all of these areas, things may be changing. American doctors and pharmacists are flocking to continuing education courses about herbs because their patients and customers demand it. Some naturopathic colleges have impressed accrediting agencies, and degree programs in natural health care continue to multiply. There is still little relief in sight for American herbalists, however, as no one has yet found an acceptable way to accredit or license herbalists in a manner that satisfies everyone. The sole exception may be in the practice of Oriental medicine, especially traditional Chinese medicine (TCM), where there are practitioners who have earned the O.M.D. degree, which is a doctorate in Oriental medicine. While this degree is far less rigorous than the training for Western medical doctors, for those looking for qualified practitioners of TCM, the O.M.D. degree may be a valuable guide.

As with so many other health decisions about herbs, there are no clear rules to follow. It is important to ask many questions of practitioners, and of their current and former patients, if possible. Questions to ask practitioners might include the following:

- What is your opinion of herbal and nutritional approaches to health care?
- Do you consider yourself knowledgeable about natural remedies?
- What role can herbs play in health care?
- Can you help your patients make informed decisions about natural health-care options?
- How much experience do you have using herbs in your practice?
- Where did you learn about herbs?
- How many hours of training in this area do you have, and from where?
- What sources of self-education have you used?
- What do you consider the best books about herbs?

These are only sample questions, of course. The point is to discover the provider's level of training, experience, and expertise on herbs, and also discern whether she or he has an open mind on the subject. You are probably best served by finding someone who is not closed to the subject of herbs, yet is also a critical thinker. The ideal mind-set for a scientist or physician is open-minded skepticism. By the way, this applies to conventional therapies as well. All too often, doctors are true believers with respect to conventional medicines, reserving their skepticism for the unorthodox. A good physician should be willing to question anything, no matter how firmly it is believed by his or her medical school instructors.

TRUSTING NATURAL REMEDIES

Whether we are considering drugs used to treat serious diseases or dietary supplements used to support and maintain health, we want assurance that all products used for health have the same attributes: safety, effectiveness, and quality. One of the most hotly debated issues on the subject of herbal medicines concerns proof of safety. For decades, medical authorities, regulators, and the media have warned that herbs are "unproven" and "unregulated." These sources claim that public safety may be at risk because herbs are not held to the same high standards of proof as are drugs. This is especially ironic considering the serious safety issues with conventional drugs.

A Look at Drug-Safety Testing

Most Americans probably believe that there is an FDA "gold standard" of research—perhaps the highest in the world—that all drugs must meet to gain approval for sale to the public. For years, opponents of herbal medicine have decried what they see as a double standard in which herbs can be sold without being proven safe and effective. The truth is, there is no gold standard for drug approval, and the double standard often works *against* herbs. Today's health professionals, along with the media and government regulators, seem to expect herbs to meet a standard of proof that has never been applied to our most common drugs.

The standards of research for approval of drugs used by Americans have actually been quite variable. According to Robert Pinco, who directed the FDA's over-the-counter drug review process, more than 75 percent of common, FDA-approved OTC medications did *not* meet a rigorous standard of evidence. Many were "grandfathered," meaning they were exempted from approval standards because they were already on the market; many more were approved based on the opinions of expert panels and not necessarily on high-quality research evidence. Some were approved without a single clinical trial and without even the most rudimentary animal-based toxicology experiments. Furthermore, the FDA itself did not conduct any research at all. Approvals were based on studies sent in by drug companies.

Only "new" drugs are required to meet the most rigorous standards, and these are usually patentable prescription drugs. The research, development, and approval process for such drugs costs more than $350 million on average and can take from 8 to 12 years. This is by far the most costly and time-consuming drug approval process in the world, but does it assure us of safe and effective medicines? According to a U.S. government study of drugs approved by the FDA over a 10-year period, more than half were found to have serious safety problems only after they were on the market. These postapproval discoveries of dangerous side

effects required many drugs to be pulled off the market and others to be restricted in use. In other words, the world's most expensive approval process failed to find serious safety problems more than half of the time. Conventional FDA-approved medications kill over 100,000 Americans annually and injure over 2 million more.[1] This does not include accidental overdoses, medication mistakes, or suicide attempts, only the problems caused by bad reactions to properly prescribed doses of the "right" medication.

Believe it or not, this discussion is not intended as an indictment of conventional medicine, of drug companies, or of the American drug-approval process. It is simply becoming increasingly important that we all set aside our biases about both synthetic and natural remedies and dispassionately consider the facts about *all* the agents we use in health care.

HERB SAFETY

There are several main types of safety evidence:

- Historical use by humans
- Laboratory toxicity testing
- Side effects observed during clinical trials
- Reports of illness or fatalities in people using the substance—called adverse event reports, or AERs

The same kinds of safety evidence apply to foods, food chemicals, dietary supplements, and drugs, with the exception of side effects. Since foods are not clinically researched, this kind of proof is not available for most foods.

The major type of evidence supporting herb safety is a long history of human use without serious problems. History of use is considered an important indicator of safety in foods, food chemicals, and old drugs. It is generally accepted that if something has a long history of human use, new safety testing is not needed. For example, food safety laws do not require any clinical or laboratory toxicology testing. Food chemicals that were already being consumed before the passage of food additive laws are also exempt from safety testing. U.S. FDA officials have testified that historical use is a legitimate basis for exempting common food chemicals from safety requirements, and apply the same logic to old drugs. They are not subject to any scrutiny at all if they are "generally recognized as safe." Herbs that have been eaten or medicinally applied for a long time are presumed safe unless proven otherwise. Internationally, the World Health Organization recommends that herbal medicines be considered safe if they have been in widespread use for lengthy periods of time without causing toxicity, and that they be assumed to possess the benefits for which they have been applied unless proven otherwise.

Many herbs have been subjected to more laboratory and clinical research than most people know. None can be considered "new" drugs, and hence should not be expected to be held to new-drug approval standards. Like OTC drugs in the United States, natural medicines were approved in Europe by expert panels, such as the German Commission E, which looked at existing research evidence and used their own expertise to make decisions about herbal remedies. Some herbs and their chemical constituents have undergone the same types of safety research as conventional drugs: animal toxicity tests designed to determine fatal doses, mutagenicity assays to predict possible cancer-causing effects (carcinogenicity) or potential to cause birth defects (teratogenicity), pharmacological profiles that explore effects on organs and tissues, and sometimes long-term feeding studies in animals to gauge the effects of extended use.

Finally, many of today's most popular herbs have been used in Europe under supervision by doctors for more than a dozen years and by millions of people. Serious problems have been rare, and there is no evidence that the large-scale use of European phytomedicines poses the kind of problems that synthetic drugs do in terms of toxic effects. Reports of herbs causing illness are infrequent, and systematic data collection processes have not detected any significant problems caused by herbs. For example, the reports of the American Association of Poison Control Centers clearly show that the leading cause of fatal poisonings is synthetic drugs, followed by cleaners and other household products.[2] Incidents involving herbs are extremely uncommon. A study conducted by the Poisons Unit in London identified only a few reports of problems with herbs that resulted in serious health consequences. The most common complaint was that herbal sedatives caused drowsiness.[3]

CONTROVERSIAL HERBS

Looking back at recent herbal controversies is just like looking back at conventional pharmaceutical and medical controversies. It seems that the problems can always be traced to the same type of agents: stimulants, sedatives, and diet pills. In the nineteenth century, doctors overprescribed the opiates morphine, heroin, and codeine; they enthusiastically promoted cocaine and marijuana into the twentieth century. In the 1960s it was amphetamines, promoted for weight loss; in the 1970s and 1980s, Valium and other habit-forming sedatives; in the 1990s, "phen-fen," also for weight loss.

In the mid-1990s, we began to see reports about abuse of ephedra (ma huang) products causing overdose reactions and possibly fatalities. The FDA and many medical authorities pointed to these problems with ephedra products as proof that herbs should be regulated as drugs. Ironically, the active compounds in ephedra are among the few herbal substances that have been scrutinized by the FDA. The FDA has already approved pure ephedra alkaloids (the active

stimulant compounds) as effective and declared them safe enough for sale without a prescription. This means that anyone in the United States can purchase ephedrine (in the form of Primatene, for example) and pseudoephedrine (as, for example, in Sudafed) at any pharmacy, grocery, or convenience store. The FDA portrayed the herbal source of these chemical compounds as a public health menace, but remained curiously silent about the pharmaceutical drugs, which are often far stronger sources of these potent stimulants. The chapter on ephedra provides some balanced information and a healthy dose of caution.

Some other herbs presenting potential safety concerns are listed here.

- **Comfrey *(Symphytum officinale)*:** Contains liver toxins called pyrrolizidine alkaloids. The degree of risk is unclear, but we do not recommend using comfrey internally.
- **Chaparral *(Larrea tridentata)*:** Reported by the FDA to have caused liver toxicity. However, a review by doctors funded by the American Herbal Products Association found insufficient evidence that chaparral caused the incidents.
- **Sassafras *(Sassafras albidum)*:** Not allowed in food products in the United States because the major constituent of its volatile oil, safrole, is carcinogenic in animals.
- **Pennyroyal essential oil *(Mentha pulegium)*:** This potent form of pennyroyal has, unfortunately, picked up a reputation as an herbal abortifacient, a substance that

could induce spontaneous expulsion of a fetus. *This is not true.* There is ample evidence that strong doses of pennyroyal oil are highly toxic, and even when used as a tea, the herb's safety is questionable. However, there is *no* evidence that pennyroyal can cause spontaneous abortion. In fact, no safe herb has this effect. Pennyroyal has been used as a repellent for fleas and other insects. Again, the essential oil is so toxic that people have accidentally killed their animals trying to use it as a flea repellent. Avoid this herb entirely.

• **Stimulant laxatives:** Some of the most abused herbs are stimulant laxatives such as senna leaf and pod, cascara sagrada, aloe latex, buckthorn, and rhubarb root. Stimulant laxatives have sometimes been used for "detoxification," and some alternative practitioners still recommend this practice. Forcing the intestines into a chemically induced frenzy is *not* a healthy thing to do, however. This type of laxative is considered to be the last resort and worst choice even for treating constipation, because of well-known side effects, especially laxative dependence. Worse still, some consumers use these herbs in the belief that they can help promote weight loss. Laxative and diuretic diet products are a sham. They can only lead to dehydration and loss of water weight, which is the most meaningless kind of weight reduction. If used regularly, stimulant laxatives cause the intestines to lose their muscle tone, creating a serious state of weakness in the digestive system. If abused,

they can also bring about electrolyte depletion, high blood pressure, and even heart attacks. For more details, see "Aloe."

• **Highly toxic plants:** Some plants are very toxic and should never be used for self-treatment. These include foxglove (*Digitalis* spp.), mayapple (*Podophyllum* spp.), belladonna *(Atropa belladonna),* and others. For more complete information, consult a book on plant medicines or poisonous plants.

HERB USE DURING PREGNANCY AND NURSING

During pregnancy and when nursing, it is critical to consider the health of the baby. We recommend great care during these sensitive times in a woman's life. While most herbs are probably safe to take during pregnancy and nursing, pregnant or nursing women should consult a health-care practitioner before using any active substances, including herbs, other dietary supplements, and especially drugs. Drugs are clinically tested in adults, not infants. Herbal phytomedicines, too, have been researched in adults. Certain herbs and many drugs have undergone laboratory testing designed to predict fetal toxicity, and these specific substances are probably relatively safe. However, there are undoubtedly shortcomings to animal and laboratory toxicity testing, so caution is advisable even if such tests have been performed.

HERBS FOR CHILDREN

Some herbs have an ancient and venerable reputation for use in children. Chamomile and fennel teas, for example, have been employed by many generations of European mothers to calm their children's stomachs. In other cases, there is clinical experience with children. For example, echinacea has been researched in clinical trials involving children. However, just as during pregnancy, we advise caution when considering herbs for children and suggest that you seek the advice of a health-care practitioner.

Herbal remedies are apparently far safer than conventional drugs, as indicated by Poison Control Center data. Accidental poisoning of small children is common with OTC drugs, especially pain medications and sleeping pills. Herbal remedies and nutritional supplements are undoubtedly also accidentally consumed by children, but rarely with harmful results. The most common cause of harm to small children from dietary supplements is iron supplements, because relatively small amounts can easily become toxic.

Strong herbs, including stimulants and stimulant laxatives, should be kept from children's reach. Herbs that are intended for conditions experienced exclusively by mature adults are, of course, inappropriate for children. These would include saw palmetto, black cohosh, and vitex.

The process of calculating herb dosages for children is similar to the method used with conventional medicines. Usually the adult herb dose is adjusted according to the weight of the child. For example, if an adult dose is 100 mg and an average adult is 60 kg (132 lb), the dose for a 30-kg (66-lb) child would be half that (60 kg divided by 30 kg), or 50 mg.

For more information, see appendix A for books that specifically address herbal medicine for children.

ALLERGIC REACTIONS

Allergic reactions to herbs are rare. However, any substance—food, drug, herb, or cosmetic—may cause certain individuals to experience allergic or *idiosyncratic* reactions, meaning unusual reactions that do not affect the majority of people. If you experience any unpleasant reaction to an herbal product (or a food, drug, or cosmetic), discontinue its use and investigate. In many cases, people mistakenly attribute an upset stomach or other minor health effect to something they have recently consumed. It is often hard to tell exactly which of the many things one has consumed might have caused the reaction. The reaction may even be unrelated to anything one ingested.

DRUG/HERB INTERACTIONS

One of the most common questions we are asked at the Herb Research Foundation concerns the potential for herbal products to interact with prescription or OTC drugs or with other herbs. Little information is available about possible herb/herb or herb/drug interactions. What many people do not realize is that very little is known about drug/drug interactions and drug/food interactions as well. Our understanding of how the hundreds of substances we consume might affect one another is in its infancy. For example, a few years ago it was discovered that grapefruit juice affects the liver enzyme system that metabolizes certain drugs. The effect is strong enough that sensitive people can overdose on the prescription drugs if they are frequently taken in combination with grapefruit juice. Since that discovery, researchers have learned that substances in broccoli, cauliflower, wheat, corn, coffee, tea, and tobacco also affect this liver enzyme system. There are certainly many other discoveries to be made in this emerging science, and some of these may involve herbs or nutritional supplements. For now, there are some known interactions, and these are detailed for each herb in Part II.

As a general rule, herbs do not interfere with the effects of conventional medications. As with drugs, though, it is wise to seek professional guidance before combining substances with similar effects. For example, taking synthetic sedatives along with alcohol or antihistamines is not recommended. For the same reason, using them with herbal sedatives may be ill advised. There is no known synergism (exaggerated enhancement of effects) between the herb

valerian and alcohol, whereas there is synergism between synthetic sedatives and alcohol. Nonetheless, we caution against it. For example, people who know how much alcohol they can handle may find that combining that amount of alcohol with herbal sedatives such as valerian or kava can produce unpredictable effects.

Some of the theoretical herb/drug interactions or contraindications mentioned in this book may eventually prove to be unwarranted. For example, taking St. John's wort along with prescription antidepressants is not recommended. However, at a meeting of the American Psychiatric Association, several psychiatrists reported that some of their patients informed them that they had been using the herb for some time, even though they were also on prescription drugs. Neither the patients nor the psychiatrists noted any adverse effects, but some of the doctors had advised their patients against self-medication while under a physician's care. For now, we recommend that you heed any and all cautions about combining herbs and conventional drugs.

DOSAGE

Throughout this book, we have attempted to provide dosage information supported by strong clinical evidence. When most research has used a particular dose or dosage range, that is the dose we list. In the event that a consistent dosage has not been tried in research, we use—and cite—official sources such as *The Complete German Commission E Monographs* (a collection of the reports from the Commission E), the *British Herbal Pharmacopoeia,* or other authoritative source. Remember that the quality of information on herbs varies greatly, and when there is limited clinical research, the dosage most likely comes from traditional or historical use and is not necessarily confirmed by modern scientific analysis.

Many herbs are safe enough that the dosage can be adjusted somewhat if needed. Those herbs that are used as common foods can generally be regarded as quite safe. For example, in using ginger to prevent motion sickness, the dose used in research was around 400 mg. This is less than a half teaspoon of powdered ginger. Obviously, there is little risk in consuming twice or three times this amount. On the other hand, the dosage limits on strong herbs such as ephedra should be respected, because overdose is possible.

Be aware that if recommended doses of an herb are not producing the desired result, increasing the dose will not necessarily produce a better result. The herb you are taking may not be the right herb for you or your condition. In fact, in some cases, there may be no appropriate amount of any herb for a particular person or condition. In other words, some conditions may not be helped by any herb, and in certain individuals, there may be *no* therapy that will be effective. As always, use common sense and consult a health-care practitioner for any serious health condition or if a condition persists.

REFERENCES

1. Lazarou J, Pomeranz B, Corey P. Incidence of adverse drug reactions in hospitalized patients. *JAMA* 1998; 279: 1200–1205.
2. Litovitz TL, Klein-Schwartz W, Dyer S, et al. 1997 annual report of the American Association of Poison Control Centers toxic exposure surveillance system. *American Journal of Emergency Medicine* 1998; 16(5): 443–497.
3. Perharic L, Shaw D, Colbridge M, et al. Toxicological problems resulting from exposure to traditional remedies and food supplements. *Drug Safety* 1994; 11(4): 284–294.

PART II

Herbs

Aloe

ALOE VERA
LILIACEAE

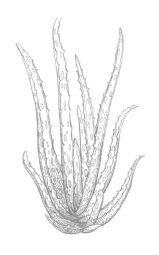

State of Knowledge: Five-Star Rating System

Clinical (human) research	✶
Laboratory research	✶✶
History of use/traditional use	✶✶✶✶
Safety record	✶✶✶
International acceptance	✶✶✶

PART USED: *Leaf gel*

PRIMARY USES

External
- *Minor burns and sunburn*
- *Wound healing*
- *Other skin conditions*

Internal
- *Diabetes (experimental)*
- *HIV infection (experimental—acemannan)*

After more than 4,000 years of traditional use, aloe vera ranks as one of the oldest medicinal plants known to humanity. Aloe was considered a "plant of immortality" by the ancient Egyptians, and legend has it that aloe gel was one of the se-cret beauty aids of the Egyptian queens Cleopatra and Nefertiti. Aloe vera gel is no less popular today, based on its well-accepted use as a skin healer and rejuvenator and, more recently, on its folk reputation as a healing tonic "juice." Aloe is one of the top ten best-selling herbs in the United States today. The gel is incorporated into countless cosmetic and medical products for the skin, and the juice made by diluting the gel is widely marketed for general "cleansing" effects and for a range of health conditions. Aloe enthusiasts claim the juice is effective in the treatment of arthritis, eczema, diabetes, stomach ulcers, digestive tract problems, constipation, and a host of other ailments. While it is possible that these are all legitimate uses of aloe gel juice, most of them are unsupported by research or have been the subject of only a few inconclusive studies.

Conflicting research results have led to confusion and skepticism about aloe's effectiveness, even regarding its well-known application for helping to heal burns and wounds. The application of aloe gel for burns and minor wounds is supported by thousands of years of traditional use for the same purpose by numerous cultures, a history that must carry at least some weight when the evidence is assessed. In tropical places where aloe grows wild, it is commonly called "the burn plant." In cooler climates, aloe vera is an attractive houseplant that doubles as a first-aid remedy for minor burns, cuts, and scrapes.

Two medicinal substances come from aloe vera, each from a different part of the plant. Soothing aloe vera gel, which comes from the center part of the leaves, should not be confused with the bitter latex—also called *drug aloe*—that comes from separate cell chambers closer to the outer rind of the leaves. (See Botany for more details on the differences between these two plant parts.) When dried, the bitter latex (also commonly known as dried leaf juice) is used as a strong stimulant laxative that may have cathartic effects, meaning that it can cause severe diarrhea and cramping when taken in large enough doses.

Although aloe bitter latex is an ingredient in many laxative formulas and is listed as an official medicine in the pharmacopoeias of a number of nations, it is not recommended for regular use as a laxative (see Safety for more information). However, cultures around the world have employed this bitter latex not only as a laxative, but also as a treatment for a variety of different ailments. Today, researchers are studying compounds isolated from aloe bitter latex to learn more about their potential health benefits. In addition, a polysaccharide compound called *acemannan,* which comes from the rind of the aloe leaf, has generated intense interest due to its antiviral potential. Studies have shown that acemannan may impair the ability of viruses, including retroviruses such as the human immunodeficiency virus (HIV), to infect healthy T-cells.

Aloe is a very complex plant that contains numerous potentially beneficial compounds. The research to date is promising. However, in spite of the plant's long history of traditional use and the substantial amount of research already conducted, no definite conclusions can yet be reached about all of the possible applications of aloe and its constituents.

HISTORY

Both aloe gel and the dried bitter latex have been used medicinally for thousands of years. A plant of ancient Africa, aloe was highly esteemed by the ancient Egyptians and has been colorfully depicted on the walls of many tombs and temples. The medicinal application of aloe in the treatment of skin infections was mentioned in Egyptian writings as early as 550 B.C. Aloe, particularly the bitter latex, also appears in the works of many ancient European physicians, including Dioscorides, Pliny the Elder, and Galen. Aloe still is employed by the Zulu of southern Africa to heal wounds and cuts on their animals. Traditionally, Zulu women have applied fresh aloe gel to their breasts when weaning their children. An important use of aloe latex in northern Africa and the Middle East has been for the treatment of diabetes.

The ancient Greeks were also enamored with aloe. Legend has it that Alexander the Great conquered the island Socotra (in the Indian Ocean) simply so that Greece could gain control of this valued commodity. Aloe was a highly prized medicinal trade item, lightweight and easy to transport, and thus spread rapidly throughout the world. In parts of China, aloe is called "jelly leaks" and has served as a treatment for eczema, dental diseases, wound healing, and as a cathartic. The plant was used similarly in the Indian Ayurvedic tradition, as well as for menstrual problems and to expel worms. Reflecting its multicultural popularity, the name *Aloe vera* stems from the Arabic word *alloeh,* which means "shining, bitter substance," and *vera,* which is Latin for "true."

Early European colonists in Africa soon learned of the benefits of aloe. By 1693, aloe bitter latex was traded in London, and soon was widely used in Europe as a laxative. As interest in the plant grew, European colonists planted aloe throughout the warm regions of the world, where it subsequently naturalized. When brought to North America by Europeans, aloe established itself in Florida. Soon the Seminole Indians of the area were availing themselves of the gel to treat burns, bee stings, and jellyfish stings.

By the early 1800s, dried aloe bitter latex became tremendously popular as a laxative in the United States and was one of the primary laxative medicines available at the time. Many laxative formulas containing aloe were included in *The United States Pharmacopoeia* for most of the nineteenth century, including one product called "Miracle Curative Pills."

INTERNATIONAL STATUS

Although aloe vera gel is considered a traditional treatment for wound healing by many cultures, it is not approved for use by any international regulatory agencies. Aloe vera bitter latex is approved for use as a stimulant laxative in the United Kingdom, France, and Germany, all of which have issued strict safety guidelines pertaining to the use of plants such as aloe, which contain laxative compounds known as anthraquinones. (For more information about the side effects of aloe bitter latex, see Safety.)

BOTANY

Although its exact origins are unclear, aloe probably originated in northern Africa. There are at least 360 members of the aloe genus, which is part of the lily family (Liliaceae). In addition to *Aloe vera,* other commonly used medicinal species include *A. ferox* and *A. perryi. (A. vera* is also sometimes known as *A. barbadensis.)* Aloe plants grow in sunny, warm, dry climates throughout the world. In Africa, some aloe species may grow as tall as trees (30 to 60 feet), whereas in the cooler climates of the Northern Hemisphere, aloe is grown as a houseplant that rarely gets taller than 2 to 3 feet. Aloes are succulent perennials made up of 99 percent water. Although dependent on moisture, the plants have the ability to withstand long periods of drought and will develop root rot if they receive too much moisture.

The base of the aloe plant is encircled by long, translucent-green leaves with spiny edges that have evolved to protect it from insects and animals. The medicinal substances in aloe come from two distinctly different leaf structures. The bitter latex that is used as a stimulating laxative is contained in a thin layer of cells, called the *pericyclic cells,* which are close to the outer part or rind of the leaf. These cells keep the latex separate from the aloe gel, an arrangement that also provides a means of protection for the aloe leaf. When a leaf is cut, the bitter latex mixes with the aloe gel to form a natural barrier that coats the cut and helps the plant retain its moisture. The extremely bitter taste of the latex and its powerful laxative action help dissuade animals and insects from eating the plant.

The milder, more commonly used part of the aloe plant is the thick, sticky gel that comes from cells in the central part of the aloe leaf, called *parenchymal cells.* These cells create vast chambers for the aloe gel, which is primarily made up of water and polysaccharides. The gel is commonly taken internally in the form of a water-diluted juice usually consisting of a minimum of 50 percent gel. Commercial aloe producers carefully drain the bitter latex from the plant to make the gel suitable for consumption. Then they evaporate the bitter yellow latex to produce a solid residue that is the drug aloe.

BENEFITS

- Helps repair skin tissue (external use)
- Reduces inflammation (external use)
- May lower blood glucose (experimental)
- May help prevent and heal stomach ulcers (experimental)

SCIENTIFIC SUPPORT

Not all of the scientific research on aloe has been positive, and much of the research conducted to date has been criticized. According to one researcher writing in 1986, "The scientific literature on aloe is very confused, with a number of contradictory reports and inconclusive experiments. There are also several properly conducted studies, but these do not always receive the recognition they deserve."[1] Another lamented, "The studies on *A. vera* gel currently available in the English language literature present an incomplete and fragmented picture. . . . In some papers the precise part of the leaf used is not emphasized. Was it the sap exuding from the pericyclic cells or the gel originating in the inner parenchymal cells?"[2]

Skin Conditions

Scientific research on the external use of aloe vera gel in the treatment of burns and wounds began in 1935. Early clinical trials showed that aloe effectively relieved the pain and inflammation caused by radiation burns and x rays. However, studies conducted since the 1940s have yielded inconsistent results. In a 1996 double-blind clinical study, aloe gel was ineffective in protecting against dermatitis (severe skin inflammation and rash) induced by radiation therapy.[3] On the other hand, there have been a number of studies both in humans and animals showing that aloe helped reduce inflammation and speed healing of wounds and burns.[1,4–6] One animal study compared the effects of two different aloe products to conventional wound-healing medications on burns, frostbite, and other tissue injuries. The investigators reported that the burn and frostbite subjects treated with aloe healed without tissue loss.[5] Good results have also been reported in the treatment of acne, fungal infections, and skin ulcers.[1,2] In addition, in one study, aloe vera cream was effective when applied to the skin in the treatment of psoriasis (see Specific Studies).[7]

Diabetes and Ulcers

Aloe has demonstrated some positive effects in the treatment of diabetes mellitus, and it appears that both aloe gel and latex may be appropriate candidates for further study. In clinical studies in people with diabetes, aloe gel was shown to significantly lower blood sugar (glucose) and triglycerides, blood fats which are often abnormally high in those with diabetes (see Specific Studies).[8,9] One study investigated the effects of aloe dried latex in five people with diabetes mellitus and in mice with experimentally induced diabetes. Aloe latex effectively lowered blood glucose in the humans, who took half a teaspoon of aloe latex once a day for 4 to 14 weeks, a dosage that was reported to be too low to cause cramping or diarrhea. In the diabetic mice, aloe latex was as effective in lowering glucose as the drug gliben-clamide.[10]

However, in an animal study using aloe vera gel, oral treatment of rats for 10 days provided no protection against the development of either gastric (stomach) lesions or diabetes mellitus.[11] In another animal study, neither aloe gel nor aloe bitter latex protected against gastric and duodenal ulcers.[12] Obviously, more research is necessary to clarify the uses of aloe in diabetes and ulcers.

Researchers currently are investigating the effects of the aloe constituents emodin and aloe-emodin on the bacterium *Helicobacter pylori,* which has been implicated in the development of gastric ulcers. Many scientists now believe that to successfully cure ulcers, *H. pylori* must first be eliminated. Preliminary studies show that emodin may destroy *H. pylori* by damaging its DNA, and in this way may help prevent and heal ulcers.[13] Aloe-emodin has also been shown to inhibit the growth of *H. pylori.*[14]

Emodin and aloe-emodin are powerful laxative compounds called *anthraquinones* isolated from aloe bitter latex. Other major anthraquinones in aloe include aloin and barbaloin. In large doses anthraquinones are cathartic, but *in vitro* studies of aloin and emodin have shown that in small amounts they have analgesic and antimicrobial effects and aid absorption in the digestive tract.[15] Commercial processing standards for aloe gel require that no more than 50 parts per million of aloin remain in an aloe gel product intended for consumption.[16]

Antiviral Effects

Acemannan, a polysaccharide compound isolated from aloe rind, has demonstrated an ability to inhibit the replication of numerous viruses, including both HIV-1 and herpes simplex.[1,17,18] It has also been shown to stimulate the activity of the immune system in people with AIDS.[19,20] Preliminary results from clinical studies have been encouraging but still inconclusive. In an early pilot study in 16 people with AIDS, 3 months of oral treatment with acemannan (up to 1,000 mg daily) was associated with a 71 percent reduction in symptoms.[21] However, a more recent placebo-controlled study in 24 people with advanced AIDS concluded that oral acemannan at a daily dose of 1,600 mg was no more effective than placebo in preventing declines in CD4 counts.[22] (Low CD4 counts signal an increase in destructive T-cells and a decrease in helper T-cells.) Some researchers believe that treatment with acemannan may be more appropriate for people in earlier stages of HIV infection.[23,24] Preliminary research has also suggested that a combination of acemannan and the drug zidovudine (AZT) may have synergistic effects that could allow HIV and AIDS patients to reduce their AZT dose.[23]

In the United States, acemannan is already approved for veterinary use as an injectable treatment for fibrosarcoma (a type of cancer) and feline leukemia, which, like AIDS, is believed to be caused by infection with a retrovirus.[23]

In addition, one clinical study of 30 people showed that canker sores healed faster in those who applied an acemannan hydrogel than in those who used a conventional medication (see Specific Studies).[25]

SPECIFIC STUDIES

Psoriasis: Clinical Study (1996)

In this double-blind, placebo-controlled study conducted in Pakistan, topical application of a 0.5 percent aloe vera cream for 4 weeks was significantly more effective than placebo in eliminating psoriasis lesions of slight to moderate severity. The 60 subjects in the study were randomly assigned to two equal groups. One group applied the aloe vera cream three times daily for 5 days a week for a maximum of 4 weeks, and the other applied a placebo cream following the same schedule. The participants, who had had psoriasis for a mean number of 8.5 years, were examined weekly to assess improvements, based on a scoring index called the Psoriasis Area and Severity Index. The researchers reported that by the end of the study, there was an 83.3 percent cure rate in the people treated with the aloe cream, compared with a 6.6 percent cure rate with placebo. The 4-week study was followed up by monthly checkups for 8 months. No relapses were reported. No side effects were observed in people using the aloe cream.[7]

Diabetes: Clinical Study (1996)

In a single-blind, placebo-controlled clinical trial performed in Thailand, people with newly diagnosed diabetes mellitus had lowered blood glucose levels after only 1 week of treatment with aloe vera gel juice. By the end of the trial, triglyceride levels were also significantly reduced. In this study, 77 people received treatment with either placebo or 1 tablespoon of aloe vera gel juice twice daily for 42 days. Weekly blood samples were taken, and participants were closely monitored by the physicians conducting the trial. Reductions in blood glucose levels were observed in individuals taking aloe after the first week of treatment, whereas the participants taking placebo had no change in blood glucose levels over the course of the trial. By the end of the study, the aloe-juice group had significantly lower blood sugar and triglyceride levels than those in the placebo group. Cholesterol levels were not affected. Only one person failed to complete the study due to diabetic complications. According to the researchers, this study confirms "the potential of aloe vera juice for use as an antidiabetic agent." The aloe juice used in the study contained 80 percent aloe gel, unidentified flavorings and preservatives, and sorbitol as a sweetener.[8]

Canker Sores: Clinical Study (1994)

In this controlled study, acemannan hydrogel was more effective than a conventional medication in accelerating lesion healing in 30 people with aphthous stomatitis (mouth ulcers commonly known as canker sores). The participants received one of three treatments: acemannan hydrogel, a freeze-dried acemannan hydrogel, or a medication called Orabase. The test medications were applied four times a day. Ulcers healed significantly faster in people treated with either acemannan hydrogel (5.89 days) or the freeze-dried acemannan hydrogel (5.70 days) compared with Orabase (7.80 days). There were no significant differences among the groups with regard to lesion size, discomfort, or redness.[25]

HOW IT WORKS

Not surprisingly, it is not yet known exactly how aloe works or which constituents are responsible for its effects, although numerous compounds have demonstrated a variety of different actions in laboratory studies. In wound healing, aloe is believed to act in two main areas: through direct effects on epithelial tissue and by stimulating immune system activity.[15] It is possible that some of the effects observed with external use may also apply when the gel is taken internally, but this is only speculation and has not yet been studied.

Aloe vera polysaccharides are believed to promote fast healing of skin tissue through anti-inflammatory, immune-stimulating, and antimicrobial effects.[7,15] *In vitro* laboratory studies showed that at the site of inflammation, polysaccharides from aloe gel inhibited the release of harmful oxidants from immune cells (neutrophils) without interfering with their beneficial actions, such as phagocytosis (the ingestion and digestion of solid substances such as other cells, bacteria, and foreign particles).[26,27] Aloe polysaccharides may also affect the immune system when taken internally.[15]

Studies indicate that aloe gel possesses analgesic (pain-relieving) properties, and, in high concentrations, kills many different bacterial and fungal organisms, including *Candida albicans, Staphylococcus aureus, Escherichia coli,* and *Pseudomonas aeruginosa,* as well as certain viruses, including herpes simplex and zoster.[15,23] Aloe has also been shown to stimulate the replication of dermal fibroblasts, which leads to an increase in collagen production and enhanced wound healing.[15] In addition, in one experiment using normal human cells and tumor cells, compounds from aloe gel promoted the attachment and growth of normal cells, but not tumor cells, and enhanced the healing of wounded cells. The authors of this study suggested that these results may help explain the healing effects of aloe on wounds and burns.[28]

Aloe's effects on the skin may also be due at least in part to high levels of amino acids found in fresh aloe gel, which contains 20 of the 22 amino acids required by the human body. Aloe also contains other substances helpful in healing the skin, including zinc, vitamin E, and vitamin C.[23] Gamma-linolenic acid and prostaglandins in aloe also play a role in its ability to help heal wounds.[23] *In vitro* laboratory studies have suggested that compounds in aloe gel may inhibit prostaglandin synthesis and inactivate bradykinin, substances involved in pain and inflammation.[2,15]

MAJOR CONSTITUENTS

Polysaccharides (including acemannan), anthraquinones (aloin, emodin, aloe-emodin, barbaloin), fatty acids (gamma-linolenic acid), prostaglandins, salicylic acid, saponins, sterols, vitamins, minerals, amino acids, lectins

SAFETY

Aloe gel and the juice made from the gel are considered safe for consumption when used appropriately.[29] The safety information in this section applies only to aloe gel and aloe gel juice, not the laxative bitter latex. See Safety Issues with Dried Aloe Latex for more information.

- **Side effects:** Used externally, leaf gel has been reported to delay wound healing following laparotomy or caesarean delivery.[29] There have been rare reports of allergy to aloe gel applied topically. Taken internally, aloe gel juice may have a laxative effect if the recommended dosage is exceeded.[30]
- **Contraindications:** None known.[29]
- **Drug interactions:** None known.[29]

Safety Issues with Dried Aloe Latex

The dried bitter aloe latex, a distinct product made from a different region of the leaves than the gel, can be an extremely potent laxative. Scientific research on dried bitter aloe latex indicates that its effect is stronger than that of senna. As a stimulant laxative, aloe vera dried latex is recommended only for occasional, short-term use in doses not exceeding 50 to 300 mg.[29] When taken in higher doses, stimulant laxatives can cause cathartic effects, such as severe diarrhea, cramping, and uterine contractions.[29]

Long-term use of stimulant laxatives such as bitter aloe can cause dependency, meaning that the body may lose its ability to have a bowel movement without the stimulation of the laxative. Chronic use of these substances can also lead to fluid loss and depletion of vital electrolytes such as potassium. Potassium loss can enhance the effects of drugs containing cardiac glycosides and affect the action of antiarrhythmic agents, causing potentially dangerous side effects for those taking heart medications.[31] Low potassium levels (hypokalemia) can also raise blood pressure and cause cardiac complications.

Aloe bitter latex and other stimulant laxatives (such as senna and cascara sagrada) should not be used during pregnancy or nursing or by children younger than 12 years. In addition, they should not be taken by people with intestinal obstruction, Crohn's disease, ulcerative colitis, appendicitis, or abdominal pain of unknown origin. Taking bitter aloe latex may cause the urine to turn red.[31]

DOSAGE

Pure aloe gel and juice products made from gel should be refrigerated to prevent spoilage. To extend shelf life, many companies add preservatives to their aloe products. Even products labeled as "pure" aloe gel may contain thickening agents, sweeteners, flavorings, and other herbs or juices. Aloe liquid concentrates may also contain large amounts of gums, lactose, and starch.[32] Consumers concerned about these issues should contact the manufacturer for more information.

Aloe gel is naturally viscous (thick) when taken from the leaf, but quickly becomes watery due to the action of enzymes in the plant. This is why companies add thickeners, including gums and starches, in an attempt to make the finished product seem more like the fresh gel. It is possible to dry aloe without releasing the enzymes, producing a powder that, when reconstituted with water, retains the original consistency of fresh aloe gel.

- **Aloe gel:** Apply externally as needed.
- **Aloe gel juice:** For internal use, take 1 or 2 teaspoons up to three times a day.
- **Bitter aloe latex:** Because it is a very stimulating laxative that can have cathartic effects, it is not recommended for general use. See Safety.

REFERENCES

1. Grindlay D, Reynolds T. The aloe vera phenomenon: a review of the properties and modern uses of the leaf parenchyma gel. *Journal of Ethnopharmacology* 1986; 16: 117–151.
2. Marshall JM. Aloe vera gel: what is the evidence? *The Pharmaceutical Journal* March 24, 1990; 360–362.
3. Williams MS, Burk M, Loprinzi CL, et al. Phase III double-blind evaluation of an aloe vera gel as a prophylactic agent for radiation-induced skin toxicity. *International*

Journal of Radiation Oncology, Biology, Physics 1996; 36(2): 345–349.

4. Udupa SL, Udupa AL, Kulkarni DR. Anti-inflammatory and wound healing properties of *Aloe vera*. *Fitoterapia* 1994; 65(2): 141–145.

5. Heggers JP, Pelley RP, Robson MC. Beneficial effects of Aloe in wound healing. *Phytotherapy Research* 1993; 7: S48–S52.

6. Bunyapraphatsara N, Jirakulchaiwong S, Thirawarapan S, et al. The efficacy of aloe vera cream in the treatment of first, second, and third degree burns in mice. *Phytomedicine* 1996; 2(3): 247–251.

7. Syed TA, Ahmad SA, Holt AH, et al. Management of psoriasis with Aloe vera extract in a hydrophilic cream: a placebo-controlled, double-blind study. *Tropical Medicine and International Health* 1996; 1(4): 505–509.

8. Yongchaiyudha S, Rungpitarangsi V, Bunyapraphatsara N, et al. Antidiabetic activity of *Aloe vera* L. juice. I. Clinical trial in new cases of diabetes mellitus. *Phytomedicine* 1996; 3(3): 241–243.

9. Bunyapraphatsara N, Yongchaiyudha S, Rungpitarangsi V, et al. Antidiabetic activity of *Aloe vera* L. juice. II. Clinical trial in diabetes mellitus patients in combination with glibenclamide. *Phytomedicine* 1996; 3(3): 245–248.

10. Ghannam N, Kingston M, Al-Meshaal IA, et al. The antidiabetic activity of aloes: preliminary clinical and experimental observations. *Hormone Research* 1986; 24: 288–294.

11. Koo MWL. Aloe vera: antiulcer and antidiabetic effects. *Phytotherapy Research* 1994; 8(8): 461–464.

12. Parmar MD, Tariq M, Al-Yahya MA, et al. Evaluation of aloe vera leaf exudate and gel for gastric and duodenal ulcer activity. *Fitoterapia* 1986; 57(5): 380–383.

13. Wang HH, Chung JG. Emodin-induced inhibition of growth and DNA damage in the *Helicobacter pylori*. *Current Microbiology* 1997; 35: 262–266.

14. Wang HH, Chung JG, Ho CC. Aloe-emodin effects on arylamine *n*-acetyltransferase activity in the bacterium *Helicobacter pylori*. *Planta Medica* 1998; 64: 176–178.

15. Atherton P. Aloe vera revisited. *British Journal of Phytotherapy* 1998; 4(4): 176–183.

16. Klabin G. The truth about Aloe vera—how to select the best Aloe vera beverage. *The Townsend Letter for Doctors* May 1992; 413–417.

17. Kemp MC, Kahlon JB, Chinnah AD, et al. *In vitro* evaluation of the antiviral effects of acemannan on the replication and pathogenesis of HIV-1 and other enveloped viruses: modification of the processing of glycoprotein precursors. *Antiviral Research* 1990; (suppl 1): 83. Abstract 84.

18. Kahlon JB, Kemp MC, Carpenter RH, et al. Inhibition of AIDS virus replication by acemannan *in vitro*. *Molecular Biotherapy* 1991; 3: 127–134.

19. Womble D, Helderman JH. Enhancement of allo-responsiveness of human lymphocytes by acemannan (Carrisyn). *International Journal of Immunopharmacology* 1988; 10(4): 967–974.

20. McDaniel HR, Combs C, McDaniel HR, et al. An increase in circulating monocyte/macrophages (M/M) is induced by oral acemannan (ACE-M) in HIV-1 pa-

tients. *American Journal of Clinical Pathology* 1990; 94(4): 516. Abstract 124.

21. McDaniel HR, Perkins S, McAnalley BH. A clinical pilot study using Carrisyn in the treatment of acquired immunodeficiency syndrome (AIDS). *American Journal of Clinical Pathology* 1987; 88: 534. Abstract.

22. Montaner JSG, Gill J, Singer J, et al. Double-blind placebo-controlled pilot trial of acemannan in advanced human immunodeficiency virus disease. *Journal of Acquired Immune Deficiency Syndromes and Human Retrovirology* 1996; 12: 153–157.

23. Murray M. *The Healing Power of Herbs.* Rocklin, CA: Prima Publishing, 1995.

24. McDaniel HR, Carpenter RH, Kemp M. Extended survival and prognostic criteria for acemannan (ACE-M) treated HIV-1 patients. *Antiviral Research* 1990; (suppl 1): 117. Abstract 147.

25. Plemons JM, Rees TD, Binnie WH, et al. Evaluation of acemannan in the treatment of recurrent aphthous stomatitis. *Wounds* 1994; 6(2): 40–45.

26. 't Hart LA, Nibbering PH, van den Barselaar MT, et al. Effects of low molecular constituents from *Aloe vera* gel on oxidative metabolism and cytotoxic and bactericidal activity of human neutrophils. *International Journal of Immunopharmacology* 1990; 12(4): 427–434.

27. 't Hart LA, van Enckevort PH, van Dijk H, et al. Two functionally and chemically distinct immunomodulatory compounds in the gel of *Aloe vera*. *Journal of Ethnopharmacology* 1988; 23: 61–71.

28. Winters WD, Benavides R, Clouse WJ. Effects of aloe extracts on human normal and tumor cells in vitro. *Economic Botany* 1981; 35(1): 89–95.

29. McGuffin M, Hobbs C, Upton R, et al., eds. *American Herbal Products Association Botanical Safety Handbook*. Boca Raton, FL: CRC Press, 1997.

30. Foster S. *101 Medicinal Herbs.* Loveland, CO: Interweave Press, 1998.

31. Blumenthal M, Busse W, Goldberg A, et al., eds. *The Complete German Commission E Monographs*. Austin, TX: The American Botanical Council; Boston: Integrative Medicine Communications, 1998.

32. Foster S. Aloe vera: every windowsill deserves one. *The Herb Companion* February/March, 1995: 49–52.

Artichoke

CYNARA SCOLYMUS

ASTERACEAE

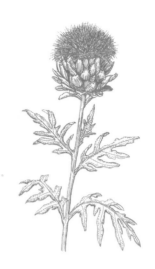

State of Knowledge: Five-Star Rating System

Clinical (human) research	✶✶
Laboratory research	✶✶✶
History of use/traditional use	✶✶✶✶
Safety record	✶✶✶✶
International acceptance	✶✶✶

PART USED: *Leaf*

PRIMARY USES

- *Indigestion in the upper intestinal tract*
- *Appetite and digestion*
- *High Cholesterol*
- *Heart and liver health*
- *Antioxidant*

To most Americans, globe artichoke is best known as an exotic-looking vegetable, not as a medicinal herb. In Europe, however, it is widely accepted as both. Like many other thistles, artichoke has a long history of use as a food and as a health-protective remedy, especially known for its effects on liver health. A close relative of milk thistle *(Silybum marianum)*, another herb well-known for its benefits to the liver, globe artichoke may provide similar antioxidant and liver-protective actions. Today, compelling clinical evidence from Germany shows that artichoke leaf extract is an effective remedy against symptoms of nonspecific upper intestinal complaints. Known collectively in Germany as *dyspeptic syndrome,* these digestive disturbances may cause abdominal pain, bloating, constipation, diarrhea, flatulence, nausea and vomiting, heartburn, loss of appetite, and other unpleasant symptoms.

While artichoke extract is officially approved in Germany only for the treatment of digestive disorders, research has revealed an additional benefit. Clinical and laboratory studies show that artichoke extract lowers elevated cholesterol, a major risk factor for heart disease. Other studies have shown that artichoke extract can prevent the oxidation of harmful low-density lipoprotein (LDL) cholesterol, which has also been implicated in the development of atherosclerosis (hardening of the arteries). Well-designed future research may prove artichoke extract to be one of the most valuable natural therapies for lowering cholesterol, preventing the build-up of atherosclerotic plaques in the blood vessels, and maintaining overall cardiovascular health.

Through its actions on the liver, artichoke has a *choleretic* effect, meaning that it stimulates the production and secretion of bile. Bile secretion is essential not only for good digestion, but also for the regulation of cholesterol levels in the blood. Traditional herbalists attribute this choleretic effect in part to the extremely bitter taste, which is thought to stimulate the production of all digestive juices, from saliva to bile. This is the idea behind the traditional "bitter tonic" or apéritif taken before meals to aid digestion. In fact, artichoke leaf is the main ingredient in the European apéritif Cynar, obviously named after the artichoke itself.

The vegetable known as artichoke and the medicinal extract actually come from two different parts of the artichoke plant. The part of the plant that is eaten is the unopened flowerhead or bud, of which the tasty artichoke heart is the base. The extremely bitter leaves that are used as medicine occur below the flowerhead, on the stem. The "leaves" that are eaten as a vegetable really are not leaves at all, but a part of the flowerhead called *bracts*.

HISTORY

A truly ancient vegetable, artichoke was first cultivated at least 2,000 years ago. The earliest accounts of the medicinal uses of artichoke come from writings of ancient Greek and Roman physicians in the fourth century B.C. and, somewhat later, from Arab medical literature. Accompanied by hieroglyphs, illustrations of artichokes are said to appear in the pictorial stories that adorned the tombs of Egyptian pharaohs, although it is unclear if these depict globe artichoke or its botanical ancestor, the cardoon (*Cynara cardunculus*).[1]

The Roman empire is credited with introducing the artichoke as a culinary delicacy as early as the first century B.C. According to historical accounts, the ancient Romans also recognized artichoke's medicinal value, praising its ability to "set the digestive fluids flowing."[1] An old Roman recipe for artichoke hearts, probably dating from the sixteenth century, describes a dish stewed in water and oil and seasoned with salt, pepper, finely chopped garlic, and peppermint leaves. Artichoke was reputed to be a favorite food of King Henry VIII of England and of the French kings and gentry of the sixteenth century. By the 1500s, artichokes were being cultivated in German gardens.[1]

Between the fourteenth and nineteenth centuries, artichoke was widely used in Europe (particularly in France and Germany) for the treatment of jaundice, liver failure, and gallbladder disease, as well as for arthritic conditions and urinary tract problems. An 1850 report in French medical literature describes the use of a cooked broth of artichoke leaves in the successful treatment of a boy with jaundice. This prompted the first serious clinical studies of artichoke leaf broth and extract, the results of which were presented to the Paris Society of Therapy in 1929.[1] Artichoke's cholesterol-lowering effects have reportedly been recognized at least since 1933.[2]

INTERNATIONAL STATUS

Artichoke leaf is listed as an approved herb in the *German Commission E Monographs,* indicated for the treatment of dyspeptic problems (indigestion).

BOTANY

Globe artichoke *(Cynara scolymus)* is in the aster family (Asteraceae), a huge plant family that is subdivided into a number of different "tribes." Artichoke is in the thistle tribe, a large group of edible plants that also includes milk thistle *(Silybum marianum)* and burdock *(Arctium lappa).* When allowed to go to flower, the artichoke plant puts forth large, spectacular blue-violet flowerheads, making it an attractive garden ornamental. The flower stems reach heights of 4 to 6 feet. The modern globe artichoke is derived from the wild artichoke, or cardoon *(Cynara cardunculus),* once widely cultivated as a food. Both globe artichoke and the cardoon are believed to have originated in Morocco or the Canary Islands.[1]

Globe artichoke is only distantly related to Jerusalem artichoke, so named because its edible tubers (roots) taste something like the heart of the globe artichoke. Jerusalem artichoke *(Helianthus tuberosa)* is a member of the Asteraceae sunflower tribe.

BENEFITS

- Increases secretion of bile
- Lowers cholesterol
- Protects liver cells from damage by free radicals and other toxins
- Inhibits oxidation of LDL cholesterol

SCIENTIFIC SUPPORT

Bile is essential for proper digestion, and inadequate bile secretion can lead to difficulty in digesting fatty foods as well as to a number of digestive disorders, including dyspeptic and irritable bowel syndromes.[3] Dyspeptic syndrome, as described by German physicians, defines nonspecific upper intestinal disturbances that may cause any number of different symptoms, including abdominal pain and bloating, nausea, vomiting, appetite disturbances, flatulence, constipation, and diarrhea, among others. Clinical studies have demonstrated artichoke's ability to enhance bile secretion and thereby greatly improve symptoms of dyspeptic syndrome and other digestive disorders.[3–6]

Adequate levels of bile are also essential for regulation of cholesterol levels. Beginning in the 1930s, numerous clinical trials have shown that artichoke extract can lower levels of serum cholesterol and triglycerides, and later studies suggest that it may improve the ratio of beneficial high-density lipoprotein (HDL) to harmful low-density lipoprotein (LDL).[4,7] Some of the older research on artichoke's cholesterol-lowering abilities focused on the isolated constituent cynarin, but more recent studies suggest that artichoke's therapeutic effects are due to the synergistic effects of a combination of compounds.[4,8]

One study specifically designed to assess artichoke's cholesterol-lowering effects demonstrated a 12.9 percent drop in triglycerides after 12 weeks of treatment in participants with the highest cholesterol levels. This trial was somewhat unique in that it tested a pressed juice of fresh artichoke leaves and flower buds, rather than an extract. Unfortunately, the study was not placebo controlled. To evaluate the effectiveness of treatment with artichoke juice, the investigators compared changes in cholesterol levels after 6 and 12 weeks of treatment with baseline measurements, and then compared their results with results achieved in other studies investigating the effects of high-dose fibrate therapy, a drug treatment for high cholesterol.[9]

Much of the evidence on artichoke's cholesterol-lowering effects comes from studies that were primarily designed to assess the plant's effectiveness in the treatment of digestive disorders. A secondary finding of one large study in people with digestive problems showed that 6 weeks of treatment resulted in a highly statistically significant drop in cholesterol and triglycerides in 302 participants whose cholesterol levels were routinely monitored during the study. The investigators also reported a slight rise in levels of HDL (see Specific Studies).[7] Another such study demonstrated a statistically significant 14.5 percent drop in total cholesterol after 6 weeks of treatment in a subgroup of 170 participants.[10]

The clinical evidence is well supported by animal studies.[4,11–13] In one controlled study of rats with experimentally induced high cholesterol, artichoke extract administered directly into the abdominal cavity produced a 45 percent reduction in cholesterol and a 33 percent reduction in triglycerides. The extract also caused a significant drop in cholesterol and triglycerides when given orally to rats eating a normal diet.[12] In addition, laboratory research shows that artichoke extract directly inhibits the production of cholesterol by the liver.

With regard to artichoke's antioxidant activity, laboratory studies have demonstrated two primary effects: protection of the liver against damage from toxins and an ability to prevent oxidation of blood fats. In *in vitro* studies using cultured liver cells, water extracts of artichoke protected cells from damage by oxidants and inhibited lipid peroxidation.[14–16] Artichoke has also been shown to prevent oxidation of harmful LDL cholesterol, which is believed to play a major role in the development of atherosclerotic disease.[4,17]

Unfortunately, not all of the clinical research on artichoke has been placebo controlled. Well-controlled research, especially research specifically designed to assess cholesterol-lowering effects, is needed.

SPECIFIC STUDIES

Digestive Disorders: Clinical Study (1996)

Standardized artichoke extract was associated with a significant improvement in a variety of digestive symptoms in this large-scale German study. The investigators also observed a highly statistically significant reduction of serum cholesterol and triglyceride

levels and a small rise in HDL levels. The main diagnoses among the 553 study participants were dyspeptic complaints, functional gallbladder problems, and constipation, most of which were classified as chronic. Both physicians and participants assessed symptom improvement following treatment with artichoke extract. After 6 weeks, doctors rated the effectiveness of artichoke extract as excellent or good in 85 percent of participants. According to subject's self-assessments, there was an average 70.5 percent reduction in symptoms. The greatest improvements were seen in incidence of vomiting (88.3 percent), nausea (82.4 percent), and abdominal pain (76.2 percent). In addition, there were improvements of 72.3 percent in loss of appetite, 71 percent in constipation, 68.2 percent in flatulence, 66 percent in meteorism (bloating of the abdomen due to gas), and 58.8 percent in dietary fat intolerance. Subjects took one to two 320-mg capsules three times a day of artichoke extract. The artichoke treatment was well tolerated, with only 1.3 percent of participants reporting side effects of bloating, weakness, and feelings of hunger.[5]

Bile Secretion: Clinical Study (1994)

Single doses of a standardized artichoke leaf extract caused a significant increase in bile secretion in this placebo-controlled, randomized crossover pilot trial in 20 men with apparently normal digestive function. The greatest increase in bile secretion occurred 1 hour after administration of artichoke extract, but differences between the artichoke and placebo groups were still evident after 3 hours. In the first part of the trial, 10 men took single doses of either six 320-mg capsules of artichoke extract or placebo, both of which were dissolved in water and administered with an intraduodenal probe directly into the gastrointestinal tract. The participants' stomachs were empty at the time the treatment was administered. In phase two, the treatment groups switched. Researchers measured bile secretion with an intraduodenal probe, starting 30 minutes after administration and continuing for 4 hours. After 30 minutes, they observed a 127 percent increase in bile secretion in men in the artichoke groups. A 151.5 percent increase was seen after 60 minutes, and after another 60 minutes, another 94.3 percent increase was recorded (each increase in relation to the first measurement). These increases, as well as those noted at 120 and 150 minutes, were all significantly higher than those seen with the inactive placebo.[3]

HOW IT WORKS

Artichoke's benefits in the treatment of digestive disorders and its cholesterol-lowering properties are both related to its effects on the liver. Of primary importance is its ability to improve the secretion of bile. In studies using cultured liver cells, artichoke leaf extract was shown to enhance bile secretion by increasing the number and size of bile vesicles within the liver.[4]

Adequate bile secretion is important not only for improving digestion, but also for regulating cholesterol levels, because bile is an important pathway for elimination of cholesterol from the body. In addition, evidence from numerous studies indicates that artichoke directly inhibits the production of cholesterol by the liver.[11,13] In one laboratory study using cultured rat liver cells, high doses of a water extract of artichoke leaf inhibited cholesterol synthesis by cells in a dose-dependent manner—in other words, the higher the dose, the greater the effect.[11]

For many years, the constituent cynarin was thought to be responsible for most of artichoke's therapeutic effects, but today researchers believe that the plant's actions are due to a combination of compounds working together.[2] Recent research suggests that the constituents cynaroside and especially luteolin are particularly important in inhibiting cholesterol synthesis by the liver.[11] There is evidence that whole artichoke extract indirectly affects cholesterol production in at least two ways, both by interfering with processes that activate cholesterol synthesis and by activating mechanisms that inhibit cholesterol synthesis.[4]

In studies investigating antioxidant effects in cultured liver cells, artichoke extract protected cells from damage in part by preventing loss of glutathione, a naturally occurring antioxidant that plays an essential role in neutralizing toxins.[14,15] If enough glutathione is lost, liver damage results.

MAJOR CONSTITUENTS

Caffeylquinic acids (including cynarin), luteolin, caffeic acid, chlorogenic acid, scolymoside, cynaroside

SAFETY

Artichoke is generally considered safe when used appropriately. A review of clinical studies on artichoke concluded that the extract was well tolerated by 95 percent of the population studied.[4]

- **Side effects:** In clinical studies, a small number of participants reported side effects such as sensations of weakness and hunger.
- **Contraindications:** Artichoke leaf extract should not be used by people with bile duct blockages. If you have gallstones, consult your doctor before using artichoke extract.[18]
- **Drug interactions:** None known.[18]

DOSAGE

- **Standardized extract:** One or two 320-mg capsules three times a day
- **Tincture (5:1):** 15 to 30 drops in a small amount of water three times a day

STANDARDIZATION

Artichoke extracts are standardized to contain 2.5 to 15 percent caffeylquinic acid.

REFERENCES

1. Mayr A, Frölich E. Two centuries of artichoke, *Cynara scolymus* [in German]. *Österreichische Apotheker-Zeitung* 1965; 19(29/30): 468–471.
2. Ernst E. The artichoke—an historical medicinal plant with perspectives for the future [in German]. *Naturamed* 1995; 10(7): 30–35.
3. Kirchhoff R, Beckers C, Kirchhoff GM, et al. Increase in choleresis by means of artichoke extract. *Phytomedicine* 1994, 1: 107–115.
4. Kraft K. Artichoke leaf extract—recent findings reflecting effects on lipid metabolism, liver and gastrointestinal tracts. *Phytomedicine* 1997; 4(4): 369–378.
5. Fintelmann V. Antidyspeptic and lipid-decreasing effects of artichoke leaf extract [in German]. *Zeitschrift Allgemeiner Medizin* 1996; 72(2): 3–19.
6. Kupke D, von Sanden H, Trinczek-Gärtner H, et al. Testing of the choleretic activity of a plant-based cholagogue [in German]. *Zeitschrift Allgemeiner Medizin* 1991; 67: 1046–1058.
7. Fintelmann V, Menssen HG. Artichoke leaf extract: current findings to the effect as a lipid-decreaser and antidyspeptic [in German]. *Deutsche Apotheker Zeitung* 1996; 136(17): 63–74.

8. Wegener T. New findings from the artichoke research [in German]. *Erfahrungsheilkunde* 1995; 1: 53.

9. Dorn M. Improvement in raised lipid levels with artichoke juice (*Cynara scolymus* L.). *British Journal of Phytotherapy* 1995/96; 4(1): 21–26.

10. Wegener T. On the therapeutic effectiveness of artichoke extract [in German]. *Zeitschrift für Phytotherapy* 1995; 16: 81.

11. Gebhardt R. Inhibition of cholesterol biosynthesis in primary cultured rat hepatocytes by artichoke (*Cynara scolymus L.*) extracts. *The Journal of Pharmacology and Experimental Therapeutics* 1998; 286(3): 1122–1128.

12. Lietti A. Choleretic and cholesterol lowering properties of two artichoke extracts. *Fitoterapia* 1977; 48(4): 153–158.

13. Gebhardt R. Artichoke extracts—*in vitro* evidence of an inhibitory effect on cholesterol biosynthesis [in German]. *Die Medizinische Welt* 1995; 46: 348–350.

14. Gebhardt R, Fausel M. Antioxidant and hepatoprotective effects of artichoke extracts and constituents in cultured rat hepatocytes. *Toxicology in Vitro* 1997; 11: 669–672.

15. Gebhardt R. Antioxidant and protective properties of extracts from leaves of the artichoke (*Cynara scolymus* L.) against hydroperoxide-induced oxidative stress in cultured rat hepatocytes. *Toxicology and Applied Pharmacology* 1997; 144: 279–286.

16. Adzet T, Camarasa J, Laguna JC. Hepatoprotective activity of polyphenolic compounds from *Cynara scolymus* against CCL4 toxicity in isolated rat hepatocytes. *Journal of Natural Products* 1987; 50(4): 612–617.

17. Fintelmann V. Clinical significance of the lipid-decreasing and antioxidative effect of *Cynara scolymus* (artichoke) [in German]. In: Loew D, Rietbrock N, eds. *Phytopharmaka II. Forschung und Klinische Anwedung.* Darmstadt, Germany: Steinkopf Publishers, 1996.

18. Blumenthal M, Busse W, Goldberg A, et al., eds. *The Complete German Commission E Monographs.* Austin, TX: The American Botanical Council; Boston: Integrative Medical Communications, 1998.

Astragalus

ASTRAGALUS MEMBRANACEUS
FABACEAE

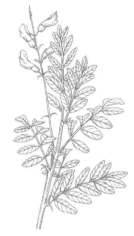

PART USED: *Root*

PRIMARY USES

- *Colds and flu*
- *Chronic respiratory problems such as bronchitis*
- *Digestive ailments (traditional)*
- *Susceptibility to infectious disease*
- *Recovery after illness*
- *General weakness and fatigue (traditional)*
- *Cancer (experimental)*

In China, the national version of a nourishing pot of chicken soup is likely to contain an ingredient that may be new to you—astragalus root. In the exotic language of traditional Chinese medicine (TCM), astragalus boosts the immune system by "stabilizing the exterior" and strengthening the "chi." The Chinese knew thousands of years ago that astragalus could strengthen our shield ("exterior") against disease and increase overall vitality (chi), long before anyone knew about bacteria, white blood cells, or the immune system.

You may already be accustomed to taking echinacea at the first sign of a cold or flu, or when people around you are getting sick. How is astragalus different? Like echinacea, Astragalus not only helps prevent colds and flu but shortens the course of a bug once it has set in. Astragalus can also be used as a long-term preventive and restorative herb, both to prevent illness and to renew energy and vitality once an acute illness has passed. Scientific evidence also suggests that astragalus may be one of the most important herbs for strengthening the immune system against serious diseases, including cancer.

HISTORY

The Chinese name for astragalus, *huang qi,* means "yellow energy," suggesting its role as an important energy-building herb. Astragalus has been used in China for thousands of years and was first mentioned in *The Divine Husbandman's Classic of the Materia Medica,* an ancient Chinese medicinal text. In TCM, astragalus is considered a treatment for frequent colds, chronic weakness of the lungs with shortness of breath, general weakness or fatigue, weak digestion, lack of appetite, diabetes, organ prolapse (sinking), stomach ulcers, nephritis (inflammation of the kidneys), and as a liver protectant and heart tonic. Astragalus has also been applied to the skin as a 10 percent ointment to treat chronic wounds and ulcers. Like most Chinese herbs, it is primarily used in combination formulas with other botanicals. For example, astragalus is often mixed with ginseng for cases of debility and fatigue.

INTERNATIONAL STATUS

Astragalus is not officially approved for use in any European nation. However, it is an of-ficial medicine in China, Japan, Thailand, Malaysia, and other Asian nations.

BOTANY

Native to northern China and Mongolia, *Astragalus membranaceus* can also be found growing wild in Taiwan, Japan, and Korea. A member of the pea family (Fabaceae), astragalus has compound leaves that grow 6 inches long, yellow flowers, and 1-inch seed pods that resemble miniature soybeans. The branched taproot is perennial and about 8 inches long at maturity. The whole plant grows up to 2 feet tall. Although some astragalus roots are collected from the wild, most are cultivated either in the United States or northeast China, a region that is known for growing some of the best-quality plants.

BENEFITS

- Strengthens many functions of the immune system
- Helps protect the liver from damage
- May have valuable anticancer effects

SCIENTIFIC SUPPORT

Much of the clinical research on astragalus is in Chinese and, unfortunately, has not yet been translated into English. A few of the available studies show that astragalus helps protect against the common cold when taken over time. In one study, 1,000 people with lowered immunity experienced fewer and less severe colds after taking astragalus either in tablet form or as a nasal spray over a 2-month period.[1] Other clinical studies have shown that astragalus helps in the treatment of chronic bronchitis.[2]

Researchers are currently studying this plant as an adjunct therapy for cancer. In China, physicians have traditionally used astragalus, ligustrum (*Ligustrum lucidum*), and other herbs to counteract the immuno-compromising effects of radiation and chemotherapy treatments.

Studies that tested injectable astragalus preparations showed positive results in treating chronic hepatitis, gastric and duodenal ulcers, viral myocarditis (inflammation of the heart muscle), and high blood pressure. More research is needed to determine whether these results are applicable to astragalus extracts and capsules as well.[1]

Astragalus and Drugs

Another area for further exploration is the possible value of combining astragalus with drug therapies in order to reduce drug toxicity and reduce or treat side effects. For example, astragalus has been employed to treat chronic leukopenia (an abnormally low white blood cell count), which often results from treatment with steroids, anticancer drugs, and other therapies.[1] In an *in vitro* study, researchers were able to use a lower dose of interleukin-2 (IL-2), a common cancer treatment, by combining the drug with astragalus. The addition of astragalus potentiated IL-2 activity 10-fold. High doses of IL-2 are associated with significant side effects.[3] In a laboratory study, astragalus also prevented liver damage induced by the common anticancer drug stilbenemide, possibly because of the astragalus constituent betaine.[4]

An example of a combination therapy in which astragalus enhanced a drug's action can be found in a study of 1,137 people prone to upper respiratory tract viruses. Overall, researchers found that a combination of astragalus and interferon prevented infection more effectively than interferon alone. In those who did develop colds, the combination successfully shortened the course of illness from 4.6 days in those taking interferon alone to 2.6 days in those taking astragalus with interferon.[2]

HOW IT WORKS

Immune-Enhancing Effects

Astragalus appears to strengthen both vital aspects of the immune system: *nonspecific immunity,* which protects against a wide range of foreign invaders, and *specific immunity,* which enlists individual antibodies to target specific invaders (*antigens*). At least three polysaccharides and two saponin constituents may be involved in these effects.

NONSPECIFIC IMMUNITY

Astragalus appears to stimulate the secretion of interferon, a protein that "interferes" with the ability of viruses to multiply by blocking their ability to reproduce themselves in cells. In a study of 28 people, astragalus given orally over a 2-month period significantly increased the production and secretion of interferon compared with controls. Remarkably, the levels of interferon remained high for 2 months after astragalus treatment ended.[2] These results have been duplicated in laboratory studies.

Astragalus also increases levels of natural killer (NK) cells, which roam the body via blood and lymph fluid, destroying a wide variety of invaders, including cancer cells and virus-infected body cells. NK cells accomplish their vital work long before antibodies are enlisted in the immune system fight.[5] Another way that astragalus stimulates immunity is by increasing levels of macrophages (literally, "big eaters"), which engulf foreign particles in lymphoid organs and connective tissue.[5]

According to animal studies, astragalus stimulates white blood cell production by promoting the maturation of these cells in bone marrow. White blood cells form a roving army that defends the body against damage by bacteria, viruses, parasites, and tumor cells. These cells have the unique ability to slip into and out of the blood vessels and thus have access to any part of the body.[6]

SPECIFIC IMMUNITY

Astragalus binds and deactivates specific foreign substances in the body (antigens) by increasing the levels of antibodies (also called *immunoglobulins*). In a clinical study with 1,000 participants, astragalus tablets and nasal sprays helped reduce the incidence and severity of colds by raising levels of immune-enhancing immunoglobulin A (IgA) and G (IgG). IgA prevents invading substances from attaching to mucous membranes in the respiratory tract and other parts of the body. IgG is the main type of antibody found circulating in the blood and is involved in most immune responses. In this study, researchers found that levels of IgA were directly correlated with the severity of cold symptoms.[1] In another clinical study, whole-plant astragalus tablets produced a rise in blood levels of IgE and IgM in 80 people. IgE helps counteract inflammation and allergies. IgM is abundant in the bloodstream and is one of the only antibodies capable of activating complement, a protein which helps antibodies to destroy harmful invaders such as bacteria.[7]

In China, astragalus is often given to elderly patients to improve declining immune function. A recent study conducted with aging mice supports this traditional use. Oral administration of astragalus to 36- and 60-week-old "elderly" mice effectively returned immune function to levels found in 10-week-old mice. Although researchers have not determined exactly how astragalus does this, they believe that it activates the function of B-cells (a type of cell that carries out antigen-specific immune responses) and enhances IgM production, both of which decline with age.[8]

Anticancer Effects

Preliminary research suggests that astragalus may also have powerful anticancer properties. In a study conducted at the University of Texas Medical Center in Houston, researchers found that a water extraction of astragalus restored or enhanced the function of T-cells (white blood cells that play specific roles in the immune system) taken from people with cancer. In some cases, astragalus stimulated the damaged cells to greater activity than found in normal cells taken from healthy individuals.[9]

In another study of people with advanced cancer, astragalus and ligustrum strengthened immunity by increasing the maturation rate of lymphocytes (immune cells that react to specific foreign invaders in the lymph nodes, spleen, and other lymphoid tissue). Astragalus also restored the activity of helper T-cells, which direct other immune cells in the body. It produced this effect by reducing excessive levels of suppressor T-cells, an action similar to that of some chemotherapy agents, but without harmful side effects.[10] However, this research was not conducted in humans or even in animals, leaving many unanswered questions about how astragalus

extracts actually work in the body. Astragalus has also been shown to increase levels of tumor necrosis factor (TNF), a type of immune cell that destroys tumors.[5]

Tonic Effects

Preliminary clinical and laboratory evidence supports the use of astragalus as a general tonic, one of its primary functions in TCM and among Western herbal practitioners. In a clinical study of 80 individuals, researchers discovered that astragalus tablets addressed several different patterns of weakness or "deficiency" in 60 percent of the participants.[7] Laboratory experiments have demonstrated positive effects on endurance, as measured by swimming tests in mice.[11] These tests measure the increase in stamina and endurance in mice swimming in cold water and are a standard test of energy-enhancing herbs.

Astragalus appears to increase oxygenation in the body by stimulating the formation of red blood cells in bone marrow.[6] Astragalus may also work as an antioxidant, protecting the body against harmful free radicals in a variety of degenerative diseases.[12] Laboratory research shows that astragalus helps defend the liver, the body's main organ of detoxification. For example, in one study, the herb shielded the liver against the harmful effects of carbon tetrachloride, a standard toxin used in testing liver-protective effects.[4]

MAJOR CONSTITUENTS

Polysaccharides (astragalan I, II, and III), saponins (astramembrannin I and II), betaine

SAFETY

Astragalus is considered a safe food herb that is extremely well tolerated.

- **Side effects:** None known.
- **Contraindications:** In traditional Chinese medicine, astragalus is not recommended for people with "deficient yin" or "excessive heat signs." In Western medical terms, this may indicate that astragalus is not appropriate during acute illness with symptoms of fever and thirst.
- **Drug interactions:** None known.

DOSAGE

In Chinese medicine, typical doses of astragalus tend to be fairly large (between 8 and 15 grams per day). Astragalus can be used in tincture or capsule form. In China, root slices that look somewhat like tongue depressors are also cooked in foods such as soups and rice, or simmered in boiling water for several hours as tea.

- **Capsules:** 400 to 500 mg, eight or nine times a day [13]
- **Tincture (1:5):** 15 to 30 drops, two times a day [13]

REFERENCES

1. Chang HM, But PPH. *Pharmacology and Applications of Chinese Materia Medica.* Vol. 2. Hong Kong: World Scientific, 1987.
2. Yunde H, Guoliang M, Shuhua W, et al. Effect of radix astragali seu hedysari on the interferon system. *Chinese Medical Journal* 1981; 94(1): 35–40.
3. Chu DT, Lepe-Zuniga J, Wong WL, et al. Fractionated extract of *Astragalus membranaceus,* a Chinese medicinal herb, potentiates LAK cell cytotoxicity generated by a low dose of recombinant interleukin-2. *Journal of Clinical and Laboratory Immunology* 1988; 26: 183–187.
4. Zhang ZL, Wen QZ, Liu CX. Hepatoprotective effects of astragalus root. *Journal of Ethnopharmacology* 1990; 30: 145–149.
5. Kajimura K, Takagi Y, Ueba N, et al. Protective effect of Astragali radix by intraperitoneal injection against Japanese encephalitis virus infection in mice. *Biological and Pharmaceutical Bulletin* 1996; 19(6): 855–859.
6. Rou M, Renfu X. The effect of radix astragali on mouse marrow hemopoiesis. *Journal of Traditional Chinese Medicine* 1983; 3(3): 199–204.
7. Chinese Academy of Medical Sciences. Effects of astragalus on immunological pa-

rameters and cAMP levels in normal humans. *Zhonghua Yixue Zazhi (National Medical Journal of China)* [Chinese]. 1979; 59(1): 23–27.

8. Kajimura K, Takagi Y, Miyano K, et al. Polysaccharide of *Astragali radix* enhances IgM antibody production in aged mice. *Biological and Pharmaceutical Bulletin* 1997; 20(11): 1178–1182.

9. Mavligit G, Ishii Y, Patt Y, et al. Local xenogeneic graft-vs-host reaction: a practical assessment of T-cell function among cancer patients. *Journal of Immunology* 1979; 123(5): 2185–2188.

10. Sun Y, Hersh EM, Lee SL, et al. Preliminary observations on the effects of the Chinese medicinal herbs *Astragalus membranaceus* and *Ligustrum lucidum* on lymphocyte blastogenic responses. *Journal of Biological Response Modifiers* 1983; 2: 227–237.

11. Willard T. *Textbook of Advanced Herbology.* Calgary, Alberta: Wild Rose College of Natural Healing, 1992.

12. Huang KC. *The Pharmacology of Chinese Herbs,* 2nd ed. Boca Raton, FL: CRC Press, 1999.

13. Foster S. *101 Medicinal Herbs.* Loveland, CO: Interweave Press, 1998.

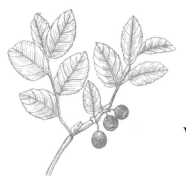

Bilberry

VACCINIUM MYRTILLUS
ERICACEAE

State of Knowledge: Five-Star Rating System

Clinical (human) research	✳✳
Laboratory research	✳✳✳
History of use/traditional use	✳✳✳
Safety record	✳✳✳✳✳
International acceptance	✳✳

PART USED: *Fruit*
PRIMARY USES

- *Eye health and vision*
- *Microcirculation*
- *Spider veins and varicose veins*
- *Capillary strengthening before surgery*

Bilberry is simply the European version of the American blueberry. It looks and tastes just like a blueberry, although wild bilberries are a bit smaller and more astringent than the table variety enjoyed by millions of Europeans, who eat the berries plain or in jams, jellies, fruit juices, and concentrates. During the Second World War, British Royal Air Force pilots reported that eating bilberry jam improved their night vision and their accuracy on night flying missions. It was not until nearly 20 years later that scientists began to study the possibility that bilberry might actually have a beneficial effect on vision. Since then, research has confirmed that bilberry can help maintain and improve eye health and may even protect against the development of serious eye diseases, including cataracts, macular (central retinal) degeneration, and possibly glaucoma. Because it strengthens tiny blood vessels called *capillaries,* it may also help in the treatment of varicose veins and hemorrhoids. Used before surgery, it may help reduce the risk of excessive bleeding.

How can a simple, tasty breakfast fruit provide such powerful medicinal protection? Bilberry contains potent antioxidants that protect and improve micro-circulation, that is, the circulation of blood through the capillaries. These antioxidant pigments, called *anthocyanosides* or *anthocyanins*, are similar to those found in red grape skins. Anthocyanosides protect cells in the circulatory system, keeping them more flexible to provide better blood flow and oxygen to capillary-rich organs such as the retina of the eye. Researchers have also found that bilberry affects enzymes responsible for energy production in the eye, which is especially important to good vision under poor light conditions, including night vision.[1,2]

Bilberry extract and bilberry constituents appear to improve circulation in young and elderly people alike. Bilberry extract may be helpful in preventing many of the vision problems associated with aging. In combination with vitamin E, it can prevent cataracts;[3] it can also prevent retinopathies (diseases of the retina), including diabetic retinopathy,[4] and possibly even ordinary nearsightedness (myopia).[5] Bilberry's ability to strengthen capillary circulation helps those who bruise easily, and bilberry extracts are even used before elective surgery to minimize bruising and excessive bleeding.[3] Increasing capillary strength also helps

in treating spider veins, varicose veins, and hemorrhoids.[6]

HISTORY

Bilberry has been recognized for its medicinal effects since the Middle Ages. It has long been valued as a nutritious fruit, and because of its high vitamin C content, as a treatment for scurvy, a disease caused by lack of vitamin C. The leaves have served as an astringent useful for treating urinary tract infections, diarrhea, and diabetes. The dried berries are also astringent and have been used for dysentery and diarrhea. The word *bilberry* comes from the Danish word *bolebar,* which means "dark berry."

In the early twelfth century, women ate bilberry fruit to promote menstruation; by the sixteenth century, Europeans were employing it for a variety of conditions, including coughs and tuberculosis, liver disorders, and bladder stones. European herbalists praised the berries as an astringent, tonic, and antiseptic. The astringent properties also made bilberry fruit helpful against inflammations and infections of the mouth and gastrointestinal tract.

Today, bilberries are a popular fruit, with an estimated 1,600 metric tons eaten each year worldwide. Sales of bilberry extract capsules were estimated at 13.3 metric tons in 1994.

INTERNATIONAL STATUS

Bilberry fruit is listed as an approved herb in the *German Commission E Monographs,* indicated for the treatment of acute, non-specific diarrhea and mild inflammation of the mucous membranes of the mouth and throat.

BOTANY

Bilberry is a small temperate-zone shrub that produces edible dark blue berries. A member of the heather family (Ericaceae), it is part of a fairly large genus containing several hundred species. The genus *Vaccinium* includes many edible berries, including blueberry *(V. angustifolium)* and cranberry *(V. macrocarpon). Vaccinium myrtillus* is a low-growing, many-branched shrub that grows from 6 inches to 2 feet tall. The tiny greenish flowers ripen into the typical dark blue berry covered with a whitish powdery coating (bloom), similar to that found on grapes.

Like other members of the heather family, bilberry prefers acidic soil and grows in wooded areas and on hillsides throughout Europe. Wild bilberry bushes tend to produce small, astringent berries, whereas the cultivated varieties are large and sweet, virtually indistinguishable from the North American blueberry. Many of the dark-colored fruits of the heather family, as well as grapes, contain antioxidant pigments called anthocyanosides (anthocyanins). The antioxidant effects of red grape pigments have been confirmed, as have the medicinal effects of cranberries and blueberries. Blueberry may produce effects similar to bilberry, but because the research has been conducted almost exclusively in Europe, American blueberries have not been extensively studied.

BENEFITS

- Improves capillary strength and flexibility
- Increases capillary blood flow (microcirculation) in eyes, hands, and feet
- Increases the generation of enzymes responsible for energy production in the eye
- Provides antioxidant benefits

SCIENTIFIC SUPPORT

French researchers began exploring bilberry's effects on the eyes in the 1960s. In these early trials, bilberry extracts and isolated anthocyanosides improved night vision and protected against vision disorders. In one of the earliest placebo-controlled studies, bilberry anthocyanosides enhanced the ability of the eyes to adapt to darkness, visual field, and sensitivity to low light in 40 people, although the dose used was not stated.[7] Several open clinical trials followed. One such trial gauged the effects of bilberry extract on night vision in 14 air traffic controllers, people whose occupation is especially light sensitive.[8] Those who took the extract for 8 days had significant improvements in the ability to adjust to dark conditions after exposure to bright light.

Another trial, 22 years later, used an electronic flash on eight normal individuals, then tracked how long it took for the macula (an area of the retina where visual perception is especially acute) to recover according to a standard optometric test device called an adaptometer. Participants showed significant improvements in their speed of adaptation to light changes after taking two 30-mg tablets of bilberry anthocyanosides per day for a week.[9] Italian research on isolated bilberry anthocyanosides also indicated that they quickly increased adaptation time. After only 2 days, researchers observed highly significant improvements in the absolute light threshold necessary for vision compared with baseline tests in 14 people taking 150 mg of anthocyanosides per day. Participants maintained the same high level of visual acuity for 3 months of treatment, after which the bilberry was discontinued. Improvements disappeared within approximately 1 month.[10]

Around the same time, in the late 1960s, scientists began looking into bilberry's protective effects on the vascular system. French researchers explored the effects of bilberry anthocyanosides on capillary fragility using a standard test called *depressurization*. Essentially, this involves placing a small cupping glass on the skin and applying a vacuum until the capillaries begin leaking blood into the skin, producing tiny spots called *petechiae*. The researchers studied "about 100 patients" with vascular disorders, including varicose and spider veins. With fairly high doses of anthocyanosides (800 to 1,200 mg per day), the participants responded well, usually experiencing a return to normal capillary resistance, often with disappearance of symptoms.[11]

SPECIFIC STUDIES

Night Vision: Clinical Study (1966)

Bilberry extract improved night vision and adaptation to darkness after exposure to glare in this open trial of 14 air traffic controllers. Air traffic controllers spend hours in a darkened room staring at radar screens and watching traffic on the runways and in the air. Their work is visually challenging, requiring their eyes to adapt quickly to darkness after exposure to bright lights. In this study, night vision was tested using a Beyne scotoptometer, which measures the threshold of nocturnal vision, that is, the dimmest image that can be distinguished. In this experiment, researchers exposed the participants to bright light for 1 minute, then tested their visual threshold 30 minutes later. All individuals were tested before beginning the experiment to establish baseline values. Then each took a bilberry extract containing 100 mg bilberry anthocyanosides and 5 mg beta-carotene at a dosage of 4 tablets per day for 8 days. The participants were retested on the day after completing the treatment period, and again 15 days later and 1 month later. They also made a subjective judgment of effects noticed on and off the job.

After treatment, participants reported vision benefits such as faster adjustment after exposure to light, not only at work but in their privates lives (for example, while driving). Air traffic controllers with good night vision before the experiment experienced minor, nonsignificant improvement, whereas those with mediocre nocturnal vision attained levels of nocturnal vision comparable with subjects with very good night vision. For the majority, the improvement was most pronounced just after completing the course of treatment, but for some, the maximum effect was seen 15 days later. The effects disappeared in all but a few cases by 30 days, indicating that the preparation does not produce a lasting benefit.[8]

Cataract Prevention: Clinical Study (1989)

A combination of bilberry extract and vitamin E prevented progression of cataracts in 97 percent of 50 people with mild senile cortical cataracts. In this randomized, double-blind, placebo-controlled trial, participants took 2 bilberry tablets twice daily (each containing 180 mg bilberry extract) and 100 mg synthetic vitamin E or placebo for 4 months. At the conclusion of the 4-month trial, 97 percent of the affected eyes in the active group showed no progression in lens opacity, whereas 3 percent worsened. In the placebo group, 77 percent had no progression of cataracts, whereas 23 percent worsened. No adverse effects were reported.[3]

Diabetic and Hypertensive Retinopathy: Clinical Study (1987)

In this double-blind, placebo-controlled clinical trial in 40 people with diabetes (87 percent of subjects) or arterial hypertension (13 percent), bilberry extract provided highly significant protection against progressive retinopathies. Physicians evaluated improvements with ophthalmoscopic measurements of retinal abnormalities. Participants took one 160-mg capsule twice daily of standardized bilberry extract or placebo for 1 month.

Of the original 40 people, 2 dropped out of each group. Of the 18 in the bilberry group, 13 had retinal abnormalities detectable by ophthalmoscopy. At the end of the trial, 1 of these 13 patients was "much improved," 9 (69 percent) were "improved," and 3 (23 percent) were unchanged. None of the placebo group showed any benefit, and all were switched to active therapy at the conclusion of the trial. Based on an additional evaluation (fluoroangiographic examination), 77 percent of the treatment group demonstrated "great improvement" or "improvement" compared with "slight improvement" in only 1 individual (6 percent) in the placebo group. People with advanced or irreversible retinal lesions, severe metabolic disorders, severe hypertension, or glaucoma were excluded from the trial.[4]

Circulatory Disorders:
Clinical Observation (1987)

Bilberry extract produced significant improvements in symptoms of circulatory disorders of the legs, including varicose veins, and also relieved hemorrhoid symptoms in 51 pregnant women. Dosage of bilberry extract was 160, 240, or 320 mg per day, depending on the severity of the symptoms. Researchers evaluated the patients for the following symptoms: pain, paresthesia (tingling), fatigability of the lower limbs, sensation of heaviness, pruritus (itching), cramps, edema (swelling), varicosities, skin pigmentation, marbling, ulceration, and burning. For venous insufficiency, results were significant by the end of the first month and highly significant by the end of the trial, at 3 months. Itching was reduced by 94 percent, tingling sensations by 87.5 percent, cramps by 80 percent, pain by 78.5 percent, and fatigability and sensation of heaviness by 60 percent. The women with hemorrhoids experienced steady and significant improvement in pain, burning, and pruritus.[6]

HOW IT WORKS

As the cells in our circulatory system age, the cell membranes become damaged by oxygen free radicals. This weakens the cells, making them less flexible and decreasing their lifespan. The antioxidants in bilberry protect two types of cells that are vital to capillary circulation: the cells that make up the capillary walls themselves, called *endothelial cells,* and the red blood cells that carry oxygen and nourishment through the capillaries to the tissues. When endothelial cells become brittle and damaged, capillaries become fragile, a condition that becomes more common with age. Capillary fragility can lead to easy bruising, spider veins, and poor circulation. Leakage of fluid from fragile capillaries manifests as inflammation. Damaged red blood cells become inflexible and are unable to squeeze through the tight spaces created by rigid capillaries. Bilberry extract increases the flexibility of the cell walls of both types of cells. This makes capillaries more distensible, that is, better able to stretch without breaking, and makes blood cells more deformable, enabling them to squeeze through tighter spaces. This combination of effects allows more blood cells, and thus more oxygen, to reach the tissues, including the retina of the eye.

Anthocyanosides also speed the recovery of *rhodopsin,* or "visual purple," which is one of the critical proteins in the rods of the eye. Rhodopsin is bleached by light and regenerated in the dark. In *in vivo* laboratory experiments, bilberry anthocyanosides were shown to dramatically speed the regeneration of rhodopsin. The mechanism is not known, but one theory is that anthocyanosides affect enzymes (including retinene-isomerase and lactate dehydrogenase) responsible for the regeneration of rhodopsin.[12,13]

Finally, bilberry extract has antiplatelet activity with an IC_{50} (inhibitory concentration, a measure of the potency of blood-thinning effect) comparable with the blood thinner dipyridamole.[14] This too can help increase microcirculation.

MAJOR CONSTITUENTS

Anthocyanosides (also called anthocyanins) and other polyphenols, cinnamic and benzoic acid derivatives, and flavonol glycosides

SAFETY

Bilberry fruit is a safe food herb with no known toxicity. No adverse effects have been reported in clinical studies. The typical dose of extract equates to around three bowls of bilberries a day, which would not be expected to cause any toxic effects.

Bilberry leaf has been used as a non-caffeinated tea substitute, has been well studied chemically, and is considered non-toxic.

- **Side effects:** None known.[15]
- **Contraindications:** None known.[15]
- **Drug interactions:** None known.[15]

DOSAGE

Standardized extract: 160 to 320 mg a day

STANDARDIZATION

Billberry extract is commonly standardized to 25 percent anthocyanosides measured as anthocyanadin.

REFERENCES

1. Cluzel C, Bastide P, Tronche P. Activités phosphoglucomutasique et glucose-6-phosphatasique de la rétine et anthocyanosides extraits de *Vaccinium myrtillus* (étude *in vitro* et *in vivo*). *Société de Biologie de Clermont-Ferrand* 1969; 163: 147–150.
2. Cluzel C, Bastide P, Wegman R, et al. Activités enzymatiques de la rétine et anthocyanosides extraits de *Vaccinium myrtillus* (lactate-deshydrogenase, a-hydroxybutyratedeshydrogenase, 6-phosphogluconate-deshydrogenase, glucose-6-phosphate-deshydrogenase, a-glycerophosphate-deshydrogengenase, 5-nucleotidase, phospho-glucoseisomerase). *Bichemical Pharmacology* 1970; 19: 2295–2302.

3. Bravetti GO, Fraboni E, Maccolini E. Preventive medical treatment of senile cataract with vitamin E and *Vaccinium myrtillus* anthocianosides: clinical evaluation [in Italian]. *Annali di Ottalmologia e Clinica Oculista* 1989; 115: 109–116.

4. Perossini M, Guidi G, Chiellini S, et al. Diabetic and hypertensive retinopathy therapy with *Vaccinium myrtillus* anthocyanosides (Tegens): double blind placebo controlled clinical trial [in Italian]. *Annali di Ottalmologia e Clinica Oculistica* 1987; 113(12): 1173–1188.

5. Virno M, Motolese E, Garofalo G, et al. Effect of bilberry anthocyanosides on retinal sensitivity of myopic patients assessed by computerized perimetry [in Italian]. *Bollettino di Oculistica* 1986; 65(7-8): 789–795.

6. Teglio L, Mazzanti C, Tronconi R, et al. *Vaccinium myrtillus* anthocyanosides (Tegens) in the treatment of venous insufficiency of lower limbs and acute piles in pregnancy [in Italian]. *Quaderni di Clinica Osterica e Ginecologica* 1987; 42(3): 221–231.

7. Jayle GE, Aubert L. The action of anthocyanin glucosides on the scoptopic and mesopic vision of the normal subject [in French]. *Thérapie* 1964; 19: 171–185.

8. Belleoud L, Leluan D, Boyer Y. Study on the effects of anthocyanin glucosides on the nocturnal vision of air traffic controllers [in French]. *Revue de Médicine Aéronautique et Spatiale* 1968; 18: 3–7.

9. Paronzini S, Indemini P. Modifications of the macular recovery tests in normal subjects after administration of anthocyanosides [in Italian]. *Bollettino de Oculistica* 1988; 67(suppl 4): 185–188.

10. Zavarise G. The effect of extended treatment with anthocyanosides on light sensitivity [in Italian]. *Annali di Ottalmologia e Clinica Oculista* 1968; 94: 209–214.

11. Coget J, Merlen JF. Clinical study on a new vascular protection agent Difrarel 20, compound of anthocyanosides extracted from *Vaccinum myrtillus* [in French]. *Phlébologie* 1968; 21(2): 221–228.

12. Bastide P, Rouher F, Tronche P. Rhodopsin and anthocyanosides. On some experimental facts [in French]. *Bulletin des Sociétés d' Ophtalmologie de France* 1968; 68: 801–807.

13. Morazzoni P, Bombardelli E. *Vaccinium myrtillus* L. *Fitoterapia* 1996; 67(1): 3–29.

14. Morazzoni P, Magistretti MJ. Activity of Myrtocyan, an anthocyanoside complex from *Vaccinium myrtillus* (VMA), on platelet aggregation and adhesiveness. *Fitoterapia* 1990; 61(13): 13–21.

15. Blumenthal M, Busse W, Goldberg A, et al., eds. *The Complete German Commission E Monographs.* Austin, TX: The American Botanical Council; Boston: Integrative Medical Communications, 1998.

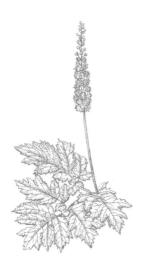

Black Cohosh

Cimicifuga racemosa
Ranunculaceae

State of Knowledge: Five-Star Rating System

Clinical (human) research	✳ ✳ ✳ ✳
Laboratory research	✳ ✳ ✳ ✳
History of use/traditional use	✳ ✳ ✳ ✳ ✳
Safety record	✳ ✳ ✳ ✳
International acceptance	✳ ✳ ✳ ✳

PART USED: *Root*

PRIMARY USES

- *Menopause*
- *Hormonal balancing*
- *Menstrual complaints (traditional)*
- *Arthritis (traditional)*

Native Americans called black co-hosh "squaw root," suggesting a rich tradition of use in maintaining women's reproductive health. For most of history, women have approached menopause with herbal therapies, ritual, and reflection, rather than synthetic hormones. Only in the past 50 years has menopause become a "disease" from the medical point of view, instead of an important life transition. Women who choose hormone-replacement therapy (HRT) increase their risk for developing breast cancer, already the leading cancer in American women. HRT may also increase the risk of endometrial cancer (cancer of the uterine lining), gallbladder disease, high blood pressure, breast tenderness, abnormal vaginal bleeding, mood changes, depression, and weight gain.

In Western countries, up to 78 percent of menopausal women experience hot flashes and 50 percent suffer from accompanying psychological disorders.[1] Fortunately, scientific research now shows that black cohosh can be just as effective as HRT in addressing physical symptoms of menopause and superior to drugs such as diazepam (Valium) in treating psychological symptoms. Today, more and more women are rediscovering black cohosh and other herbs to ease the transition through the "change of life." In fact, currently only about 15 percent of American women use HRT during menopause.

HISTORY

The Cherokees and Iroquois used black cohosh root for menstrual cramps, rheumatism, backache, coughs, fever, snakebite, as a gargle for sore throats, and as a mild sedative. The root was an official drug in *The United States Pharmacopoeia* from 1820 to 1936, and was even championed by the American Medical Association during the 1850s. By the mid-nineteenth century, black cohosh was one of the main ingredients in Lydia E. Pinkham's Vegetable Compound, a popular herbal formula for female complaints. The Eclectic physicians, a prominent group of medical doctors who used herbs and other natural therapies between 1880 and 1930, also prescribed the root for rheumatism and other inflammatory conditions, muscle soreness, respiratory problems, nervous system conditions, headaches, and as a cardiac tonic and digestive aid. Black cohosh was taken to stimulate contractions and to soothe false ones during the last weeks of pregnancy, and for pain and nervous tension following birth. Another common name for black cohosh is "bugbane," which reflects the traditional use of the strong-smelling flowers as an insect repellent.

In China, Japan, Korea, and Russia, indigenous species of *Cimicifuga* were employed for gynecological purposes as well. By the late nineteenth century, black cohosh found its way to Germany, along with other popular American plants such as saw palmetto and echinacea. During the 1950s, scientific research began in earnest as German doctors sought a safer, scientifically proven alternative to HRT, which was already causing serious side effects.

INTERNATIONAL STATUS

Black cohosh is approved by Germany's Commission E for menopausal complaints as well as dysmenorrhea (painful or difficult menstruation). It is also approved for use in the United Kingdom.

BOTANY

The Native American name "black cohosh" refers to the rough, black appearance of the roots. Native to North America, *Cimicifuga racemosa* can be found growing on hillsides in the moist eastern forests of the United States, from southern New England and Wisconsin into the Deep South. Five other species of *Cimicifuga* grow wild in America, in addition to three rare species occasionally seen in the western states. There are 13 additional species in Asia and just one that is native to Europe.

Like goldenseal, black cohosh is a member of the buttercup family (Ranunculaceae). The plant blooms from May to August, putting forth long graceful wands of small, showy, white flowers. During the flowering season, the 3- to 8-foot plants are visible from a distance in their forest homes. The roots are harvested in the fall after the fruits have ripened. Black cohosh should not be confused with blue cohosh *(Caulophyllum thalictroides),* an unrelated plant that may present more safety concerns.

A Word About Sustainability

Because of the root's growing popularity, wild populations of black cohosh are now considered at risk of commercial over harvesting in some locales. In 1998, one midsize broker was reportedly purchasing 10,000 dry pounds of black cohosh weekly, an amount equal to approximately 140,000 plants per week. This represents just a small fraction of the black cohosh being harvested for medicinal use. Unlike goldenseal, the majority of wild-harvested black cohosh is exported to European markets. As of 1999, conservationists are still pushing the U.S. Fish and Wildlife Service for a listing in the Convention for International Trade in Endangered Species of Wild Fauna and Flora (CITES) in order to prevent this valuable, potentially threatened plant from being shipped out of the country without a permit. Currently, black cohosh is mainly harvested from American forests, although some commercial cultivation has begun in Europe.[2]

You can help protect this important medicinal plant by growing black cohosh in your own yard. Often cultivated as an ornamental, the plant grows fairly easily in many different environments, producing roots that are ready to harvest in 2 to 4 years. Although black cohosh prefers shady areas, it generally tolerates more sunlight than goldenseal. (For more information on growing black cohosh, contact United Plant Savers; see appendix E.) More important, when buying black cohosh products, look for those made from cultivated sources and support the companies that use such sources. Growing herbs commercially allows greater control over potential adulterants or accidental misidentification, saves wild populations, and supports farmers.

BENEFITS

- Reduces physical symptoms of menopause: hot flashes, night sweats, headaches, heart palpitations, dizziness, vaginal atrophy, and tinnitus (ringing in the ears)
- Relieves psychological symptoms of menopause: insomnia, nervousness, irritability, and depression

- Improves difficult menstrual cycles by balancing the hormones and reducing uterine muscle spasms (experimental)
- May help relieve arthritis due to its anti-inflammatory properties (experimental)

SCIENTIFIC SUPPORT

Since the mid-1950s, there have been at least 20 clinical trials of black cohosh involving more than 3,000 women. Most of these studies have been German and have focused on the herb's use in menopause. Their results show that black cohosh extract is significantly more effective than placebo and comparable with hormone-replacement therapy in relieving menopause symptoms. A large multicenter study of 629 participants found that black cohosh was effective in at least 80 percent of women within 6 to 8 weeks.[3]

The main measure of improvement used in the studies was the Kupperman Menopausal Index, which assesses the following 10 symptoms: hot flashes, sweating, insomnia, nervousness and irritability, depression, vertigo (dizziness), poor concentration, arthritic pain, headache, and heart palpitations. Additional research shows that black cohosh has a beneficial effect on vaginal walls that are thinning.[4,5] Preventing this vaginal atrophy is an especially important quality-of-life issue for sexually active postmenopausal women. The research cited in Specific Studies also demonstrates positive effects in women who have had hysterectomies and in those making a transition from synthetic HRT to black cohosh.

Menopausal women who take black cohosh may also benefit from the plant's potential value in the prevention of osteoporosis, according to preliminary Japanese research. Two Asian *Cimicifuga* species, *C. heracleifolia* and *C. foetida,* significantly inhibited bone resorption and increased bone mineral density in laboratory studies. Researchers have not determined whether these effects are due to possible phytoestrogen content (compounds that have effects on hormonal function), suppression of parathyroid hormones, or direct prevention of bone turnover.[6] However, this research may or may not apply to *Cimicifuga racemosa,* the species used in Western medicine.

SPECIFIC STUDIES

Menopause Symptoms: Clinical Study (1985)

Standardized black cohosh extract was just as effective as synthetic estrogen (Premarin) in reducing the physical symptoms of menopause in a randomized, open trial. In addition, black cohosh was comparable with both estrogen and diazepam (Valium) in improving psychological complaints. The study included 60 menopausal women, aged 45 to 60, who took either 40 drops of standardized black cohosh extract twice daily, 0.6 mg conjugated estrogen daily, or 2 mg diazepam daily for 12 weeks. Within the first 4 weeks, women in both the black cohosh and hormone-therapy groups experienced an improvement in symptoms such as hot flashes, night sweats, and heart palpitations, according to the Modified Menopausal Index. They also demonstrated a thickening of the vaginal lining, as measured by the Karyopyknotic and Eosinophilic Indices. More marked effects were evident at 12 weeks. In terms of psychological complaints, all three groups showed comparable improvement of symptoms such as nervousness and depression, as measured by the Self-Assessment Depression Scale, the Hamilton Anxiety Scale, and the Clinical Global Impressions Scale. Researchers concluded that black cohosh is the remedy of choice for treating mild to moderate menopausal complaints, especially in light of long-term risks associated with drug therapies.[5]

Transition from Hormone Therapy: Clinical Study (1987)

Researchers found that a majority of menopausal women could make a successful transition from synthetic hormone therapy to black cohosh in a relatively short period of time. The study included 50 women who had been taking hormone-replacement treatment for menopause symptoms. Over 50 percent of the women (28 total) were able to switch to black cohosh extract without a need for additional hormone injections. Over a 6-month period, 21 other women needed an additional hormone injection, and 1 woman required two more injections. No side effects were reported in this study.[7]

Menopause Symptoms After Hysterectomy: Clinical Study (1988)

Standardized black cohosh extract was just as effective as three synthetic hormone therapies in relieving menopause symptoms in 40 women who had undergone hysterectomy. During the 6-month randomized study, subjects took either standardized black cohosh extract (4 mg twice daily), estriol (1 mg Ovestin daily), conjugated estrogens (1.25 mg Presomen daily), or combined estrogen-gestagen therapy (1 tablet Trisequens daily). All of the women were under the age of 40 and had at least one intact ovary. In all four treatment groups, most of the participants were symptom free by the end of the study, as measured by the Kupperman Menopausal Index.[8]

HOW IT WORKS

Estrogen-like Activity

Since 1932, when researchers began conducting animal experiments using black cohosh, they have hypothesized that black cohosh contains isoflavones, or "phytoestrogens," that may increase estrogen levels by binding to estrogen receptors in the body.[9] More recently, however, a few researchers have begun questioning the long-held assumption that black cohosh contains phytoestrogens. Recent animal experiments concluded that black cohosh has no estrogenic effects, because it did not affect uterine or vaginal tissue in the way that estrogens normally do.[10] In addition, isoflavones are generally rare in plant families other than the Fabaceae, a family that includes soy and red clover, but not black cohosh. Although black cohosh was originally believed to contain the isoflavone formononetin, more recent research has called this into question.[11] It may be some time before the controversy is resolved. (For more information about phytoestrogens, see "Soy" and "Red Clover.")

Luteinizing Hormone– Lowering Effect

Most women are aware that estrogen levels drop during menopause, but the accompanying rise in luteinizing hormone (LH) is less well known. Both of these hormonal changes have been linked to physical and psychological symptoms of menopause. In clinical studies, researchers have directly connected surges of LH in menopausal women with hot flashes, through measurements of changes in skin temperature.[12] Clinical research shows that black cohosh lowers LH levels in menopausal women, presumably by acting on the anterior pituitary gland, which regulates ovarian hormones.[13] Black cohosh's ability to decrease LH levels may or may not be related to its possible estrogenic activity. A recent laboratory study proposes that declines in LH levels are due to interference with neurotransmitters, rather than an estrogenic effect.[14]

Anti-Inflammatory Effects

Recent Japanese research sheds some light on the traditional American use of black cohosh for inflammatory problems like arthritis. Scientists found that two Asian *Cimicifuga* species, *C. heracleifolia* and *C. dahurica,* inhibit interleukin-8, significantly reducing levels of neutrophils, cells that promote and regulate inflammatory reactions. Ferulic acid and isoferulic acid are the two constituents thought to be responsible for black cohosh's anti-inflammatory action.[15]

MAJOR CONSTITUENTS

Triterpene glycosides (actein, 27-deoxyactein, and cimicifugoside) and flavonoids

SAFETY

Black cohosh is generally regarded as safe when used appropriately.[16]

The German drug regulatory agency known as the BGA feels that black cohosh is safe for use in women with estrogen-sensitive cancers as well as in uterine bleeding, liver/gallbladder disease, pancreatitis, endometriosis, uterine fibroids, and fibrocystic breast disease, conditions that generally rule out synthetic hormone replacement.

Although Commission E recommends limiting black cohosh use to 6 months, there is no scientific or historical evidence to support this restriction. Some experts feel that the German organization based their guidelines on the lack of long-term safety studies, not on any direct evidence of harm. Traditionally, black cohosh was used for periods much longer than 6 months, and there is no contemporary evidence of toxicity or major adverse effects.

- **Side effects:** Minor stomach upset has been reported on occasion.[17]
- **Contraindications:** Black cohosh should not be used during pregnancy. In very large amounts, it may cause dizziness, headache, nausea, impaired vision, vomiting, and impaired circulation.[17]
- **Drug interactions:** None known.[16] Possible interactions with hormone-replacement therapy are unknown. Consult a health-care practitioner if you are currently taking HRT and would like to switch to black cohosh.

DOSAGE

The dosage of standardized extract tested in clinical studies was 2 tablets twice daily, equivalent to 4 mg triterpenes or 40 drops of standardized tincture twice daily. In clinical studies, most women began to see results within 4 weeks. Although black cohosh acts more slowly than hormone-replacement therapy, it also has far fewer side effects and risk factors. Black cohosh is most effective when used as a liquid extract, tablet, or capsule, rather than as a tea.

- **Standardized extract:** 2 tablets twice a day, or 40 drops of standardized tincture twice a day
- **Capsules/tablets:** one 500- to 600-mg tablet or capsule three times a day[18]
- **Tincture:** 40 drops, one to two times a day

STANDARDIZATION

Black cohosh is typically standardized to 1 mg of triterpenes (calculated as 27-deoxyactein) per tablet.

REFERENCES

1. Jarry H, Gorkow CH, Wuttke W. Treatment of menopausal symptoms with extracts of *Cimicifuga racemosa: In vivo* and *in vitro* evidence for estrogenic activity [in German]. *Phytopharmaka Forschung* 1995; 99–112.

2. Cech RA. Balancing conservation with utilization: restoring populations of commercially valuable medicinal herbs in forests and agroforests. *United Plant Savers Newsletter* Winter 1999: 1–4.

3. Stolze H. An alternative to treat menopausal complaints [in German]. *Gynäkologie* 1982; 3(1): 14–16.

4. Stoll W. Phytopharmacon influences atrophic vaginal epithelium: double-blind study—*Cimicifuga* vs. estrogenic substances [in German]. *Therapeutikon* 1987; 1: 23–30.

5. Warnecke G. Influencing menopausal symptoms with a phytotherapeutic agent [in German]. *Die Medizinische Welt* 1985; 36: 871–874.

6. Li JX, Kadota S, Li HY, et al. Effects of *Cimicifugae* rhizoma on serum calcium and phosphate levels in low calcium dietary rats and on bone mineral density in ovariectomized rats. *Phytomedicine* 1996/1997; 3(4): 379–385.

7. Pethö A. Menopausal complaints: change-over of a hormone treatment to a herbal gynecological remedy practicable? [in German]. *Arztliche Praxis* 1987; 38(47): 1551–1553.

8. Lehmann-Willenbrock E, Riedel HH. Clinical and endocrinologic examinations concerning therapy of climacteric symptoms following hysterectomy with remaining ovaries [in German]. *Zentralblatt für Gynakologie* 1988; 110: 611–618.

9. Jarry H, Harnischfeger G. Studies on the endocrine effects of the contents of *Cimicifuga racemosa*. 1. Influence on the serum concentration of pituitary hormones in ovariectomized rats. *Planta Medica* 1985; 51(1): 46–49.

10. Gruenwald J. Standardized black cohosh (*Cimicifuga*) extract clinical monograph. *Quarterly Review of Natural Medicine* Summer 1998; 117–125.

11. Struck D, Tegtmeier M, Harnischfeger G. Flavones in extracts of *Cimicifuga racemosa*. *Planta Medica* 1997; 63: 289.

12. Meldrum DR, Tataryn IV, Frumar AM, et al. Gonadotropins, estrogens and adrenal steroids during menopausal hot flash. *Journal of Clinical Endocrinology and Metabolism* 1980; 50(4): 685–689.

13. Düker EM, Kopanski L, Jarry H, et al. Effects of extracts from *Cimicifuga racemosa* on gonadotropin release in menopausal women and ovariectomized rats. *Planta Medica* 1991; 57: 420–424.

14. Einer-Jensen N, Zhao J, Andersen KP, et al. Cimicifuga and Melbrosia lack oestrogenic effects in mice and rats. *Maturitas* 1996; 25: 149–153.

15. Hirabayashi T, Ochiai H, Sakai S, et al. Inhibitory effect of ferulic acid and isoferulic acid on murine interleukin-8 production in response to influenza virus infections *in vitro* and *in vivo*. *Planta Medica* 1995; 61: 221–226.

16. Blumenthal M, Busse W, Goldberg A, eds. *The Complete German Commission E Monographs*. Austin, TX: American Botanical Council; Boston MA: Integrative Medical Communications, 1998.

17. McGuffin M, Hobbs C, Upton R, et al., eds. *American Herbal Products Association Botanical Safety Handbook*. Boca Raton and New York: CRC Press LLC, 1997.

18. Foster S. *101 Medicinal Herbs*. Loveland, CO: Interweave Press, 1998.

Boswellia

BOSWELLIA SERRATA
BURSERACEAE

State of Knowledge: Five-Star Rating System

Clinical (human) research	✶✶
Laboratory research	✶✶✶
History of use / traditional use	✶✶✶✶
Safety record	✶✶✶✶
International acceptance	✶✶✶

PART USED: *Resin*

PRIMARY USES

- *Anti-inflammatory*
- *Rheumatoid arthritis*
- *Ulcerative colitis (experimental)*

Boswellia serrata, a tree found in hilly areas of India, is a close relative of frankincense. Frankincense *(Boswellia carteri)* was one of the gifts of the three wise men in the Bible, and *Boswellia serrata* provides another gift—an important Ayurvedic remedy long used in the treatment of rheumatoid arthritis and other inflammatory conditions. This remedy comes from an extract of the resin of *Boswellia serrata* and is used in India not only for inflammatory conditions but also for lung diseases, diarrhea, reproductive disorders, ulcers, and a host of other ailments. For millions of people with arthritis, boswellia may offer symptomatic relief without harsh side effects—a gift of improved quality of life.

Both boswellia and frankincense have been used by many cultures since antiquity. The two plants contain many of the same compounds, including boswellic acids, believed to be their most important anti-inflammatory compounds. Modern research, however, has focused on boswellia. Today, standardized boswellia extract is widely sold in India and Europe as a popular over-the-counter anti-inflammatory remedy.

Rheumatoid arthritis is not completely understood, and because the condition is chronic the conventional medications used to treat it must be taken long term to keep symptoms under control. They also often have unpleasant and potentially dangerous side effects. Nonsteroidal anti-inflammatory drugs (NSAIDs), frequently prescribed to relieve arthritis symptoms, can cause gastrointestinal irritation, ulceration, and hemorrhage as well as kidney damage. Sulfasalazine, another type of anti-inflammatory drug, and other arthritis drugs, such as corticosteroids, pose even more serious risks.

Boswellia, on the other hand, causes none of these unwanted side effects, and the results of several clinical studies suggest it may have value in relieving pain, stiffness, and inflammation. Boswellia's successful track record in treating arthritis in traditional medicine, together with promising results from recent studies, suggests that the herb has potential in the treatment of other inflammatory conditions, including bowel problems such as Crohn's disease and ulcerative colitis.

HISTORY

Sallai guggal is the traditional Ayurvedic name for the gum resin of the *Boswellia serrata* tree. Ayurvedic practitioners regard this preparation as an effective therapy for a number of inflammatory diseases, including rheumatoid arthritis, osteoarthritis, and cervical spondylitis (an inflammatory arthritic condition of the spine). In traditional Ayurvedic medicine, boswellia has also been administered to treat chronic lung conditions, diarrhea, and menstrual disorders. A paste made of the gum resin has been applied to ulcers, boils, and other skin problems.[1] Today, a preparation of the standardized extract called *Sallaki* is used in India for the treatment of chronic arthritis.[2] Boswellia extract is also currently marketed in Germany, Switzerland, and other European countries.

Olibanum, the gum resin from frankincense *(B. carteri)* also has pharmacological effects because it contains boswellic acids, but *B. serrata* has been the subject of much more medical research.[2]

INTERNATIONAL STATUS

Boswellia is not officially approved for use in Europe.

BOTANY

Boswellia serrata and its close relative *B. carteri* (frankincense) are members of the botanical family Burseraceae, plants known for the resin ducts in their bark. *Boswellia serrata* is a shrub or small tree with thick, aromatic bark and small, white, fragrant flowers. The tree can grow as tall as 12 feet, attaining a width of up to 4 feet at the base of the trunk. It is found in dry, hilly areas of India. *Sallai guggal* is the Indian name for the gum resin collected from the bark of the tree. When the bark is cut, a milky liquid flows out and hardens on the branches or ground. This solid is then collected and processed into various preparations.[1,3]

BENEFITS

• Reduces inflammation associated with rheumatoid arthritis and certain bowel disorders

SCIENTIFIC SUPPORT

Research into the uses of *Boswellia serrata* in the treatment of inflammatory conditions has focused on constituents called *boswellic acids*. These compounds are also found in the resin of *B. carteri* (frankincense), and some of the research refers to the resins of the two plants interchangeably. Most sources, however, distinguish boswellia resin as the one used medicinally. The term *olibanum* has been used to describe the resin collected from either of the two trees, but today, commercially available preparations containing boswellic acids and claiming the health benefits of boswellia are made from the resin of *B. serrata*.

At least one well-designed clinical study supports the therapeutic action of an herbal preparation containing boswellia in relieving arthritis pain.[4] Other uncontrolled human studies also suggest the effectiveness of a standardized boswellia extract in reducing arthritis symptoms.[5] In one clinical study investigating the effects of boswellia gum resin extract on ulcerative colitis, the herbal preparation was found to be at least as effective as the synthetic drug sulfasalazine.[6] Virtually all of the clinical studies point out that boswellia preparations cause none of the side effects associated with conventional drugs for arthritis, which may include stomach irritation and ulceration, headache, nausea, vomiting, and skin irritations.

In addition to this limited clinical research, animal studies have demonstrated the anti-inflammatory action and safety of boswellia and boswellic acids.[2,7–10] One study suggested that boswellic acids may mildly suppress the immune system, but the investigator concluded that the anti-inflammatory effects are not connected to a generalized immune suppression.[11]

Finally, one laboratory study proposes that boswellic acids may protect against chemically induced hepatitis (liver inflammation) in the same way that they decrease other forms of inflammation.[12]

SPECIFIC STUDIES

Rheumatoid Arthritis: Review of Clinical Studies (1996)

This overview of 11 German clinical studies reported that compared with placebo, standardized boswellia extract produced a significant reduction in swelling and pain, often reduced morning stiffness, and resulted in an overall improvement in general health and well-being for people with rheumatoid arthritis. Some participants were able to decrease their intake of NSAIDs during treatment with the boswellia extract. The clinical studies involved a total of 260 people who had not responded well to conventional treatments. Researchers utilized several different clinical approaches to evaluate improvements, including assessments of pain, swelling, and sensitivity. The boswellia capsules tested in the studies each contained 400 mg and in most studies were given in dosages of 3 capsules two or three times a day. On the basis of the study results, the author concluded that the boswellia extract is a safe, useful replacement or supplement for other therapies used in the treatment of rheumatoid arthritis. The long-term effects of boswellia extract on the progression of joint disease are unclear, as they are for conventional therapy.[5]

Ulcerative Colitis: Clinical Study (1997)

Boswellia gum resin extract was as effective as the synthetic drug sulfasalazine in causing remission of ulcerative colitis symptoms in this open clinical trial involving 42 people with grade II or III ulcerative colitis. Patients received treatment with either 350 mg boswellia extract three times a day or sul-

fasalazine (1 gram three times daily) over a 6-week period. At the conclusion of the study, people in both treatment groups reported improvement in a range of symptoms, including abdominal pain and loose stools. Patients with grade II colitis appeared to respond more favorably to treatment with boswellia than did those with grade III colitis. A diagnostic procedure performed after the study showed significant improvement in the pathological grading of the disease. Seventy-five percent of grade III patients in both treatment groups improved to grade 0 (normal colonic tissue) or grade I (minor changes in tissue appearance). Overall, 82 percent of patients receiving boswellia and 75 percent of those taking sulfasalazine experienced remissions. Six of the 34 boswellia recipients (18 percent) complained of side effects of burning, nausea, and a feeling of gastrointestinal "fullness." Researchers concluded that although boswellic acids did not prove to be superior to sulfasalazine, they were at least as effective.[6]

Arthritis: Clinical Study (1991)

A randomized, double-blind, placebo-controlled, crossover study of 42 people with arthritis demonstrated the effectiveness and safety of a traditional Ayurvedic preparation that included the stem of *Boswellia serrata*. People taking the formula reported significant improvement in pain and disability; other measurements, including grip strength and morning stiffness, reflected favorable but nonsignificant changes. However, x-ray and erythrocyte sedimentation rate (two diagnostic measures used to assess the stage and type of arthritis) did not show any significant changes for either the study or control group, suggesting that the herbal formula had no effect on the progression of the disease. Overall, at the end of the study, 93 percent of the participants said they preferred the herbal formula to placebo. Eight individuals complained of nausea, abdominal pain, or skin irritation during treatment with the herb mixture, but none of these side effects was severe enough to cause them to stop taking the remedy. Other ingredients in the formula were ashwagandha *(Withania somnifera)* and turmeric *(Curcuma longa),* both of which have demonstrated anti-inflammatory effects in other studies, as well as a zinc complex. The investigators concluded that boswellia may work together with the other herbs in the preparation to produce relief of arthritis symptoms.[4]

HOW IT WORKS

The anti-inflammatory activity of boswellia has been attributed to its ability to interrupt leukotriene synthesis. Leukotrienes are known to be involved in the initiation and progression of the symptoms of inflammation in many diseases, such as colitis, Crohn's disease, psoriasis, and chronic rheumatism.[13] At least two studies suggest that boswellic acids appear to specifically block the leukotriene precursor 5-lipoxygenase without interfering with other biochemical pathways.[8,13]

MAJOR CONSTITUENTS

Triterpenic acids, including alpha-, beta-, and gamma-boswellic acids

SAFETY

Boswellia is considered safe when used appropriately.[14] Its safety for pregnant and nursing women has not been investigated.

- **Side effects:** In at least two studies using boswellia to treat ulcerative colitis, some participants (less than 18 percent) complained of gastrointestinal symptoms, but these were mild and did not require discontinuation of the remedy.
- **Contraindications:** None known.
- **Drug interactions:** None known.

DOSAGE

In most clinical studies investigating effects on arthritis, the dosage of boswellia standardized extract (400-mg capsules) was 3 tablets two or three times a day.[5]

- **Standardized extract:** Three 400-mg capsules two or three times a day

STANDARDIZATION

Boswellia extracts are standardized to contain 60 to 65 percent boswellic acids.

REFERENCES

1. Kapoor LD. *CRC Handbook of Ayurvedic Medicinal Plants.* Boca Raton, FL: CRC Press, 1990.

2. Ammon HPT, Safayhi H, Mack T, et al. Mechanism of anti-inflammatory actions of curcumine and boswellic acids. *Journal of Ethnopharmacology* 1993; 38: 113–119.

3. Leung AY. *Encyclopedia of Common Natural Ingredients Used in Food, Drugs, and Cosmetics.* New York: John Wiley & Sons, 1980.

4. Kulkarni RR, Patki PS, Jog VP, et al. Treatment of osteoarthritis with a herbomineral formulation: a double-blind, placebo-controlled, cross-over study. *Journal of Ethnopharmacology* 1991; 33: 91–95.

5. Etzel R. Special extract of *Boswellia serrata* (H 15) in the treatment of rheumatoid arthritis. *Phytomedicine* 1996; 3(1): 91–94.

6. Gupta I, Parihar A, Malhotra P, et al. Effects of *Boswellia serrata* gum resin in patients with ulcerative colitis. *European Journal of Medical Research* 1997; 2(1): 37–43.

7. Singh GB, Singh S, Bani S. Anti-inflammatory actions of boswellic acids. *Phytomedicine* 1996; 3(1): 81–85.

8. Ammon HPT. Salai guggal—*Boswellia serrata:* from a herbal medicine to a specific inhibitor of leukotriene biosynthesis. *Phytomedicine* 1996; 3(1): 67–70.

9. Singh GB, Atal CK. Pharmacology of an extract of salai guggal ex-*Boswellia serrata,* a new non-steroidal anti-inflammatory agent. *Agents and Actions* 1986; 18(3/4): 407–412

10. Singh GB, Bani S, Singh S. Toxicity and safety evaluation of boswellic acids. *Phytomedicine* 1996; 3(1): 87–90.

11. Sharma ML, Kaul A, Khajuria A, et al. Immunomodulatory activity of boswellic acids (pentacyclic triterpene acids) from *Boswellia serrata. Phytotherapy Research* 1996; 10(2): 107–112.

12. Safayhi H, Mack T, Ammon HPT. Protection by boswellic acids against galactosamine/endotoxin-induced hepatitis in mice. *Biochemical Pharmacology* 1991; 41 (10): 1536–1537.

13. Safayhi H, Mack T, Sabieraj J, et al. Boswellic acids: novel, specific, nonredox inhibitors of 5-lipoxygenase. *The Journal of Pharmacology and Experimental Therapeutics* 1992; 261(3): 1143–1146.

14. McGuffin M, Hobbs C, Upton R, et al., eds. *American Herbal Products Association Botanical Safety Handbook.* Boca Raton, FL: CRC Press, 1997.

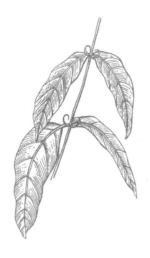

Cat's Claw

UNCARIA TOMENTOSA
AND U. GUIANENSIS
RUBIACEAE

***

State of Knowledge: Five-Star Rating System

Clinical (human) research	✳
Laboratory research	✳✳
History of use/traditional use	✳✳✳
Safety record	✳✳
International acceptance	✳✳

***

PART USED: *Root bark, stem*

PRIMARY USES

- *Immune stimulation (experimental)*
- *Inflammation (experimental)*

Intrigued by stories of a rainforest vine being used in South American folk medicine to treat cancer, European researchers and physicians in the 1970s began experimenting with extracts of the plant to learn more about how it worked. Rumors of cat's claw's promise in the treatment of a number of serious conditions reached North America by the early 1990s. Virtu-ally unknown in the United States before this time, by 1997, cat's claw was the seventh best-selling herb in the country. Today, manufacturers' claims for cat's claw supplements run the gamut from disease prevention to cancer treatment, including uses for arthritis, asthma, ulcers, chemotherapy side effects, stomach ulcers, hemorrhoids, abscesses, wounds and other skin problems, menstrual problems, recovery from childbirth, and even contraception.

Needless to say, few of these claims fall into the category of legal structure/function claims for dietary supplements in the United

States. More important, it is particularly difficult to separate hype from fact about cat's claw because no clinical studies have yet confirmed its effectiveness or safety. Laboratory research has demonstrated that cat's claw possesses immune-stimulating and anti-inflammatory properties, and the plant has shown some experimental evidence of anticancer effects. In Germany and Austria, where standardized cat's claw extract is a pharmaceutical available by prescription only, physicians use the herb to help stimulate immune system function in people with cancer.

However, to date, all of the reports of cat's claw's effectiveness against disease in humans are of an anecdotal nature, meaning that they are based on word-of-mouth claims made by practitioners or individuals who have used the herb, not on controlled studies. This is not to say that cat's claw is ineffective, but simply that more research is needed before conclusions can be drawn about the most appropriate uses of this rainforest herb.

HISTORY

Cat's claw is a valued remedy of native healers of the upper Amazon basin. In the traditional medicine system of the Ashéninka Indians of Peru, healers hold that disease may arise from disorders of a person's spiritual being, and cat's claw plants are thought to be inhabited by good spirits. Therefore, the use of cat's claw in healing is relegated to priests, who believe the plant can help regulate the relationship between the physical and spiritual being.[1]

There is little written history on the traditional applications of cat's claw, but ethnobotanists have gathered important information through interviews with native healers of Peru, who use a water extract of cat's claw bark to treat cancer, arthritis, liver disorders, stomach ulcers and other digestive problems, skin conditions, and inflammation. The plant has also been traditionally employed as a contraceptive. To prevent disease, people drink a cup of water-based cat's claw extract every week or two. Much larger amounts are administered to treat disease.

Cat's claw is a popular folk remedy for the treatment of cancer among other South American peoples as well, particularly Brazilians. They believe it to be especially useful as a treatment for cancers of the urinary tract.

INTERNATIONAL STATUS

In Germany and Austria, standardized cat's claw extracts are regulated as pharmaceuticals, available by prescription only.[2]

BOTANY

Cat's claw (*uña de gato* in Spanish) is a type of large, climbing, woody tropical vine called a *liana*. The vine gets it common name from the long hooklike spines it uses to pull itself upright on trees in its home in the Amazonian rainforest. There are at least 50 members of the genus *Uncaria,* most of which are vines that grow in tropical regions of Asia, Africa, and South America. Cat's claw is a member of the madder family (Rubiaceae), a large family of plants that also includes the herb cleavers *(Galium aparine).*

The two species of cat's claw that are most widely used medicinally are *U. guianensis,* which is preferred in Europe, and *U. tomentosa,* which makes up most of the supply sold in the United States. In traditional South American medicine, the two species are considered interchangeable.

Nearly all of the world's supply of cat's claw is harvested from the wild in Peru and Brazil. Although there are reports of sustainable harvest and cultivation, some conservation groups fear that commercial over harvesting will threaten cat's claw populations and have a negative impact on its rainforest ecosystem.

Two Different Types of *U. tomentosa*

Recently, researchers discovered that there are two different chemotypes of *U. tomentosa,* meaning that although they are of the same species, the plants differ in their chemical makeup. This is an important point, because the two chemotypes of *U. tomentosa* are

reported to differ greatly in their content of alkaloids, believed to be the most active compounds in cat's claw. One chemotype contains mostly pentacyclic alkaloids, a group of chemicals that have been shown to have immune-stimulating properties, whereas the other chemotype contains mostly tetracyclic alkaloids, which are thought to affect the central nervous system and to counteract the immune-stimulant effects of the pentacyclic alkaloids.[3] This variance could have important implications for the therapeutic use of cat's claw. The only way to tell the difference between the two chemotypes is through chemical testing, making a good case for the standardization of cat's claw products to contain less than 0.02 percent tetracyclic alkaloids.[4]

BENEFITS

- Stimulates immune system function (experimental)
- Reduces inflammation (experimental)

SCIENTIFIC SUPPORT

To date, no clinical studies have demonstrated the effectiveness of cat's claw for any of the conditions for which it is commonly used or promoted. Reportedly, clinical studies underway in Europe and South America are investigating the value of cat's claw in HIV infection and cancer, but so far no results have been published. European physicians prescribe standardized cat's claw extract to stimulate the immune system in people with cancer. Anecdotal reports describe success in treating allergies, AIDS, arthritis, ulcers, Crohn's disease, diverticulitis, ulcers, and many other serious conditions, but once again, these claims are not supported by any solid clinical research.

However, a limited number of test-tube experiments have demonstrated effects that could account for some of the herb's therapeutic uses. In the laboratory, cat's claw's best-documented effects have been immune-stimulating, anti-inflammatory, and antimutagenic actions. In addition, the plant has shown some antioxidant activity.

In one interesting laboratory study, extracts of cat's claw bark as well as a number of isolated constituents inhibited mutagenicity (genetic changes that could lead to cancer) in bacteria, a test that is commonly used to assess the anticancer potential of experimental substances. In the same study, the researchers found that cat's claw extract dramatically lowered the level of mutagens in the urine of a cigarette smoker. The two men in this study, one a smoker and one a nonsmoker, each drank a decoction (water extract) of cat's claw daily for 15 days. The researchers suggested that this antimutagenic activity could be due to antioxidant effects. The cat's claw decoction was made by boiling cat's claw bark in water for about 3 hours.[5]

In another preliminary laboratory study, six alkaloid compounds isolated from cat's claw bark inhibited the growth of human leukemia cells without affecting normal bone marrow cells, leading the researchers to suggest that cat's claw may have potential in the treatment of acute leukemia.[6]

Other studies have demonstrated that cat's claw constituents may enhance the activity of the immune system. One such study showed that alkaloid compounds from cat's claw encouraged *phagocytosis,* an important process by which the immune system attacks and destroys invading disease-causing organisms.[7] Cat's claw has also shown some antiviral activity.[8]

HOW IT WORKS

Current science knows little about the way in which cat's claw works, but researchers have identified a number of alkaloid compounds that appear to play a role in its immune-stimulating, anti-inflammatory, and antimutagenic effects.

Evidence from *in vitro* research shows that the oxindole alkaloids isopteropodine, pteropodine, isomitraphylline, and isorynchophylline can enhance phagocytosis.[7] Of six oxindole alkaloids tested for their ability to hinder the growth of human leukemia cells, uncarine F was the most active.[6] A quinovic acid glycoside from cat's claw root bark demonstrated anti-inflammatory effects *in vitro*.[9] In addition, a procyanadin compound called cinchonain was shown to inhibit 5-lipoxygenase, suggesting that this constituent may also contribute to cat's claw's anti-inflammatory effects.[10] As with many herbs, researchers speculate that the activity of cat's claw extract is likely due to the actions of a number of compounds working together.

MAJOR CONSTITUENTS

Pentacyclic oxindole alkaloids (pteropodine, isopteropodine, isomitraphylline, uncarine F), tetracyclic oxindole alkaloids (rhynchophylline, isorhynchophylline), quinovic acid glycosides, procyanidins, triterpenoid saponins

SAFETY

Although there have been no reports of significant toxicity with cat's claw, not enough is known about the plant to make definitive conclusions about its safety. The information presented here is based on anecdotal reports from practitioners using cat's claw in a clinical setting.[11]

- **Side effects:** No information available.
- **Contraindications:** Because of cat's claw's traditional application as a contraceptive, its use in pregnancy is not advised. Some sources recommend against taking cat's claw in conditions that involve the immune system, such as AIDS, multiple sclerosis, tuberculosis, and organ transplantation.[2,11] Cat's claw is not recommended for use in children or while nursing.
- **Drug Interactions:** No research-based information is available on the potential of cat's claw to cause drug interactions. However, in Europe, physicians do not use cat's claw in combination with vaccines, insulin, hormone therapies, or fresh blood plasma.[2,11]

DOSAGE

- **Capsules:** Up to nine 500- to 600-mg capsules a day.[2]
- **Decoction:** Simmer 1 tablespoon powdered root for 45 minutes in 1 quart of water. Take 1 teaspoon in hot water in the morning, before breakfast.[2]
- **Tincture:** 20 to 40 drops up to five times a day.[2]

STANDARDIZATION

Some manufacturers standardize cat's claw products to contain 3 percent total oxinadole alkaloids (including isopteropidine) and 15 percent total polyphenols.

REFERENCES

1. Keplinger K, Laus G, Wurm M, et al. *Uncaria tomentosa* (Willd.) DC—ethnomedical use and new pharmacological, toxicological and botanical results. *Journal of Ethnopharmacology* 1999; 64: 23–24.

2. Foster S. *101 Medicinal Herbs.* Loveland, CO: Interweave Press, 1998.

3. Laus G, Keplinger K. Radix Uncariae tomentosae (Willd) DC—a monographic description [in German]. *Zeitschrift für Phytotherapie* 1997; 18: 122–126.

4. Foster S, Tyler V. *Tyler's Honest Herbal,* 4th ed. New York and London: The Haworth Herbal Press, 1999.

5. Rizzi R, Re F, Bianchi A, et al. Mutagenic and antimutagenic activities of *Uncaria tomentosa* and its extracts. *Journal of Ethnopharmacology* 1993; 38: 63–77.

6. Stuppner H, Sturm S, Geisen G, et al. A differential sensitivity of oxindole alkaloids to normal and leukemic cell lines. *Planta Medica* 1993; 59 (suppl): A583.

7. Wagner H, Kreutzkamp B, Jurcic K. Alkaloids of *Uncaria tomentosa* and their phagocytosis enhancement activity [in German]. *Planta Medica* 1985; 51: 419–423.

8. Aquino R, De Simone F, Pizza C. Plant metabolites, structure and in vitro antiviral activity of quinovic acid glycosides from *Uncaria tomentosa* and *Guettarda platypoda*. *Journal of Natural Products* 1989; 52(4): 679–685.

9. Aquino R, De Feo V, DeSimone F, et al. Plant metabolites. New compounds and anti-inflammatory activity of *Uncaria tomentosa*. *Journal of Natural Products* 1991; 54(2): 453–459.

10. Wirth C, Wagner H. Pharmacologically active procyanidines from the bark of *Uncaria tomentosa*. *Phytomedicine* 1997; 4(3): 265–266.

11. McGuffin M, Hobbs C, Upton R, et al., eds. *American Herbal Products Association Botanical Safety Handbook.* Boca Raton, FL: CRC Press, 1997.

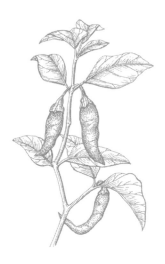

Cayenne

CAPSICUM ANNUUM
SOLANACEAE

State of Knowledge: Five-Star Rating System

Clinical (human) research	✳ ✳ ✳
Laboratory research	✳ ✳ ✳ ✳
History of use/traditional use	✳ ✳ ✳
Safety record	✳ ✳ ✳
International acceptance	✳ ✳ ✳

PART USED: *Fruit*

PRIMARY USES

- *Painful or itchy skin conditions such as psoriasis, shingles, diabetic neuropathy, and postmastectomy pain (topical cream)*
- *Circulatory system health (traditional)*

With its intense heat and a name that literally means "to bite," you might not expect cayenne to have potent pain-relieving properties. Surprisingly, clinical studies show that a topical cream made with *capsaicin,* the ingredient that makes cayenne hot, is safe and effective for reducing the pain and itching associated with many disorders. This is an important breakthrough, especially for long-term or chronic pain, which is often very difficult to treat. Conditions such as psoriasis and shingles frequently do not respond to conventional drugs, including steroids and tranquilizers, leaving people with few treatment options. The success of these drugs is also limited by serious side effects and the potential for dependency. Fortunately, many people have obtained considerable relief in clinical trials that tested capsaicin creams against discomfort caused by postsurgical and diabetes-related nerve damage, psoriasis, and many other conditions.

Traditionally, cayenne has added spice to many cuisines around the world, including those of South America, southeast Asia, China, southern Italy, and Mexico. These countries have also valued cayenne for its benefits to the circulatory system. Cross-cultural studies suggest that heart disease is less common in countries such as Thailand, where locals consume large amounts of cayenne pepper. In Thailand, people eat roughly 5 grams of cayenne each day, one of the highest per capita consumption rates in the world. Although clinical studies have not been conducted in this area, laboratory research suggests that cayenne acts as an antioxidant and reduces cholesterol levels, platelet aggregation (the tendency of the blood to clot abnormally), and plaque build-up in the arteries. For those who favor less spicy fare, cayenne is also available in capsule form.

HISTORY

Cayenne peppers date back thousands of years, to the civilizations of South America and the West Indies. In these tropical areas, hot peppers (also called chili peppers) help people stay cooler through a mechanism that stimulates the part of the brain that regulates body temperature. The ancient Mayans also used cayenne to treat mouth sores and inflamed gums. In the fifteenth century, Christopher Columbus brought pepper seeds back to Italy from the new world. The plant quickly spread to Africa and India, and by 1650 it was being cultivated throughout northern Europe.

Cayenne was a traditional treatment for fevers, asthma, impaired circulation, sore throats, respiratory tract infections, digestive problems, constipation, toothaches, and even certain cancers. Traditional herbalists often use it as a catalyst in herbal formulas, to speed the absorption and circulation of other herbs in the body.

Some Like it Hot

Hot pepper sauces are now the best-selling condiment in America—even more popular than tomato catsup. People who like hot food just can't seem to get enough of it. The theory about fiery foods is that they stimulate the release of endorphins, the body's natural painkillers, producing a sort of high.

INTERNATIONAL STATUS

A 0.075 percent capsaicin cream is approved as an over-the-counter drug in both the United States and Canada. Topical preparations are also approved by Germany's Commission E for painful muscle spasms in the shoulders, arms, and spine.

BOTANY

Although Christopher Columbus initially confused this fiery pepper with a variety of black pepper, he quickly discovered his mistake! Cayenne is actually related to eggplant, sweet peppers, and tomatoes—all members of the nightshade family (Solanaceae). Other common relatives range from mild sweet paprika to blazing hot jalapeños and *Capsicum frutescens,* the type of cayenne pepper used to make Tabasco sauce.

Cayenne is a shrubby perennial plant that grows to 3 feet or taller. Native to South America, cayenne peppers are now cultivated in sunny, tropical places around the world. In temperate zones, they generally grow just as successfully as tomatoes and eggplants.

BENEFITS

- Blocks the transmission of pain and itching by nerve fibers in the skin
- May aid digestion by increasing blood flow to the stomach and intestinal tract (traditional)
- May stimulate circulation, lower cholesterol levels, and balance blood pressure (traditional/experimental)

SCIENTIFIC SUPPORT

In numerous clinical studies, a topical cream containing 0.025 or 0.075 percent capsaicin has proven helpful in treating many painful and itchy skin disorders, including psoriasis (a chronic skin disorder characterized by itching, scaling, redness, and other symptoms), shingles (a systemic herpes infection), diabetic neuropathy (a type of nerve pain suffered by at least 50 percent of people with diabetes), and postmastectomy pain (pain following partial or complete removal of the breast).

Preliminary research suggests that capsaicin cream may also be effective in relieving the severe, stabbing pain associated with trigeminal neuralgia, a disorder that affects the largest nerve in the face. Improvement was generally apparent after several days of applying the cream three times daily.[1] Similarly, capsaicin may alleviate the pain of cluster headaches, as shown in a placebo-controlled double-blind study. When results were assessed after 8 and 15 days of treatment, those who received capsaicin ointment in the nostril for 7 days reported less severe cluster headaches than those receiving placebo.[2] Cayenne has even been given successfully for mouth pain due to chemotherapy or radiation, in the form of capsaicin-laced taffy.[3]

Capsaicin creams also show promise in reducing the pain of arthritis. One double-blind, placebo-controlled, randomized study showed that a 0.075 percent capsaicin cream reduced tenderness and pain associated with osteoarthritis by roughly 40 percent over a 4-week period. The researchers noted the need for longer studies with a larger number of subjects in order to determine whether capsaicin might reduce symptoms further. To date, studies on rheumatoid arthritis have failed to include enough subjects to draw meaningful conclusions.[4]

Another area needing further study is the use of capsaicin cream for fibromyalgia, a difficult-to-treat condition characterized by achy pain, tenderness, and stiffness of muscles, tendons, and soft tissue. One double-blind study showed that a 0.025 percent capsaicin cream reduced tenderness and increased grip strength during the 4-week treatment period. There was no improvement in pain severity or quality of sleep, but the researchers believe that further studies with a more potent capsaicin cream might produce better results in these areas as well.[5]

Does Cayenne Help or Hurt Your Stomach?

Researchers have not yet reached any definite conclusion on this burning issue. However, some clinical research challenges the commonly held view that hot peppers aggravate stomach ulcers. In 1988, a study in the *Journal of the American Medical Association* reported that eating highly spiced meals did not contribute to gastrointestinal damage.[6] More recently, a comparison of chili-eating habits between 103 peptic ulcer patients and 87 healthy individuals found that people who ate more chili peppers actually had a lower incidence of ulcers.[7] Likewise, a study with duodenal ulcer patients found no difference

in healing rates between those who consumed chilis and those who did not.[8]

There is some evidence that cayenne may even offer some protection against ulcers. An in vitro study found that capsaicin inhibited the growth of *Helicobacter pylori,* a type of bacteria associated with ulcer formation.[9] A clinical trial on a different aspect of stomach health showed that chili protected against stomach injury associated with aspirin use. In the study, people who took 20 grams of chili (the equivalent of one whole chili pepper) followed by 600 mg aspirin half an hour later had significantly less damage to the stomach lining than those who took aspirin alone.[10] However, until there is more conclusive research in this area, those with ulcers should probably still be cautious about overindulging in spicy foods.

Population studies comparing the effects of chili consumption in cultural groups with high and low dietary intake of chilis have produced conflicting results. Some studies found an ulcer-protective effect in cultures that consume generous amounts of chilis. On the other hand, a population study in Mexico actually linked high chili consumption to an increased risk for gastric cancer.[11] However, researchers always caution against placing too much stock in epidemiological (population) studies, which are known to have a high potential for bias and other factors that could confound results. As with most things, moderation is probably the key to keeping your stomach happy.

SPECIFIC STUDIES

Postsurgical Nerve Pain: Clinical Study (1997)

A 0.075 percent capsaicin cream was significantly more effective than placebo in easing postsurgical nerve pain in 99 cancer survivors during a 16-week randomized, placebo-controlled, crossover study. During the first 8 weeks, half of the patients applied the capsaicin cream four times daily, while the second group used a placebo cream. After 8 weeks, the patients switched treatment groups. The average pain reduction was 53 percent in the cayenne group and only 17 percent in the placebo group after 8 weeks of treatment. The benefits of the capsaicin cream during the first 8 weeks continued throughout the following 8-week placebo period, suggesting a carry-over effect. At the end of the study, participants were asked which treatment was most effective: They chose the capsaicin treatment by a 3-to-1 margin. Side effects in the cap-saicin group included skin burning, redness (which decreased as the study progressed), and coughing, but the withdrawal rate in the capsaicin group was no higher than that of the placebo group.[12]

Psoriasis: Clinical Study (1993)

A 0.025 percent capsaicin cream was far superior to placebo in treating moderately severe psoriasis in a 6-week double-blind multicenter study of 197 people. Before entering the study, the majority of participants had been using steroid therapy with little success. All subjects were required to discontinue topical steroid medications 1 week before the study began and systemic steroids 8 weeks before. By week 4, the capsaicin group showed significant improvement, as measured by the physicians' global evaluations and combined psoriasis severity scores. By the end of the study, 66 percent of the capsaicin patients reported relief, compared with only 49 percent in the placebo group. Side effects in the capsaicin group included a burning or stinging sensation, mild coughing, sneezing, and tearing of the eyes—symptoms that diminished or disappeared in most patients over the course of the study. Out of 197 participants, 36 withdrew from the capsaicin group due to side effects, compared with 22 from the placebo group.[13]

Diabetic Neuropathy: Clinical Study (1991)

A 0.075 percent capsaicin cream was significantly more effective than placebo in relieving pain while improving sleep quality and pain-free walking distance in 49 patients with moderate to very severe diabetes-related nerve pain. During the 8-week double-blind study, participants used either a 0.075 percent capsaicin cream or a placebo cream four times per day. All other topical medications were discontinued at least 1 week prior to the study, and no new oral pain relievers were allowed during the treatment period. By the eighth week of treatment, 90 percent of the capsaicin group reported pain reduction, with a 49 percent average decrease in pain intensity and a 66 percent reduction in overall pain. Although the placebo group also improved modestly, this benefit ceased after the first 2 weeks. Sixty-one percent of the capsaicin group and 19 percent of the placebo group experienced a burning sensation, leading five patients in the capsaicin group and two in the placebo group to withdraw before the end of the study. Side effects, such as a local burning sensation and sneezing, generally disappeared during the first 2 weeks.[14]

HOW IT WORKS

Effects on Pain

As a topical cream, capsaicin helps relieve pain by depleting local supplies of a neurotransmitter called *substance P*, which transmits pain and itching signals from the nerves in the skin to the spinal cord. Researchers have found a link between many painful disorders and unusually high levels of substance P in the nerve fibers. Unlike other local anesthetics, cayenne does not block impulses to all of the nerve fibers. Research shows that it blocks type C fibers, which are strictly related to pain, leaving the sense of touch, temperature, and pressure intact.[14]

Capsaicin is thought to decrease inflammation by reducing vasodilation (widening of blood vessels). Patients with psoriasis often develop dilated, elongated, convoluted, and leaky veins long before lesions appear on the skin. Capsaicin may help relieve this underlying problem.[15] Research shows that capsaicin also increases the production of collagenase and certain prostaglandins that reduce both pain and inflammation.[16,17]

So why does capsaicin cream initially cause a burning and stinging sensation? Scientists have found that capsaicin first encourages the release of substance P, which produces the characteristic local burning reaction (and the hot taste sensation when taken internally). Subsequently, it hinders the body's ability to make more substance P. The end result is that after 4 or 5 days of use, burning sensations diminish, and so does the pain. People who use topical capsaicin creams gradually get accustomed to the heat, in the same way that fans of spicy food do.[18]

Circulatory Effects

To date, no clinical trials have investigated cayenne's traditional use for circulatory problems. However, promising results from numerous laboratory studies suggest that cayenne may help protect against heart disease. A rich source of antioxidants, cayenne contains vitamins A, C, and E and other substances that help protect the body against harmful free radicals, which are oxygen compounds that can damage cell membranes. Experimental research shows that cayenne reduces blood cholesterol (especially harmful low-density lipoprotein [LDL] cholesterol levels) and triglycerides, possibly by decreasing cholesterol absorption in the intestines and by increasing its excretion through the bile.[19]

Laboratory studies show that cayenne decreases platelet aggregation (abnormal blood clotting), another risk factor for heart disease. It is believed that cayenne does this by inhibiting synthesis of thromboxanes, substances that promote blood clotting.[19] In a cross-cultural study, researchers also found increased fibrinolytic activity (the breakdown of fibrin, a blood-clotting protein) in Thais who ate chiles daily, compared to whites living in Thailand who consumed a traditional American diet.[20] Laboratory studies show that cayenne also reduces fat deposits in the arteries by increasing the levels of liver enzymes involved in breaking down fat.[21]

Major Constituents

Capsaicin; vitamins A, C, and E

Safety

Cayenne is generally recognized as safe for use (GRAS) by the FDA and has a long history of consumption as a food. Wash hands thoroughly after applying capsaicin creams, and do not apply additional heat. When handling fresh hot peppers, use gloves to protect your skin from capsaicin's irritating, non-water-soluble effects. Since it is oil soluble, capsaicin can be removed from the skin using a cloth dipped in vegetable oil or a vinegar bath.

- **Side effects:** When applied topically, capsaicin often causes a temporary burning sensation. As long as the cream is applied frequently, this effect usually subsides within a few days. In clinical studies, a few people also reported sneezing and tearing of the eyes. Internal use may cause gastrointestinal irritation in sensitive individuals when taken in excessive amounts.[22]
- **Contraindications:** Not for use on injured skin, open wounds, or near the eyes.[23]
- **Drug interactions:** There are no known drug interactions with topical capsaicin creams.[23]

Dosage

According to studies, substantial pain relief with capsaicin creams may require 2 or more weeks of committed use. Germany's Commission E recommends that the external use of capsaicin creams be limited to 2 days, with a 14-day time lapse between applications.[23] However, this is contradicted by clinical evidence and by the *Physicians' Desk Reference,* which note that continued treatment produces the best results while actually reducing the rate of side effects.

External use

- **Cream (0.025 or 0.075 percent capsaicin):** Apply to affected areas up to four times a day.

Internal use

- **Capsules/tablets:** 400 to 500 mg, up to three times a day[24]
- **Tincture:** 5 to 10 drops in water.[24]

REFERENCES

1. Fusco BM, Alessandri M. Analgesic effect of capsaicin in idiopathic trigeminal neuralgia. *Anesthesia and Analgesia* 1992; 74: 375–377.

2. Marks DR, Rapaport A, Padla D, et al. A double-blind placebo-controlled trial of intranasal capsaicin for cluster headache. *Cephalalgia* 1993; 13: 114–116.

3. Berger A, Henderson M., Nadoolman W, et al. Oral capsaicin provides temporary relief for oral mucositis pain secondary to chemotherapy/radiation therapy. *Journal of Pain and Symptom Management* 1995; 10(3): 243–248.

4. McCarthy GM, McCarty DJ. Effect of topical capsaicin in the therapy of painful osteoarthritis of the hands. *The Journal of Rheumatology* 1992; 19: 604–607.

5. McCarty DJ, Csuka M, McCarthy G, et al. Treatment of pain due to fibromyalgia with topical capsaicin: a pilot study. *Seminars in Arthritis and Rheumatism* 1994; 23(6)(suppl 3): 41–47.

6. Graham DY, Smith JL, Opekun AR. Spicy food and the stomach: evaluation by videoendoscopy. *Journal of the American Medical Association* 1988; 260(23): 3473–3475.

7. Kang JY, Yeoh KG, Chia HP, et al. Chili: protective factor against peptic ulcer? *Digestive Diseases and Sciences* 1995; 40(3): 576–579.

8. Kumar N, Vij JC, Sarin SK, et al. Do chiles influence healing of duodenal ulcer? *British Medical Journal* 1984; 288: 1803–1804.

9. Jones NL, Shabib S, Sherman PM. Capsaicin as an inhibitor of the growth of the gastric pathogen *Helicobacter pylori*. *FEMS Microbiology Letters* 1997; 146: 223–227.

10. Yeoh KG, Kang JY, Yap I, et al. Chili protects against aspirin-induced gastroduodenal mucosal injury in humans. *Digestive Diseases and Sciences* 1995; 40(3): 580–583.

11. López-Carillo L, Hernández Avila M, Dubrow R. Chili pepper consumption and gastric cancer in Mexico: a case-control study. *American Journal of Epidemiology* 1994; 139 (3): 263–271.

12. Ellison N, Loprinzi CL, Kugler J, et al. Phase III placebo-controlled trial of capsaicin cream in the management of surgical neuropathic pain in cancer patients. *Journal of Clinical Oncology* 1997; 15(8): 2974–2980.

13. Ellis CN, Berberian B, Sulica VI, et al. A double-blind evaluation of topical capsaicin

in pruritic psoriasis. *Journal of the American Academy of Dermatology* 1993; 29: 438–442.

14. Scheffler NM, Sheitel PL, Lipton MN. Treatment of painful diabetic neuropathy with capsaicin 0.075 percent. *Journal of the American Podiatric Medical Association* 1991; 81(6): 288–293.

15. Bernstein JE, Parish LC, Rapaport M, et al. Effects of topically applied capsaicin on moderate and severe psoriasis vulgaris. *Journal of the American Academy of Dermatology* 1986; 15: 504–507.

16. Partsch G, Matucci-Cerinic M. Effect of capsaicin on the release of substance P from rheumatoid arthritis and osteoarthritis synoviocytes *in vitro*. *Annals of the Rheumatic Diseases* 1990; 49(8): 653.

17. Partsch G, Matucci-Cerinic M, Marabini S, et al. Collagenase synthesis of rheumatoid arthritis synoviocytes: dose-dependent stimulation by substance P and capsaicin. *Scandinavian Journal of Rheumatology* 1991; 20(2): 98–103.

18. Donofrio P, Walker F, Hunt V, et al. Treatment of painful diabetic neuropathy with topical capsaicin: a multicenter, double-blind, vehicle-controlled study. *Archives of Internal Medicine* 1991; 151: 2225–2229.

19. Wang JP, Hsu MF, Teng CM. Antiplatelet effect of capsaicin. *Thrombosis Research* 1984; 36: 497–507.

20. Visudhiphan S, Poolsuppasit S, Piboonnukarintr O, et al. The relationship between high fibrinolytic activity and daily capsicum ingestion in Thais. *The American Journal of Clinical Nutrition* 1982; 35: 1452–1458.

21. Kawada T, Hagihara K-I, Iwai K. Effects of capsaicin on lipid metabolism in rats fed a high fat diet. *Journal of Nutrition* 1986; 116: 1272–1278.

22. McGuffin M, Hobbs C, Upton R, et al., eds. *American Herbal Products Association Botanical Safety Handbook*. Boca Raton and New York: CRC Press LLC, 1997.

23. Blumenthal M, Busse W, Goldberg A, eds. *The Complete German Commission E Monographs*. Austin, TX: American Botanical Council; Boston, MA: Integrative Medical Communications, 1998.

24. Foster S. *101 Medicinal Herbs*. Loveland, CO: Interweave Press, 1998.

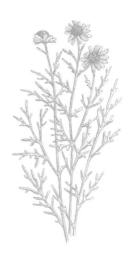

Chamomile

MATRICARIA RECUTITA
ASTERACEAE

State of Knowledge: Five-Star Rating System

Clinical (human) research	✱✱
Laboratory research	✱✱
History of use/traditional use	✱✱✱✱
Safety record	✱✱✱
International acceptance	✱✱✱✱

PART USED: *Flower*

PRIMARY USES

- *Mild sedative effects*
- *Skin irritations and inflammations (topical)*
- *Digestive upset*
- *Menstrual cramps*
- *Stomach ulcers*

According to traditional Slovakian folklore, one should bow with respect when standing before a chamomile plant, out of deference to its healing powers.[1] In Germany, where chamomile enjoys great popularity as a beverage and a medicine, it is often called *alles zutraut,* meaning "capable of anything."[1] Chamomile is used extensively on nearly every continent for the treatment of a wide range of ailments, from stomach upset and ulcers to inflamed skin and mucous membranes. Because of its widespread acceptance, chamomile is currently listed as an official drug in the pharmacopoeias of 26 countries. However, in spite of its international acceptance, chamomile has been the subject of only a few clinical studies, which provide some support for the herb's usefulness in inducing relaxation, soothing colic, treating wounds and skin conditions, and easing symptoms of colds and flu.

Although it is one of America's favorite herbal tea ingredients, chamomile has its most enthusiastic following in Europe, where chamomile tea is served in most restaurants and hotels and is widely used as a mild sedative both for adults and fussy children. In addition to its sedative effects, chamomile helps relieve spasms of smooth muscle tissue, making it useful for gastrointestinal and menstrual cramps. A popular children's herb, chamomile has a long history of use for easing symptoms of colds and flu, calming upset stomachs, and soothing colicky babies.

In Europe, chamomile is also considered a valuable remedy in the treatment of stomach ulcers. According to Rudolf Fritz Weiss, M.D., a well-known German doctor, "the remedy of choice is chamomile" for inhibiting inflammation and promoting the long-term healing of ulcers. "Chamomile does not merely give symptomatic relief in these cases, but directly effects a cure, influencing the pathological process," he writes. Dr. Weiss notes that fairly large doses of chamomile should be used over an extended period of time to effectively heal an ulcer.[2] Studies have confirmed that chamomile can prevent and treat stomach ulcers in laboratory animals, but this application has not yet been clinically tested in humans.

Externally, chamomile flowers have a strong traditional reputation for helping to heal wounds, inflammations, and other skin conditions. Outside the United States, chamomile preparations are added to medicinal baths to soothe hemorrhoids and to treat gynecological problems.

HISTORY

References to the healing properties of chamomile abound in the written histories of many cultures, from Europe and North America to Asia, Africa, and South America. The Egyptians associated chamomile with the sun and used it to treat fevers. Ancient Greek and Indian physicians prescribed chamomile for headaches as well as kidney, liver, and bladder conditions. In England, it has been applied in the treatment of a wide range of health problems, including digestive difficulties, general aches and pains, fevers, congestive heart failure, and menstrual irregularities. In North America, chamomile has been administered to promote wound healing and to treat women's reproductive disorders. Modern South Africans use chamomile for colic, diarrhea, and a host of other ailments.

Chamomile also has a long history of use as a cosmetic herb, especially valued as a rinse to bring out the highlights of blonde hair. Chamomile essential oil, which is distilled from the flowerheads, contains a compound called *azulene* that gives the oil a deep azure blue color.[3] Chamomile essential oil is a popular ingredient of perfumes, shampoos, lotions, salves, mouthwashes, and soaps, and is used to flavor beverages, desserts, candies, and liqueurs.[4]

INTERNATIONAL STATUS

Chamomile is listed as an official drug in the pharmacopoeias of 26 countries, including Germany, Belgium, France, and the United Kingdom. Germany's Commission E approved chamomile for external use for skin and mucous membrane irritations, bacterial skin diseases (including those of the mouth and gums), and inflammations of the anogenital region; for internal use against spasms and inflammatory conditions of the gastrointestinal tract; and as an inhalation to relieve respiratory inflammation and irritation. In Belgium, chamomile is recommended for the treatment of digestive disorders and for external use in skin problems. In France, it is approved in topical use as well as for internal use in certain digestive disorders, including spasmodic colitis.

BOTANY

Matricaria recutita (German chamomile) is a small annual herb in the aster family (Asteraceae). Chamomile is native to southern and eastern Europe and western Asia, but its range now also includes Australia, the United Kingdom, and the United States. The plant is commonly found in acidic soils in many areas, including mountains, open fields, and roadsides. A popular garden herb, chamomile grows best in a sunny location in well-drained, sandy soil. The plant may reach a height of 3 feet, with feathery leaves and delicate, daisylike white and yellow flowerheads. If left undisturbed, the plant will reseed itself and spread readily.

Two species, both commonly known as chamomile, have been used medicinally: German chamomile (*Matricaria recutita*, often called *Chamomilla recutita* or *Matricaria chamomilla*) and Roman or English chamomile (*Chamaemelum nobile*, also known as *Anthemis nobilis*). The two plants are botanically related, seem to have been used somewhat interchangeably throughout history, and have some constituents in common. Modern research, however, has focused on *M. recutita*.

Chamomile's mild, pleasant, applelike fragrance is reflected in its name, which comes from the Greek words *kamai melon*, meaning "ground apple." A related wild species, *Matricaria matricarioides*, is commonly called pineapple weed because of its light, fruity scent. This plant has been used in folk medicine for many of the same purposes as German chamomile, including relief of flatulence, stomach and menstrual cramps, and cold symptoms. It has also been applied externally as a wash for sores and itchy skin conditions.[5]

BENEFITS

- Produces antispasmodic effects on smooth muscle, particularly the gastrointestinal tract

- Possesses mild sedative and anti-anxiety properties
- Acts as an anti-inflammatory for skin, mucous membranes, gums, and mouth conditions
- Helps protect against the development of stomach ulcers, possibly by strengthening the mucosal layer or by preventing histamine release (implicated in the formation of stress ulcers)

SCIENTIFIC SUPPORT

Clinical Research

Despite centuries of traditional medicinal use, there have been surprisingly few well-controlled clinical studies investigating chamomile's sedative, anti-inflammatory, and antispasmodic effects. One such 1993 study offers some support for chamomile's traditional reputation as a folk remedy for treating infant colic (a painful condition believed to be caused by intestinal spasms), although the herbal preparation tested contained a number of other herbs in addition to chamomile.[6] In a small study from the 1970s, 10 of 12 patients undergoing a cardiac diagnostic procedure fell into a deep sleep shortly after drinking chamomile tea—an unexpected result of a study designed to investigate the effects of chamomile on the heart.[7] In a 1990 study of people with colds or flu, chamomile dramatically reduced the severity of symptoms

for those who inhaled steam containing chamomile extract.[8]

Chamomile has also shown benefits in the treatment of skin abrasions, but not all clinical studies have been conclusive. In one single-blind controlled study, a cream prepared from chamomile extract produced some improvement in radiation-induced skin irritations when applied topically, although this effect was not statistically significant.[9] In another double-blind study, chamomile extract significantly improved healing after dermabrasion for tattoo removal (an operative procedure performed with abrasive materials), speeding healing by enhancing the drying of oozing wounds in 14 people.[10]

Laboratory Research

Even though chamomile's excellent traditional reputation is only partially confirmed by studies in humans, laboratory studies provide some support for its wide range of effects, including antispasmodic, sedative, anti-inflammatory, wound-healing, and anti-ulcer effects. In one experiment comparing the effects of chamomile extract with those of the anti-inflammatory drug benzydamine, topical application of chamomile to the ear produced a reduction of edema (swelling) similar to that seen with the drug.[11] Chamomile has also demonstrated sedative effects in the laboratory. In one 1995 study, a water extract of chamomile was effective in reducing anxiety in mice.[12] Another study confirmed that chamomile causes mild depression of the central nervous system, resulting in drowsiness and reduced movement.[13] Antispasmodic effects were demonstrated in at least one laboratory study, the results of which showed that an alcohol extract of chamomile reduced contractions caused by histamine or acetylcholine.[14]

In a number of animal studies, chamomile and the constituent bisabolol have shown protective effects against the development of stomach ulcers. In these studies, bisabolol both protected against development of ulcers and enhanced ulcer healing.[15,16]

SPECIFIC STUDIES

Infant Colic:
Clinical Study (1993)

In a study of 69 infants, colic symptoms disappeared in 57 percent of babies who drank an antispasmodic herbal tea formula, according to assessments made by parents. The tea consisted of chamomile, vervain *(Verbena officinalis),* licorice *(Glycyrrhiza glabra),* fennel *(Foeniculum vulgare),* and lemon balm *(Melissa officinalis).* Thirty-three infants took the herbal tea powder dissolved in water (the amount of the powder was not specified) and 36 infants received placebo. During the first 7 days of the randomized, double-blind, placebo-controlled trial, no treatment was administered, but during the next 7 days, the babies were treated when colic symptoms were observed. Doses of up to 150 ml were given, no more than three times daily.

At the end of the study, colic was completely relieved in significantly more infants in the treatment group than in the placebo group (19 infants compared with 9). The colic improvement score, based on the number of nighttime awakenings and the frequency and length of crying spells, was also significantly better in the tea group than the placebo group. No adverse reactions were observed. Fennel and lemon balm are also known to possess antispasmodic actions. The investigators suggest that future studies should include larger numbers of infants and test individual herbs for their effects in relieving colic. As drawbacks to the current study, they pointed out its short duration and the fact that assessments were made only by parents, not by physicians.[6]

Cardiac Disease:
Clinical Study (1973)

The most striking result from this small study was the fact that 10 of the 12 patients undergoing a cardiac catheterization procedure fell into a deep sleep within 10 minutes of drinking chamomile tea. During the trial, which was designed to investigate the herb's effects on the heart, chamomile demonstrated no cardiac effects except a slight increase in average brachial artery pressure. However, shortly after drinking 6 ounces of chamomile tea, 10 of the 12 patients fell asleep and remained asleep until the catheter was removed. Based on the dramatic sedative effects observed in this trial, the researchers suggested that the hypnotic (sleep-inducing) properties of chamomile would be a rich area for further study.[7]

Common Cold: Clinical Study (1990)

Participants in this study reported that their cold symptoms improved after treatment with a steam inhalation containing chamomile extract. The higher the dosage of chamomile, the more benefit was reported. The 47 subjects were divided into four groups. Three groups (consisting of 15, 16, and 16 people) received treatment with a steam inhalation containing various doses of an alcohol extract of chamomile; the control group of 13 subjects inhaled steam containing nothing but alcohol. The participants were instructed to inhale the steam slowly and deeply for 10 minutes, keeping their heads covered with a towel.

The subjects assessed the severity of their symptoms immediately before treatment and at regular intervals for up to 2 hours after treatment. People who received the highest dose of chamomile extract (39 ml in 1,000 ml hot water) reported the greatest benefit, and improvement in all groups was reported within 15 minutes of beginning treatment. Effects peaked between 30 and 120 minutes after treatment started, but de-clined after 2 to 3 hours. Nearly 40 percent of the people in the group receiving the highest dose of chamomile said they felt dizzy at first, but no other side effects were reported.[8]

HOW IT WORKS

In laboratory experiments, whole-plant chamomile extract and many different chamomile constituents have shown medicinal effects. Two groups of compounds in chamomile are believed to be responsible for most of the herb's properties: the essential oil constituents and the flavonoids. Some of the most important constituents in the essential oil are bisabolol, bisabololoxides A and B, and azulenes, all of which have anti-inflammatory and antispasmodic effects. The most active chamomile flavonoids include apigenin and luteolin.[17]

Bisabolol and, to a lesser extent, bisabololoxides A and B, have shown anti-inflammatory properties and the ability to relax smooth muscle tissue in many animal studies. In such studies, bisabolol also protected against ulcer development and shortened the healing time of ulcers.[15,16] Possible mechanisms for this protective activity include strengthening the mucosal layer of the stomach[15] and decreasing the secretion of pepsin.[18]

Azulene and chamazulene have also demonstrated anti-allergenic activity.[3] Researchers believe that azulene helps prevent the allergic response by blocking the discharge of histamine from body tissues. Although the mechanism of action is not entirely clear, it is thought that azulene triggers the pituitary-adrenal system which, in turn, releases cortisone, a hormone that inhibits histamine production.[3]

Laboratory studies suggest that the flavonoid apigenin eases anxiety by binding to benzodiazepine receptors in the brain, promoting antianxiety and mild sedative effects without affecting the muscles. However, it is unlikely that apigenin is the only constituent responsible for chamomile's sedative effects.[12] Apigenin also demonstrates some anti-inflammatory activity, most likely by inhibiting some of the processes that control inflammatory responses. Cells that line the blood vessels release substances called *cytokines,* which are important in initiating and maintaining inflammatory responses. Apigenin appears to block part of the pathway activated by cytokines.[19]

Other chamomile flavonoids, as well as coumarins, have been shown to relax smooth muscle tissue and to possess some antibacterial and antiviral activity.[3] In addition, whole-plant chamomile extract has demonstrated mild antispasmodic activity in at least one study, but no conclusions were drawn as to its mechanism of action.[14] Chamomile is reported to accelerate wound healing both by reducing inflammation and by promoting tissue granulation and regeneration.[20]

MAJOR CONSTITUENTS

Essential oil (sesquiterpenes including bisabolol, azulene, and chamazulene); flavonoids (including apigenin and luteolin); coumarins

SAFETY

Chamomile is on the U.S. FDA list of herbs that are generally recognized as safe (GRAS).

During the early 1980s, there was an isolated report of anaphylactic (allergic) shock possibly related to chamomile tea consumption; subsequently, warnings about chamomile were issued by the FDA. However, millions of people consume chamomile each year, and only five documented cases of chamomile allergy have been reported. In each of these cases, the individual experiencing the allergic reaction recovered completely.[21] Some sources caution people who suffer from allergies to ragweed or other aster family plants to avoid chamomile. This warning, which has also been suggested for echinacea and other aster family plants, is not supported by clinical evidence. The concept of cross-sensitization is highly controversial among allergy specialists. In the case of chamomile, the popularity of the tea suggests that many hay fever sufferers have consumed it without problems.

- **Side effects:** None known.
- **Contraindications:** Some sources advise those who have experienced allergic reactions to ragweed or to other members of the Asteraceae family to avoid chamomile, but clinical support for this warning is lacking. In Germany, products are required to carry a warning advising against the use of chamomile near the eyes.
- **Drug interactions:** None known.[22]

DOSAGE

For the treatment of ulcers, German physician Rudolf Fritz Weiss, M.D., recommends large and frequent doses of concentrated chamomile extract or tea, taken over a longer period of time than for other purposes. Dr. Weiss advises taking 30 drops of chamomile fluid extract in a glass of warm water, or 2 to 3 teaspoons of highly concentrated chamomile tea in water.[2] Dosages for other uses are summarized in the following list of preparations.

- **Standardized extract:** Up to six 300- to 400-mg capsules a day[1]
- **Tincture:** 10 to 40 drops, three times a day[1]
- **Tea:** One-half to 1 teaspoon of dried flowers steeped in a cup of hot water, three to four times a day[1]

- **Sitz bath:** Approximately 100 grams (about a quarter pound) of chamomile flowers steeped in a quart of hot water, and then strained[21]
- **Bath:** Approximately 100 grams (about a quarter pound) of chamomile flowers steeped in a gallon of hot water, and then strained[21]

STANDARDIZATION

Chamomile extracts typically are standardized to 1 percent apigenin and 0.5 percent essential oil.

REFERENCES

1. Foster S. *101 Medicinal Herbs.* Loveland, CO: Interweave Press, 1998.
2. Weiss RF. *Herbal Medicine.* Portland, OR: Medicina Biologica, 1988.
3. Mann C, Staba EJ. The chemistry, pharmacology, and commercial formulations of chamomile. In: Craker LE, Simon JE, eds. *Herbs, Spices, and Medicinal Plants.* Vol. I. Phoenix, AZ: Oryx Press, 1986.
4. Duke JA. *CRC Handbook of Medicinal Herbs.* Boca Raton, FL: CRC Press, 1985.
5. Foster S, Duke J. *Eastern/Central Medicinal Plants.* Boston: Houghton Mifflin Company, 1990.
6. Weizman Z, Alkrinawi S, Goldfarb D, et al. Efficacy of herbal tea preparation in infantile colic. *The Journal of Pediatrics* 1993; 122: 650–652.

7. Gould L, Reddy CVR, Gomprecht RF. Cardiac effects of chamomile tea. *Journal of Clinical Pharmacology* 1973; 13(11/12): 475-479.

8. Saller R, Beschorner M, Hellenbrecht D, et al. Dose-dependancy of symptomatic relief of complaints by chamomile steam inhalation in patients with common cold. *European Journal of Pharmacology* 1990; 183: 728–729.

9. Maiche A, Gröhn P, Mäki-Hokkonen H. Effect of chamomile cream and almond ointment on acute radiation skin reaction. *Acta Oncologica* 1991; 30: 395–396.

10. Glowania HJ, Rauilin C, Swoboda M. The effect of chamomile in healing wounds: a clinical, double-blind study [in German]. *Zeitschrift für Hautkrankheiten* 1987; 17(62): 1262–1271.

11. Tubaro A, Zilli C, Redaelli C, et al. Evaluation of anti-inflammatory activity of a chamomile extract after topical application. *Planta Medica* 1984; 51: 359.

12. Viola H, Wasowski C, Levi de Stein M, et al. Apigenin, a component of *Matricaria recutita* flowers, is a central benzodiazepine receptors-ligand with anxiolytic effects. *Planta Medica* 1995; 61: 213–216.

13. Della Loggia R, Traversa U, Scarcia V, et al. Depressive effects of *Chamomilla recutita* (L.), Rausch, tubular flowers on central nervous system in mice. *Pharmacological Research Communications* 1982; 14(2): 153–162.

14. Forster HB, Niklas H, Lutz S. Antispasmodic effects of some medicinal plants. *Planta Medica* 1980; 40(4): 309–319.

15. Szelenyi I, Isaac O, Thiemer K. Pharmacological experiments with compounds of chamomile/III. Experimental studies of the ulcer-protective effect of chamomile [in German]. *Planta Medica* 1979; 35: 218–227.

16. Isaac O, Thiemer K. Biochemical studies on camomile components/III. *In vitro* studies about the antipeptic activity of (–)-alpha-bisabolol. *Arzneimittel-Forschung* 1975; 25(9): 1352–1354.

17. Brinker F. *Eclectic Dispensatory of Botanical Therapeutics*. Vol. 2. Sandy, OR: Eclectic Medical Publications, 1995.

18. Thiemer K, Stadler R, Isaac O. Biochemical studies of chamomile constituents. I. Anti-peptic effect of chamomile extract and sodium 1, 4-dimethyl-7-isopropylazulen sulfonic acid [in German]. *Arzneimittel-Forschung/Drug Research* 1972; 22(6): 1086–1087.

19. Gerritsen ME, Carley WW, Ranges GE, et al. Flavonoids inhibit cytokine-induced endothelial cell adhesion protein gene expression. *American Journal of Pathology* 1995; 147(2): 278–292.

20. Carle R, Issac O. Effect and effectiveness. A commentary on the monograph of *Matricaria flos* (chamomile blooms) [in German]. *Zeitschrift für Phytotherapie* 1987; 8: 67–77.

21. McCaleb R. Chamomile: the world's most soothing herb. *Better Nutrition for Today's Living* September 1993; 48–51.

22. Blumenthal M, Busse W, Goldberg A, et al., eds. *The Complete German Commission E Monographs*. Austin, TX: The American Botanical Council; Boston, MA: Integrative Medical Communications, 1998.

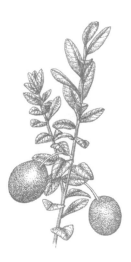

Cranberry

VACCINIUM MACROCARPON
ERICACEAE

State of Knowledge: Five-Star Rating System

Clinical (human) research	✶✶
Laboratory research	✶✶✶
History of use/traditional use	✶✶✶✶
Safety record	✶✶✶✶
International acceptance	✶✶

PART USED: *Fruit*

PRIMARY USES

- *Mild urinary tract infections*
- *Urinary tract health*

Cranberry juice is often the first remedy to which people turn at the early signs of urinary tract infection, and with good reason. Long valued for its beneficial actions in the urinary tract, this popular "folk remedy" finally is getting the strong scientific recognition it deserves. Clinical studies have confirmed that drinking cranberry juice can help prevent the development of urinary tract infections in people who are prone to them, and re-

searchers have identified the plant compounds in cranberry that are responsible for this action. We now know that these compounds work to prevent disease-causing bacteria from getting a foothold in the urinary tract. More recent research has shown that the same compounds may prevent bacteria in the mouth from sticking together and forming dental plaque, suggesting a possible use for cranberry compounds in maintaining gum health.

Many people know that cranberry juice can bring fast relief of symptoms once a urinary tract infection has set in. These infections cause extremely unpleasant symptoms, including burning during urination and increased urinary frequency. Women are more likely than men to get urinary tract infections; researchers estimate that from 10 to 20 percent of women will experience a urinary tract infection at some time in their lives.[1] Women older than 65 seem to be especially prone to this type of infection.[2]

Although cranberry juice may help relieve symptoms, no clinical studies have yet confirmed the effectiveness of cranberry in curing urinary tract infections. If left untreated, urinary tract infections can worsen and lead to other health problems. If you think you have a urinary tract condition, consult your health-care practitioner.

HISTORY

Northern European settlers who came to eastern North America coined the name *crane-berry* because of the resemblance of the flower stamens to the bill of a crane. By the mid-1600s this name had become *cranberry,* first noted in a letter by a Cape Cod missionary in 1647.[3]

Cranberry has a long history of practical and therapeutic uses. In addition to consumption as a food, cranberries were employed medicinally by several Native American tribes and in early American medicine. Among other uses, early American settlers used cranberries to diminish the intensity of gallbladder attacks, and Native Americans added the berries to poultices on open wounds. The traditional applications of cranberry have also included treatments for ailments of the stomach, liver, and blood, and, most notably, urinary tract disorders. Cranberry's high vitamin C content also made it a useful preventive remedy against scurvy.

Historical accounts describe a foodstuff known as *pemmican,* which was made by Native Americans in the region that is now New England. Consisting of dried deer meat, fat, and mashed cranberries, it resisted spoilage and could be stored for weeks. The deep red juice of the cranberry served as a dye for rugs and blankets. Today, cranberry's ample supply of vitamin C and its appealing, tangy flavor help to explain the popularity of cranberry products in millions of American households.

INTERNATIONAL STATUS

Cranberry is not officially approved for use in any European nation.

BOTANY

Native to North America, cranberry is a member of the plant genus *Vaccinium,* which also includes blueberry *(V. angustifolium)* and bilberry *(V. myrtillus).* Hardy and resilient, the cranberry plant can live more than 100 years in conditions that would kill other plants. Cranberry grows wild in a wide band covering the eastern portion of North

America, extending from Canada to the southeastern United States. A member of the heather family (Ericaceae), cranberry is a low-lying vine that prefers ample water, acidic soils, and low temperatures. Cranberries are grown commercially in bogs and marshes in the Pacific Northwest, Massachusetts and several mid-Atlantic states, Wisconsin, some parts of Canada, and Chile. The vines produce short-lived pink flowers in late spring.

BENEFITS

- Helps prevent urinary tract infections
- Inhibits bacteria from attaching to the walls of the urinary tract
- Prevents different species of bacteria from forming dental plaque in the mouth

SCIENTIFIC SUPPORT

Several clinical studies have shown that daily consumption of cranberry can help prevent the bacterial colonization that can cause urinary tract infection. At least one study suggests that cranberry juice may clear existing infection in addition to preventing new infection.[2] In addition, a limited amount of research has shown that cranberry supplements (capsules) may help reduce the frequency of urinary tract infections for women troubled by frequent recurrences.[4]

Scientists have shown that cranberry's power to prevent urinary tract infection and relieve symptoms comes from its ability to keep disease-causing bacteria from adhering to the walls of the urinary tract, thereby reducing the risk of infection. *Escherichia coli* bacteria (commonly known as *E. coli*) are believed to cause more than 80 percent of all urinary tract infections.[5] Research has shown that antioxidant pigments called *proanthocyanidins* as well as the fructose in cranberry juice impair the ability of certain types of *E. coli* to affix themselves to the cells that line the walls of the urinary tract.[6,7] In an earlier laboratory study, cranberry juice inhibited adherence of 60 percent of all *E. coli* bacterial strains tested.[8]

There has been a small amount of research into other possible uses for cranberry. One laboratory study suggests that the proanthocyanidin portion of cranberry extract (and other *Vaccinium* species such as blueberry and lingonberry) may have anti-cancer activity.[9] Another laboratory experiment showed that cranberry has antioxidant effects. In the study, flavonoid compounds from cranberry prevented the oxidation of low-density lipoprotein (LDL) cholesterol, which has been linked to heart disease.[10]

Finally, an interesting study showed that one constituent of cranberry may help prevent different types of gingival (gum) bacteria from sticking to each other, a process called *coaggregation*. Coaggregation is an important step in the formation of dental plaque, and researchers believe that substances that block this step can help improve oral hygiene.[11]

SPECIFIC STUDIES

Prevention of Urinary Tract Infection: Clinical Study (1994)

A double-blind, placebo-controlled clinical study published in the *Journal of the American Medical Association* showed that regular intake of cranberry juice cocktail significantly reduced the frequency of bacteriuria (bacteria in the urine) and pyuria (pus in the urine, indicating mild infection) in elderly women after 4 to 8 weeks of regular cranberry beverage intake. The 153 women in this 6-month study drank 300 ml daily of cranberry juice cocktail or a synthetic placebo drink with a similar flavor but no cranberry content.[2]

Prevention of Urinary Tract Infection: Clinical Study (1991)

In a clinical study in 28 nursing home residents, cranberry juice cocktail prevented urinary tract infections in 19 of the participants. The remaining 9 individuals all had significant counts of Gram-negative bacteria in their urine. The participants drank 4 to 6 ounces of cranberry juice cocktail almost daily for 7 weeks. The researchers concluded that cranberry juice may act more as a preventive than a curative agent against urinary tract infections.[12]

Prevention of Bacterial Adhesion: Laboratory Study (1998)

This laboratory study built on previous research that showed that cranberry works by preventing bacteria from sticking to the walls of the urinary tract. The study provides evidence that cranberry compounds called proanthocyanidins are responsible for preventing the adherence of disease-causing P-fimbriated *E. coli* to the urinary tract lining (see How It Works for an explanation of fimbriae). Fruits (such as blueberry) from the same genus *(Vaccinium)* exhibited similar activity, whereas other fruits and vegetables did not.[13]

Prevention of Coaggregation of Gum Bacteria: Laboratory Study (1998)

A constituent of cranberry juice, identified only as "a high molecular-weight nonprotein constituent of the juice," reversed the coaggregation (bonding between different bacterial species) of 58 percent of the gingival bacterial strains tested. Dental plaque begins to form when certain types of bacteria *(Streptococci, Actinomyces)* adhere to substances normally found on tooth surfaces. Plaque accumulates as other bacteria latch on to the initial colonies. Therefore, substances that prevent bacteria from sticking to one another could interrupt the progression of dental plaque formation. The results of this study thus suggest that cranberry may help in the prevention or management of some gum diseases. However, the researchers noted that the high sugar content of commercially available cranberry juice cocktails makes them inappropriate as promoters of good oral hygiene.[11]

HOW IT WORKS

For many years, researchers believed that cranberry's effects on urinary tract health came from its ability to lower the pH of urine, creating an inhospitable environment for bacterial growth. Yet as early as 1967, a study showed that the effects of cranberry juice on urine pH were temporary, suggesting that making urine more acidic was not its main mechanism of action.[14]

Later studies provided evidence that compounds in cranberry prevent bacteria, especially different types of *E. coli,* from sticking to the cells that line the urinary tract. These bacteria normally attach themselves to urinary tract cells by using specialized fibers called *fimbriae.* Proanthocyanidins in cranberry are responsible for keeping one kind of disease-causing *E. coli* bacteria (called P-fimbriated *E. coli*) from attaching to the urinary tract walls, according to a study published in *The New England Journal of Medicine* in 1998. The same researchers showed that other closely related fruits, such as blueberry, worked in a similar fashion, whereas other fruits and vegetables did not.[13] Cranberry also contains fructose, which prevents the adherence of type 1 *E. coli* to the urinary tract.[7]

MAJOR CONSTITUENTS

Proanthocyanidins, flavonoids, fructose, vitamin C

SAFETY

Cranberry has been safely used as a food for centuries, and is considered safe for consumption when used in reasonable doses by average consumers.

- **Side effects:** None known.
- **Contraindications:** None known.
- **Drug interactions:** None known.

DOSAGE

Cranberry juice cocktails typically consist of approximately one-third pure juice. The high sugar content of commercially available cranberry juice cocktails may bother some people. Unsweetened cranberry juice cocktails are available in many health-food stores, and cranberry is also available as a dietary supplement in the form of dried cranberry powder capsules. Six capsules are approximately equivalent to 3 ounces of cranberry juice cocktail.[15] If you think you have a urinary tract infection, consult a health-care practitioner.

- **Capsules:** 9 to 15 capsules a day (400 to 500 mg each)

• **Juice:** 4 to 6 ounces of cocktail a day as a preventive; up to 32 ounces as treatment

REFERENCES

1. Fowler JE. Urinary tract infections in women. *Urologic Clinics of North America* 1986; 13(4): 673–683.

2. Avorn J, Monane M, Gurwitz JH, et al. Reduction of bacteriuria and pyuria after ingestion of cranberry juice. *Journal of the American Medical Association* 1994; 271(10): 751–754.

3. Siciliano AA. Cranberry. *HerbalGram* 1996; 38: 51–54.

4. Walker EB, Barney DP, Mickelsen JN, et al. Cranberry concentrate: UTI prophylaxis (letter). *The Journal of Family Practice* 1997; 45(2): 167–169.

5. Schmidt DR, Sobota AE. An examination of the anti-adherence activity of cranberry juice on urinary and nonurinary bacterial isolates. *Microbios* 1988; 55: 173–181.

6. Ofek I, Goldhar J, Sharon N. Anti-*Escherichia coli* adhesion activity of cranberry and blueberry juices. In: Ofek I, Kahane I, eds. *Toward Anti-Adhesion Therapy for Microbial Diseases.* New York: Plenum Press, 1996: 179–183. Advances in Experimental Medicine and Biology; No. 408.

7. Zafriri D, Ofek I, Adar R, et al. Inhibitory activity of cranberry juice on adherence of type 1 and type P fimbriated *Escherichia coli* to eucaryotic cells. *Antimicrobial Agents and Chemotherapy* 1989; 33(1): 92–98.

8. Sobota AE. Inhibition of bacterial adherence by cranberry juice: potential use for the treatment of urinary tract infections. *The Journal of Urology* 1984; 131: 1013–1016.

9. Bomser J, Madhavi DL, Singletary K, et al. *In vitro* anticancer activity of fruit extracts from *Vaccinium* species. *Planta Medica* 1996; 62: 212–216.

10. Wilson T, Porcari JP, Harbin D. Cranberry extract inhibits low-density lipoprotein oxidation. *Life Sciences* 1998; 62: 24 (PL381–PL386).

11. Weiss EI, Lev-Dor R, Kashamn Y, et al. Inhibiting interspecies coaggregation of plaque bacteria with a cranberry juice constituent. *Journal of the American Dental Association* 1998; 129: 1719–1723.

12. Gibson L, Pike L, Kilbourn JP. Effectiveness of cranberry juice in preventing urinary tract infections in long-term care facility patients. *The Journal of Naturopathic Medicine* 1991; 2(1): 45–47.

13. Howell AB, Vorsa N, Marderosian AD, et al. Inhibition of the adherence of P-fimbriated *Escherichia coli* to uroepithelial-cell surfaces by proanthocyanidin extracts from cranberries (letter). *New England Journal of Medicine* 1998; 339(15): 1085–1086.

14. Kahn HD, Panariello VA, Saeli J, et al. Effect of cranberry juice on urine. *Journal of the American Dietetic Association* 1967; 51: 251–254.

15. Foster S, Tyler V. *Tyler's Honest Herbal:* 4th ed. New York and London: Haworth Herbal Press, 1999: 127–129.

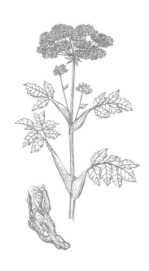

Dong Quai

ANGELICA SINENSIS
APIACEAE

State of Knowledge: Five-Star Rating System

Clinical (human) research	✳
Laboratory research	✳✳✳
History of use / traditional use	✳✳✳✳
Safety record	✳✳✳✳
International acceptance	✳✳✳✳

PART USED: *Root*

PRIMARY USES

- *Painful menstruation (traditional)*
- *Premenstrual syndrome (traditional)*
- *Irregular menstrual cycles (traditional)*
- *Delayed or absent periods (traditional)*
- *Anemia or weakness (traditional)*
- *Menopause (traditional)*
- *Cardiovascular health (experimental)*
- *Liver support (experimental)*

Often called "the female ginseng," dong quai eclipsed even ginseng's reputation in China centuries ago. More recently, the plant's popularity has grown in the United States despite a lack of clinical research by Western scientists. Much of the information on dong quai comes from the complex system of traditional Chinese medicine (TCM) and from Asian laboratory and clinical studies conducted since the 1960s. From this context, an icon of Chinese medicine emerges—a gentle, warming, nourishing root that has been used to strengthen and regulate women's reproductive function for over 2,000 years. Like many Chinese herbs, the use of dong quai is generally not well understood in the West. In the United States, it is often sold as a single-herb remedy, whereas in China it is almost never taken by itself. Traditionally, dong quai is blended with other herbs in teas, soups, and dishes such as "danggui duck" that support and balance a woman's system over time.

Dong quai has been the subject of just one Western clinical study on menopause, which led to disappointing results. Several promising studies have been conducted in China on menstrual problems and uterine prolapse (sinking), although few details have been translated into English. Some researchers, including well-known medicinal plant expert Albert Leung, Ph.D., maintain that proving dong quai's benefits to women's reproductive health through clinical studies may be difficult because of the plant's subtle tonic effects.[1] Given its reputation, dong quai should not be dismissed because of a lack of clinical evidence. Future studies could answer many questions by testing the root in combination with other Chinese herbs over an adequate period of time, using criteria that can detect the plant's more subtle effects.

HISTORY

In China, dong quai is called *tang kuei* (or *dang gui*), which means "proper order." As a blood tonic, the root is used to restore balance in a woman's reproductive system by toning the uterus, nourishing the blood, and stimulating healthy circulation. It also strengthens the heart, liver, and lungs. Dong quai was mentioned in Chinese medical texts as early as A.D. 588, where it is recommended for "deficient blood," a condition characterized by dizziness, a pale face and lips, weak vision, lethargy, heart palpitations, dry skin, menstrual irregularities, pale tongue, and a thready pulse. The plant's warming action is typically used for chronic and deficient (weakened) conditions, which are considered "cold," rather than acute problems, which are classified as "hot." Similarly, dong quai is an appropriate herb for those who tend to be introverted or "yin" (cold) in temperament and constitution, rather than more extroverted and "yang" (hot).

In TCM, dong quai has historically been used for menstrual problems and anemia, as a postpartum tonic, and as an aphrodisiac. The plant is also said to have "fetus-calming" properties and is sometimes prescribed with other herbs to assure a healthy pregnancy and a smooth delivery. Dong quai is said to relieve pain caused by abnormal blood clotting in cases of bruising, menstrual clots, and uterine fibroids. The root is also used for high blood pressure, angina, headaches, bronchial asthma, chronic bronchitis, hepatitis, diabetes, cirrhosis, chills, constipation, and as a mild sedative. Chinese practitioners also inject doses of dong quai into acupuncture points to relieve pain. Although primarily a female herb, men can also take dong quai to "build the blood."

Dong quai's warming, tonic properties are believed to be even stronger when the root is cooked in soups, teas, and other dishes. It is traditionally added to chicken soup, with or without astragalus *(Astragalus membranaceus)*, and consumed over a 4-day period during recovery from illness or to improve poor circulation. Four Things Soup, the most widely prescribed women's tonic in China, is made of equal parts dong quai, peony *(Peonia albiflora)*, rehmannia *(Rehmannia glutinosa)*, and ligusticum *(Ligusticum sinense)*. An even tastier recipe combines one dong quai root with six Chinese jujube dates *(Ziziphus jujuba)*. The herbs are simmered in 3 cups of water until the mixture has cooked down to 1 cup. A half cup of this tea is consumed by many Asian women daily. Whole dong quai roots can also be lightly steamed, sliced into pieces the thickness of a penny, dried, and eaten in quantities of one to two pieces each day.

Dong quai has a much shorter and less illustrious history in the West. It was introduced into Western medicine in 1899 by the German company Merck and sold as a liquid extract or tablet for menstrual problems. Today, dong quai is the fourteenth best-selling herb in the United States market.

INTERNATIONAL STATUS

Dong quai is not officially approved for use in any European nation. However, it is an official medicine in China, Japan, Korea, and other Asian countries.

BOTANY

A member of the celery (Apiaceae) family, dong quai grows in cool, moist, shady areas with rich soil, from sea level to altitudes of 8,000 feet. Native to China, the plant is primarily cultivated in its homeland, as well as in Japan and Korea, instead of harvested from the wild. Some of the highest-quality roots come from the Yunnan and Gansu provinces in southwestern China, where dong quai has been grown for 1,500 years.

Dong quai is a biennial or perennial with smooth purplish stems that reach heights of 3 to 7 feet. The umbels of white flowers bloom from May to August. Dong quai roots are harvested in the fall of the third year and then peeled, sliced, and dried in the shade. The most potent roots are said to be large, sweet, and pungent tasting, with a creamy white interior. American herbalist Rosemary Gladstar describes the root slices as "delicately carved pieces of ivory."

Dong quai's species name, *sinensis*, refers to its origin in China. Although closely related to the Western plant angelica *(Angelica archangelica)*, the two plants are not interchangeable. Dong quai and angelica share some similar properties in treating women's problems, but angelica is stronger and intended for shorter-term use. The Chinese occasionally substitute the Western plant lovage *(Levisticum officinale)* for dong quai.

BENEFITS

- Regulates bleeding, reduces pain, and relaxes the uterus in cases of menstrual cramps, due to its antispasmodic and blood-building properties
- Helps balance irregular menstrual cycles
- Encourages blood flow when periods are delayed or absent
- Helps build the blood in anemia

SCIENTIFIC SUPPORT

Most of the research on dong quai has been conducted in China and Japan since the early 1960s. Although research has consisted mainly of laboratory studies, the findings do support many of dong quai's traditional uses. Several clinical trials also show promise, although they have not been fully translated into English.

A single clinical study from the United States found dong quai to be no more effective than placebo in relieving a variety of menopausal symptoms, including vaginal atrophy (thinning of the tissue that lines the vagina).[2] Although the American study was randomized, double-blind, and placebo controlled, the overall design was lacking in several important ways. The researchers' objective was to determine whether dong quai had estrogenic effects, as measured by hormone-dependent changes in the vaginal lining. The negative outcome is not surprising in light of the fact that Asian researchers have long known that the plant does not affect hormone levels. The authors also admit that "use of dong quai alone (in this study) can be criticized because traditional Chinese practitioners never prescribe dong quai alone." They go on to state that a mixture of dong quai, peony, ligusticum, atractylodes (Atractylodes lancea), and poria (Poria cocos) was previously found to reduce menopausal problems by more than 70 percent in 43 women. Impressive improvements in menstrual cramps and amenorrhea (lack of menstruation) have also been seen when dong quai was used by itself.[3]

Preliminary research suggests that dong quai has strong antitumor activity and an immune-stimulating effect in animals. Several studies show that a polysaccharide constituent in the root increases the ability of natural killer cells, macrophages, and other immune cells to destroy tumors. Researchers continue to study its potential as an adjunct tumor therapy and a possible treatment for AIDS.[4] Dong quai has also demonstrated anti-allergenic activity. Studies show that it helps prevent production of allergy-related antibodies (IgE) and provides protection against capillary permeability, an important factor in allergic reactions.[3,5]

Another area of current research is dong quai's potential as a pain reliever. In China, the root is commonly given as an injection into acupuncture points in the treatment of many different types of pain. In one Chinese clinical trial, it effectively reduced postoperative pain in 105 patients who had just had chest surgery.[3,6] Laboratory studies suggest that dong quai has potent anti-inflammatory properties, as well as pain-relieving effects that are 1.7 times as strong as aspirin.[7]

SPECIFIC STUDIES

Menopause: Clinical Study (1997)

Dong quai was no more effective than placebo in increasing the thickness of the vaginal and uterine linings and reducing other symptoms of menopause in a randomized, double-blind, placebo-controlled study of 71 women. During the 6-month study, participants took either 3 capsules of dong quai three times daily (equivalent to 4.5 g of root) or placebo. The dong quai capsules were standardized to 0.5 mg/kg of ferulic acid. Assessments at 6, 12, and 24 weeks showed no statistically significant change in blood levels of the hormones estradiol and estrone or in the cells of the vagina and endometrium (uterine lining). Patients in the dong quai and placebo groups reported a similar improvement of 25 to 30 percent in scores on the Kupperman Menopausal Index based on 10 common menopause symptoms. Minor side effects such as burping, gas, and headache were reported just as frequently in the placebo group as the herb group. The researchers concluded that dong quai does not have estrogenic effects and is not effective by itself in treating menopause complaints.[2]

HOW IT WORKS

Effects on the Menstrual Cycle

Researchers believe dong quai helps relieve menstrual cramps because of its relaxing effect on the uterus. Depending on how the root is prepared, dong quai can have a relaxing or a more toning and mildly stimulating effect on the uterus, according to laboratory studies. In most of its forms (raw, as an alcohol extract, or as a tea), dong quai reduces spasms in the uterus, possibly due to its volatile oil content. When a more stimulating preparation is desired, the root can be simmered in an uncovered pot to boil away the relaxing volatile oils.[8]

The plant's overall benefits to the female reproductive system may be due to its effects on the liver, rather than to an estrogenic effect. In traditional Chinese medicine, the liver is considered to be one of the chief organs that regulates the menstrual cycle.[9,10] Dong quai also works by increasing blood circulation to the uterus and relieving pelvic congestion (poor circulation in the pelvic area).[8,11] In animal studies, other tonic effects include an increase in DNA content and glucose metabolism in the uterus, leading to a healthy growth of uterine tissue, and protective effects on the liver.[12] The constituents currently thought to contribute to dong quai's blood-enriching properties are polysaccharides, rather than vitamin B_{12}, as was previously believed.[5]

Liver-Protective Effects

Laboratory studies show that dong quai strengthens liver function by increasing the liver's ability to use oxygen, while preserving glycogen (stored energy in the liver) and glutathione, a potent antioxidant that helps protect the organ from destructive free radicals.[13] Dong quai also guards the liver against a variety of toxic substances, such as carbon tetrachloride.[9]

Cardiovascular Benefits

Laboratory research shows that dong quai helps lower blood pressure by dilating the peripheral blood vessels. For this reason, it has also been used to treat glaucoma, a buildup of pressure in the eye.[14] At the same time, dong quai strengthens the heart's pumping action, slows the pulse rate, and relaxes cardiac muscle.[8] It helps prevent abnormal blood clotting (platelet aggregation) by preventing the release of serotonin (5-hydroxytryptophan, or 5-HTP) and ADP (adenosine diphosphate), which can cause blood to become sticky, and by inhibiting arachidonic acid metabolism. These effects are thought to be due to the root's coumarin and ferulic acid content.[5,6,11,13]

Dong quai also helps relieve smooth muscle spasms in the arteries and increase blood flow, as a result of stimulation of acetylcholine receptors and beta-adrenergic receptors, respectively.[5] Researchers have also demonstrated that the plant helps reduce cholesterol and fat deposits in the arteries.[13] Some of dong quai's cardiovascular effects are likely due to its ability to increase the body's utilization of vitamin E.[5]

Effects on the Respiratory System

Researchers believe dong quai's relaxing effects on bronchial smooth muscle are due to the constituents butylidenphthalide and ligustilide. In a Chinese clinical study of 50 patients with chronic obstructive pulmonary disease, an oral extract of dong quai improved the patients' ability to breathe after 50 to 60 days of treatment. The extract successfully increased the forced expiratory volume from 43 percent before treatment to 56 percent after treatment, while significantly decreasing mortality rates.[6]

MAJOR CONSTITUENTS

Ferulic acid, polysaccharides, butylidenephthalide, ligustilide, coumarins

SAFETY

Dong quai is considered reasonably safe, even when used long term.

- **Side effects:** Side effects are rare. In high amounts, dong quai could cause excessive menstrual bleeding and increase the body's overall bleeding time.
- **Contraindications:** Do not use this herb during pregnancy. Although in Chinese medicine, dong quai has traditionally been used by pregnant women, this requires the supervision of a qualified health-care practitioner.[15] Because dong quai is warming to the body, traditional Chinese medical texts caution against using it during acute ("hot") illnesses and by those who tend to be extroverted or "yang" (hot).[9] Dong quai should not be used by those with excessive menstrual flow or diarrhea or during menstruation. When using dong quai to treat menstrual cramps, the herb is usually taken as a tonic for many months, with a break during menstruation itself.[11,16]
- **Drug interactions:** Dong quai should not be used in combination with anticoagulant drugs.

DOSAGE

- **Capsules/tablets:** 500 to 600 mg up to six times a day[17]
- **Tincture (1:5):** 5 to 20 drops, up to three times a day[17]
- **Tea:** 1 cup, two to three times a day[17]

STANDARDIZATION

Dong quai is not currently available as a standardized extract.

REFERENCES

1. Leung AY. *Better Health with (Mostly) Chinese Herbs and Foods.* New Jersey: AYSL Corporation, 1995.
2. Hirata JD, Swiersz LM, Zell B, et al. Does dong quai have estrogenic effects in postmenopausal women? A double blind, placebo-controlled trial. *Fertility and Sterility* 1997; 68(6): 981–986.
3. Chang HM, But PPH. *Pharmacology and Applications of Chinese Materia Medica.* Vol 1. Hong Kong: World Scientific, 1986.
4. Choy YM, Leung KN, Cho CS, et al. Immunopharmacological studies of low molecular weight polysaccharide from *Angelica sinensis. American Journal of Chinese Medicine* 1994; 22(2): 137–145.
5. Noe JE. *Angelica sinensis:* a monograph. *Journal of Naturopathic Medicine* 1997; 7(1): 66–72.
6. Qi-bing M, Jing-yi T, Bo C. Review article: advances in the pharmacological studies of radix *Angelica sinensis* (oliv) diels (Chinese danggui). *Chinese Medical Journal* 1991; 104(9): 776–781.
7. Tanaka S, Kano Y, Tabata M, et al. Effects of "Toki" (*Angelica acutiloba* Kitagawa) extracts on writhing and capillary permeability in mice (analgesic and antiinflammatory ef-

fects) [in Chinese]. *Yakugaku Zasshi* 1971; 91(10): 1098–1104.

8. Teeguarden R. *Chinese Tonic Herbs.* United States: Kodansha America Inc., distributed by Farrar, Straus & Giroux, 1984.

9. Bensky D, Gamble A, Kaptchuk T. *Chinese Herbal Medicine Materia Medica.* Seattle, WA: Eastland Press, 1986.

10. Johnston A. Dang gui: never use it alone. *Village Herbalist* 1995; 1: 8.

11. Zhu DPQ. Dong quai. *American Journal of Chinese Medicine* 1987; 15(3-4): 117–125.

12. Hsu HY, Chen YP, Shen SJ, et al. *Oriental Materia Medica: A Concise Guide.* Long Beach, CA: Oriental Healing Arts Institute, 1986.

13. Huang KC. *The Pharmacology of Chinese Herbs.* Boca Raton and London: CRC Press, 1999.

14. Yoshihiro K. The physiological actions of tang-kuei and cnidium. *Bulletin of the Oriental Healing Arts Institute* 1985; 10(7): 269–278.

15. McGuffin M, Hobbs C, Upton R, et al., eds. *American Herbal Products Association Botanical Safety Handbook.* Boca Raton, FL: CRC Press, 1997.

16. Tierra M. *The Way of Herbs.* New York: Simon & Schuster, Pocket Books, 1990.

17. Foster S. *101 Medicinal Herbs.* Loveland, CO: Interweave Press, 1998.

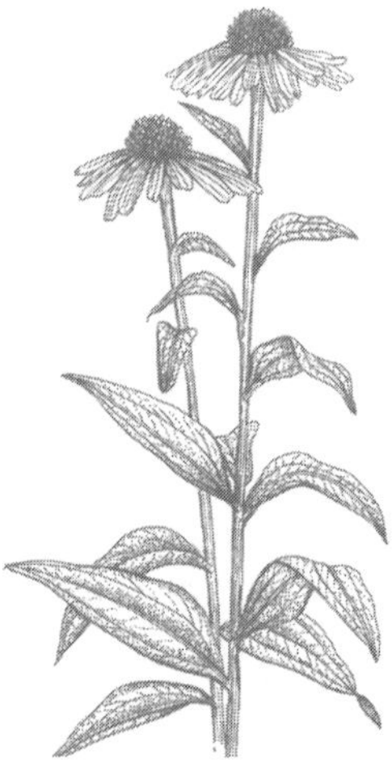

Echinacea

Echinacea spp.
Asteraceae

State of Knowledge: Five-Star Rating System

Clinical (human) research	✶✶✶
Laboratory research	✶✶✶✶
History of use/traditional use	✶✶✶✶
Safety record	✶✶✶✶
International acceptance	✶✶✶

Part Used: *Root, flower, leaf, seed*

Primary Uses

- *Immune system function*
- *Colds and flu*
- *Other minor infections*
- *Wounds, psoriasis, and eczema (external use)*

Echinacea, the purple coneflower, is the most widely used herb for stimulating the function of the immune system. Without a doubt, it is also America's favorite herbal remedy, topping the list of best-selling herbs since 1996. Although echinacea may be a novelty to many modern Americans, its current popularity has historical precedent. Native Americans of the Great Plains region used echinacea more than any other medicinal plant, and during the 1920s, it was the most widely prescribed remedy of the American Eclectic physicians, a group of medical doctors who practiced during the late nineteenth and early twentieth centuries. After the introduction of antibiotics, echinacea was all but forgotten in American medicine, despite the fact that antibiotics are actually ineffective against viral infections, including most colds. Today, however, with concerns about the dangers of antibiotic overuse on the rise, echinacea extracts can once again be found in medicine cabinets across the country.

Millions of Americans and Europeans now use echinacea as their primary therapy for colds, flu, minor infections, and general immune-boosting effects. European physicians prescribe the herb for minor infections and even use it in injectable form for a number of more serious conditions. Topical echinacea preparations are used in the treatment of wounds, burns, eczema, psoriasis, herpes infections, and other skin conditions.

This native North American herb is supported by an impressive record of laboratory and clinical research. According to the evidence, echinacea increases the nonspecific activity of the immune system. In other words, unlike a vaccine, which is active only against a specific disease, echinacea stimulates the overall activity of certain immune cells responsible for fighting infections. Unlike antibiotics, which are directly lethal to disease-causing bacteria, echinacea makes the body's own immune cells more efficient in attacking bacteria, viruses, and abnormal cells.

The best-studied and most widely used species of echinacea are *Echinacea purpurea, E. angustifolia,* and, to a somewhat lesser extent, *E. pallida.* There has been a great deal of speculation and some research aimed at determining which of these species delivers the most potent immune-stimulating effects, but there have been few conclusive results. The research has been complicated by a number of factors, including variations in the types of preparations and plant parts tested and even uncertainty about which

species were actually tested in the studies. Currently, the consensus among experts is that the three species can be used interchangeably. There is no scientific evidence to support the notion that wild *E. angustifolia* is a stronger or otherwise superior remedy to cultivated *E. purpurea.* Researchers found that root and aerial (above-ground) parts of *E. purpurea* and *E. angustifolia* were roughly equivalent in activity *in vitro* (in laboratory studies) and *in vivo* (in the body).

HISTORY

Echinacea has a rich tradition among Native Americans of the Great Midwest Plains region, who used it medicinally more than any other plant. At least 14 different tribes utilized their local echinacea species for conditions ranging from coughs, colds, sore throats, and infections to toothaches, inflammations, wounds, and snakebites. The plant was even used by the Dakotas as a veterinary medicine for horses.

In the late 1800s, settlers to the area learned about echinacea from Native Americans and began to apply it medicinally for many of the same purposes. In 1885, the medicinal virtues of echinacea were brought to the attention of pioneering American pharmacist John Uri Lloyd by a Nebraskan doctor, H.C.F. Meyer, who was marketing a patent medicine called "Meyer's Blood Purifier" that he claimed was effective in the treatment of nearly all disorders. By 1920, echinacea preparations were the most popular remedies sold by Lloyd Brothers Pharmacists, Inc., who produced the line of medicines used by the American Eclectic physicians. The long list of conditions for which the Eclectics prescribed echinacea included abscesses, chronic bronchitis, diabetes, psoriasis and eczema, wounds, cancer, and many infectious diseases such as malaria, syphilis, typhoid pneumonia, chickenpox, and measles. *Echinacea angustifolia* and *E. pallida* were both listed in *The United States Pharmacopoeia* in 1916, where they remained until 1950. Echinacea was introduced to Europe around the turn of the twentieth century, and has been widely studied, used, and grown there since the 1930s.

INTERNATIONAL STATUS

In the *German Commission E Monographs,* the pressed juice of *Echinacea purpurea* herb is recommended as supportive therapy for colds and chronic infections of the respiratory and lower urinary tract. *E. purpurea* is also indicated for external use in the treatment of poorly healing wounds and chronic ulcerations. The Commission E recommends *Echinacea pallida* root as supportive therapy for influenzalike infections. *E. angustifolia* root is approved in the United Kingdom for the treatment of chronic viral and bacterial infections, mild septicemia (blood poisoning), and skin complaints, including boils.

BOTANY

Native to North America, echinacea plants are members of the aster (Asteraceae) family. Most commonly known as coneflower, echinacea is also called by various other local names in different parts of the United States, including snakeroot, red sunflower, Indian head, and black Sampson. Nine species of *Echinacea* grow in North America, all east of the Rocky Mountains. In general, members of the *Echinacea* genus are large, sturdy, drought-tolerant perennials with spectacular daisylike flowerheads. The flowerheads of most species vary in color from purple to white. The common name *coneflower* comes from the distinctive conelike shape of the center portion of the flowerhead (the disk). Before habitat loss and large-scale commercial harvesting reduced their numbers, echinacea plants formed vast colonies throughout the Great Plains region.

Echinacea purpurea, commonly called the purple coneflower, is a familiar garden plant that is well loved for its hardiness and its large, stunning flowerheads, which may grow to 6 inches across and vary in color from deep purplish-pink to white. The natural range of *E. purpurea* extends from Ohio to Iowa and south from Louisiana to Georgia. *E. purpurea* usually stands about 3 feet tall but may reach heights of up to 6 feet. Of the three most popular medicinal *Echinacea* species, *E. purpurea* is the easiest to cultivate and yields more plant material in a shorter period of time.

E. angustifolia, or narrow-leaved coneflower, is a shorter, less rugged plant that grows to heights of about 2 feet. *E. angustifolia* has smaller, usually paler pink flowers than *E. purpurea* and narrow, lance-shaped leaves. The natural range of *E. angustifolia* is from Saskatchewan, Canada, to Minnesota in the United States, and south to Texas and Tennessee.

E. pallida is similar to *E. angustifolia,* but sturdier and slightly taller, reaching heights of 3 feet. As the species name *pallida* suggests, its flowers are paler in color than those of other species. The flowerheads are further distinguished by their long, drooping ray flowers. This species, commonly called the pale coneflower, occurs naturally from the midwestern United States southeast to Louisiana, Alabama, and Georgia. Under cultivation, *E. pallida* produces larger roots than *E. angustifolia.*

There is currently large-scale cultivation of *E. angustifolia* and *E. pallida* in Europe, which began as early as the 1930s. Cultivation of echinacea, particularly *E. purpurea,* is also underway in the United States, Canada, and Germany.

A number of plant conservation organizations have joined forces to raise public awareness and develop workable strategies to protect this treasured American native

An Urgent Need for Conservation

Unfortunately, echinacea's popularity has a dark side. Although *E. purpurea* is not difficult to grow, commercial cultivation has not yet caught up with the huge worldwide demand for the herb. Consequently, much of the world's supply of echinacea is still harvested from wild plant stands in the central United States, and populations are dwindling swiftly. Conservationists, herbalists, and other plant lovers are increasingly alarmed at the rate at which wild echinacea is disappearing from areas of former abundance in Montana, Nebraska, North and South Dakota, Kansas, Oklahoma, and Missouri. Unauthorized collection—in other words, poaching— is taking place on public and private land, tribal lands, and even nature preserves. In the winter 1999 issue of the *United Plant Savers Newsletter,* a Native American woman in North Dakota said of the poaching on her reservation, "They drive through fences, dig holes, don't cover them, and drive off with car trunks full."[1]

plant and its delicate prairie ecosystem (see Herb Conservation Organizations in appendix E). In 1999, representatives and senators from North Dakota passed a bill that makes unauthorized removal or possession of *E. purpurea* or *E. angustifolia* a class A misdemeanor, subject to a penalty of up to $10,000 and confiscation of any vehicle used to transport illegally harvested echinacea. To do your part to protect echinacea, make every effort to avoid products labeled "wildcrafted" or "wild-harvested" and instead seek products from organically cultivated sources.

BENEFITS

- Stimulates phagocytosis
- Increases the number and activity of immune cells
- Shortens the duration of colds and flu
- Aids in the treatment of wounds and other skin problems

SCIENTIFIC SUPPORT

More than 350 scientific studies document the clinical applications, pharmacology, and chemistry of echinacea. The most consistently proven effect of the herb is in stimulating *phagocytosis,* an important function of the immune system. This means that echinacea enhances the activity of the immune system by encouraging white blood cells and other immune cells to attack and destroy invading organisms. Echinacea's ability to stimulate immune function has been demonstrated both in laboratory studies and in human subjects.[2-4]

Most of the research on echinacea has been carried out in Germany. Clinical studies have shown that when taken at the first sign of infection, echinacea shortens the duration of cold and flu symptoms and lessens the likelihood that a minor infection will de-velop into a full-blown cold. Other clinical studies support echinacea's traditional reputation for effectiveness in the treatment of wounds and other skin problems. In a large, uncontrolled clinical study of 4,598 people, an echinacea ointment was 85 percent effective in treating wounds, inflammatory skin conditions, eczema, leg ulcers, burns, and herpes simplex infections.[5] Another study suggests that echinacea may be useful in the treatment of recurrent vaginal yeast infections.[6] A number of compounds in echinacea have shown an ability to protect collagen against the effects of potentially damaging substances known as free radicals, suggesting that echinacea may have value in defending skin against sun damage.[7] Echinacea given by injection has shown some promise in the supportive treatment of colorectal and liver cancers.

However, not all echinacea research has yielded positive results. In some studies, echinacea failed to demonstrate a protective effect against upper respiratory tract infections in study participants. For example, in one American study designed to test the effectiveness of echinacea in preventing respiratory tract infection, *E. purpurea* and *E. angustifolia* root extracts were not significantly more protective than placebo. The 302 study participants took either placebo, *E. purpurea,* or *E. angustifolia* continuously for a period of 12 weeks. The dosage used was 50 drops twice daily. The investigators noted when participants contracted respiratory tract infections, how many infections occurred, and how many participants had side effects. They observed no significant differences among the groups. Nonetheless, people in the echinacea groups felt that they derived more benefit from their treatment than did those in the placebo group.[8]

One difference between this study and other, more positive studies was the manner in which echinacea was used. In the negative study, healthy people took echinacea continuously, as a preventive remedy. In the studies in which echinacea demonstrated positive effects in shortening the duration of colds and flu, participants were instructed to start taking echinacea at the first sign of infection. This use is more consistent with the way in which echinacea has been used traditionally in the treatment of infections.

SPECIFIC STUDIES

Acute Colds: Clinical Study (1997)

In this double-blind, placebo-controlled trial, treatment with a pressed juice preparation of *E. purpurea* at the first sign of infection was effective in shortening the duration of colds. People taking echinacea recovered from their colds twice as fast as those taking placebo. In addition, fewer of those taking echinacea developed a "real" cold with full-blown symptoms. The 120 study participants, randomly divided into two groups, took either 20 drops of the echinacea preparation or placebo in water every 2 hours for the first day, after which they took 20 drops three times daily for up to 10 days. Only 40 percent of those taking echinacea developed a "real" cold, compared with 60 percent in the placebo group. Among the participants who had full-blown cold symptoms, the median time to improvement was 4 days for those taking echinacea, compared with 8 days for placebo. No adverse effects were reported. All of the people enrolled in the study had experienced at least three respiratory infections within the past 6 months.[9]

Acute Colds: Clinical Study (1998)

This double-blind, placebo-controlled study, carried out under the direction of a Swedish infectious disease specialist, showed that *E. purpurea* extract was significantly superior to placebo in reducing cold symptoms. The 119 infection-prone study subjects were randomized to take either placebo or echinacea at the first sign of infection and to continue for up to 8 days. The dosage of echinacea used was 2 tablets three times daily of *E. purpurea* extract consisting of 95 percent aerial (above-ground) parts and 5 percent root. Based on assessment of 12 typical cold symptoms, echinacea was significantly more effective than placebo in reducing symptoms. A similar number of mild adverse effects occurred in the echinacea and placebo groups.[10]

Upper Respiratory Tract Infections: Clinical Study (1997)

In this double-blind study involving 160 people with current upper respiratory tract infections, a liquid alcohol extract of *E. pallida* root was significantly superior to placebo in shortening the duration of illness. In addition, in the echinacea group, lymphocytosis and neutrophil counts—important markers of immune function—returned to normal much more quickly, correlating closely with the symptomatic improvement. The 80 people in the echinacea group took 900 mg (90 drops) of echinacea extract for 8 to 10 days, and the other 80 participants took an identical dose of a placebo preparation. The subjects' frequency of upper respiratory tract infection in the past 3 years had no impact on the effectiveness of treatment with echinacea.[11]

Acute Colds: Clinical Study (1992)

In this double-blind, placebo-controlled study, freshly pressed *E. purpurea* juice was more effective than placebo in preventing colds in 108 people who were highly susceptible to upper respiratory tract infections. Fewer of the people taking echinacea developed colds, and for those who did get sick, the interval of time between colds was longer (40 days for echinacea, as opposed to 25 for placebo). In addition, in 78.6 percent of echinacea recipients who developed colds, the symptoms were less severe. The

dosage of echinacea pressed juice used in this study was 4 ml twice daily. People who had shown evidence of weakened immune system function at the beginning of the study appeared to derive the most benefit from preventive treatment with echinacea.[12]

HOW IT WORKS

The immune system utilizes two basic approaches in defending the body against disease. These can be described simply as *specific* and *nonspecific immune defenses*. These two types of defenses work together to track down and destroy disease-causing invaders, such as bacteria, but each works in a somewhat different way. For a specific immune response, the immune cells must recognize specific invaders in order to destroy them. Immune cells called *lymphocytes* (including B-cells, T-cells, and natural killer cells) are involved in specific immune responses. Vaccines work by stimulating the function of specific immune defenses.

Echinacea, on the other hand, stimulates the nonspecific activity of the immune system. Nonspecific immune defenses do not require the immune cells to recognize invaders. Instead, invaders are destroyed by functions such as fever, release of antiviral proteins called interferons, and phagocytosis, the process by which nonspecific immune cells engulf and destroy disease-causing organisms and abnormal cells. Stimulation of phagocytosis is one of echinacea's best-documented effects. Echinacea increases the number and activity of immune cells called macrophages, granulocytes, and leukocytes, all of which are directly involved in phagocytosis, and stimulates the production of interferon and tumor necrosis factor. In addition, echinacea inhibits the action of an enzyme called *hyaluronidase,* which is produced and used by bacteria to help them gain access to healthy cells. Echinacea's benefits in helping to heal wounds are believed to be related to its ability to stimulate fibroblast production and to hinder the production of hyaluronidase by the human body, two actions which help in wound healing.

No single constituent has been identified as echinacea's "active ingredient." The polysaccharide compounds are believed to play a key role in echinacea's immune-stimulating and anti-inflammatory actions, but a number of other compounds in the plant have also demonstrated effects on immune function. Researchers believe that a combination of constituents work together to produce immune stimulation. Cichoric acid is one compound that all three of the major echinacea species have in common. In laboratory studies, cichoric acid enhanced phagocytosis, inhibited hyaluronidase, and protected collagen from free radical damage.[4] Heteroxylan (a polysaccharide) and alkamides also stimulated phagocytosis. Studies demonstrated that another polysaccharide constituent, arabinogalactan, improved phagocytosis and promoted the release of tumor necrosis factor.[4,13] Echinacin B has been shown to promote tissue granulation in wounds.[14]

Some manufacturers standardize their echinacea preparations to echinacoside, although echinacoside has shown no immune-stimulating activity in studies.[4,13,15] Therefore standardized levels of echinacoside cannot be considered a guarantee of therapeutic potency.[13,15]

MAJOR CONSTITUENTS

Caffeic acid derivatives (including cichoric acid and echinacoside), polysaccharides (including arabinogalactan and heteroxylan), lipophilic compounds (polyacetylenes and alkamides)

SAFETY

Echinacea is considered an extremely safe herb with no known toxicity.

- **Side effects:** None known.[16]
- **Contraindications:** According to Commission E, echinacea should not be used by people who have diseases such as tuberculosis, leukoses, collagenosis, multiple sclerosis, AIDS, HIV infection, and other autoimmune disorders.[16] However, this recommendation has been challenged on the grounds that echinacea's primary

effect is stimulation of phagocytosis, and so would not be expected to exacerbate these diseases. Echinacea has demonstrated no adverse effects in people with any of the conditions listed previously.[17]

- **Drug interactions:**
  None known.[16,18]

DOSAGE

Many clinical studies suggest that echinacea is most effective when used at the first sign of infection, when symptoms first become apparent. Taking repeated small doses throughout the day may be better than taking larger, less frequent doses. The *German Commission E Monographs* recommends that continuous use of echinacea be limited to no longer than 8 weeks.

- **Capsules:** 500 to 1,000 mg three times a day
- **Tincture:** 15 to 30 drops two to five times a day
- **Pressed juice:** 6 to 9 ml a day in divided doses

STANDARDIZATION

Some manufacturers standardize echinacea extract to 4 to 5 percent echinacoside. Some standardize to phenolics, which include cichoric acid.

REFERENCES

1. Crawford, G. Echinacea, prairies, and rural life on fire . . . "help!" A North Dakota report. *United Plant Savers Newsletter* 1999; winter: 20–21.
2. Jurcic K, Melchart D, Holzmann M, et al. Two proband studies for the stimulation of granulocyte phagocytosis through *Echinacea* extract-containing preparations [in German]. *Zeitschrift für Phytotherapie* 1989; 10: 67–70.
3. Bräunig B, Dorn M, Limburg E, et al. *Echinacea purpureae* radix for strengthening the immune response in flu-like infections [in German]. *Zeitschrift für Phytotherapie* 1992; 13: 7–13.
4. Bauer R. Echinacea: biological effects and active principles. In: Lawson LD, Bauer R, eds. *Phytomedicines of Europe*. Washington, DC: American Chemical Society, 1998: 141–157.
5. Viehmann VP. Experiences with a skin salve containing echinacea [in German]. *Erfahrungsheilk* 1978; 27: 353–358.
6. Coeugniet E, Kühnast R. Relapsing candidiasis: adjuvant immune therapy with different Echinacin® dosage forms [in German]. *Therapiewoche* 1986; 36: 3352–3358.
7. Facino RM, Carini M, Aldini G, et al. Echinacoside and caffeoyl conjugates protect collagen from free radical-induced degradation: a potential use of *Echinacea* extracts

in the prevention of skin photodamage. *Planta Medica* 1995; 61(6): 510–514.

8. Melchart D, Walther E, Linde K, et al. Echinacea root extracts for the prevention of upper respiratory tract infections. *Archives of Family Medicine* 1998; 7: 541–545.

9. Hoheisel O, Sandberg M, Bertram S, et al. Echinagard treatment shortens the course of the common cold: a double-blind, placebo-controlled trial. *European Journal of Clinical Research* 1997; 9: 261–268.

10. Brinkeborn R, Shah D, Geissbühler S, et al. Echinaforce® in the treatment of acute colds [in German]. *Schweizer Zeitschrift Ganzheits Medizin* 1998; 10: 26–29.

11. Dorn M, Knick E, Lewith G. Placebo-controlled, double-blind study of *Echinaceae pallidae radix* in upper respiratory tract infections. *Complementary Therapies in Medicine* 1997; 5(1): 40–42.

12. Schöneberger D. The influence of immune-stimulating effects of pressed juice from *Echinacea purpurea* on the course and sever-

ity of colds [in German]. *Forum Immunologie* 1992; 8: 2–12.

13. Bone K. Echinacea: what makes it work? *MediHerb* 1997; 3(2): 19–23.

14. Bauer R. Echinacea drugs—effects and active ingredients [in German]. *Zeitschrift für ärztliche Fortbildung (Jena)* 1996; 90(2): 111–115.

15. Foster S, Tyler V. *Tyler's Honest Herbal,* 4th ed. New York and London: The Haworth Herbal Press, 1999.

16. Blumenthal M, Busse W, Goldberg A, et al., eds. *The Complete German Commission E Monographs.* Austin, TX: The American Botanical Council; Boston: Integrative Medical Communications, 1998.

17. Bone K. Echinacea: when should it be used? *European Journal of Herbal Medicine* 1998; 3(3): 13–17.

18. McGuffin M, Hobbs C, Upton R, et al., eds. *American Herbal Products Association Botanical Safety Handbook.* Boca Raton, FL: CRC Press, 1997.

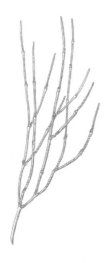

Ephedra

EPHEDRA SPP.
EPHEDRACEAE

State of Knowledge: Five-Star Rating System

Clinical (human) research	★★
Laboratory research	★★★
History of use/traditional use	★★★★
Safety record	★★
International acceptance	★★

PART USED: *Stem, branches*

PRIMARY USES

- *Mild to moderate asthma*
- *Allergies and hay fever*
- *Weight loss (in certain cases)*

The controversy surrounding ephedra is enough to raise almost anyone's blood pressure. After 5,000 years of safe use in China, the sale of ephedra is currently threatened in Texas and at least nine other American states. How did a revered Chinese herb acquire such notoriety? Much of the problem stems from irresponsible marketing of recreational ephedra products as a means for achieving euphoria, "cosmic consciousness," and better sex. These products, such as Herbal Ecstasy, Ultimate Xphoria, Cloud Nine, and many others, combine large amounts of ephedra with caffeine into what many consider a prescription for potentially serious side effects, including high blood pressure, heart rate irregularities, insomnia, nausea and vomiting, and even heart attacks and strokes.

In the United States, ephedra is also commonly used for weight loss, another practice that seems a world away from traditional Asian application. Scientific research does show that ephedra may play a role in weight loss when taken over short periods—if sluggish metabolism is the cause of excess weight. However, many people are relying on ephedra as a magic pill, without incorporating essential lifestyle changes such as healthy diet and exercise. Others may be taking too much ephedra for too long, leading to weakened adrenal glands and other side effects.

Traditionally, ephedra has been used for respiratory problems such as asthma and hay fever. To avoid serious side effects, Chinese doctors prescribe whole-plant ephedra in combination with other herbs according to a person's constitution. In the West, over-the-counter (OTC) medicines for sinusitis, nasal congestion, and asthma contain the isolated ephedra constituents ephedrine and pseudoephedrine (usually in synthetic form), which may increase the risk of side effects.

Wise modern use of ephedra requires respect for the plant's power as well as an understanding of how it has been safely used in traditional medicine. It is possible to find herbal allergy formulas in health-food stores that contain ephedra in whole-plant form. If you're thinking about trying ephedra for any reason, it is a good idea to visit a health-care practitioner to find out how to do it safely and effectively.

HISTORY

Ephedra is the botanical name for a plant traditionally called *ma huang,* meaning "yellow astringent" in Chinese. Considered a warming and stimulating "yang" herb, ephedra disperses cold and strengthens the lung "chi" (vital energy). It has been used for respiratory problems such as bronchial asthma, coughing, wheezing, rhinitis, hay fever, and emphysema since 220 B.C. According to Chinese medicine, ephedra diverts energy from the inside of the body to the surface. For this reason, in traditional medicine it is not given to people with weak constitutions and is always combined with other herbs that help counteract negative effects. Because it encourages sweating, ephedra is also taken for colds, fevers, and malaria. A less familiar use is for rheumatoid arthritis, which may respond to ephedra's circulation-stimulating activity. The plant has also been used for epilepsy and certain types of headaches.

In North America, Native Americans used several milder indigenous ephedra species. They took ephedra to treat colds, headaches, urinary system problems, enterorrhagia (bleeding in the intestinal tract), and sexually transmitted diseases. When the early American pioneers adopted ephedra, the plant became so well known for treating syphilis that one species was dubbed *Ephedra antisyphilitica.* Later, when the Mormon leader Brigham Young toasted the new state of Utah with a cup of American ephedra tea, the plant acquired the more pious name "Mormon tea." The early Eclectic physicians used ephedra for colds, kidney disorders, and as a treatment for asthma, in combination with expectorant herbs such as licorice *(Glycyrrhiza glabra)* and grindelia *(Grindelia* spp.).

Ephedra was the first Chinese herb from which researchers produced an active constituent that is now widely used in Western medicine. In 1923, a Chinese researcher teamed up with a German pharmacologist, leading to the first isolation of the alkaloids ephedrine and pseudoephedrine by the German company Merck. By the 1930s, these constituents had been incorporated into a variety of OTC cold and allergy medicines.

INTERNATIONAL STATUS

Ephedra is approved by Germany's Commission E for respiratory problems with mild bronchospasm. It is an official medicine in China and other Asian countries.

BOTANY

One of the world's oldest plants, ephedra is a distant relative of two other ancient and well-known medicinal plants—ginkgo and horsetail. The most popular commercial species, *Ephedra sinica* and *E. equisetina,* are from China; *E. gerardiana* comes from India. Other species thrive in the warmer regions of South America, Pakistan, Tibet, and the Mediterranean. The American deserts are home to nine species and two hybrids, including *Ephedra americana* (American ephedra), *E. nevadensis* (Mormon tea), and *E. viridis* (desert tea).

The Greek word *ephedra* means "climbing," which describes the plant's affinity for climbing across dry, rocky soil. Ephedra shrubs grow 1 to 4 feet tall, branching out into many-jointed limbs. At each joint or node there are two to three dry, scalelike leaves. During June or July, the plant is covered with small white flowers that turn into red fruits, and later into two-seeded cones. As the perennial plants age, their color changes from green to yellowish-brown and the alkaloid level declines. Ephedra is traditionally harvested before the first frost because the alkaloid content is highest in the summer and fall. In general, *Ephedra sinica* tends to contain the highest amount of ephedrine, whereas Mormon tea *(E. nevadensis)* contains little or none. Ephedra's strong pinelike fragrance and astringent, bitter taste is not a favorite with hungry wildlife.

BENEFITS

- Helpful in acute allergy flare-ups and mild asthma attacks
- Helpful for raising the metabolic rate and aiding weight loss in certain individuals
- Useful as a short-term approach while one is exploring holistic, long-term solutions to respiratory or weight problems

The Highs and Lows of Ephedra Regulation in the United States

On June 4, 1997, the Food and Drug Administration (FDA) proposed banning products such as Herbal Ecstasy and Cloud Nine, which are marketed as "herbal alternatives" to illegal street drugs—a move that won wholehearted support from responsible members of the supplement industry. However, the FDA's other recommendations on ephedra remain more controversial. Currently, the government agency allows the open sale of 24-mg tablets of ephedrine for asthma, for use up to four times daily. The FDA is now proposing a maximum single dosage of 8 mg total ephedrine alkaloids, a maximum daily dosage of 24 mg, and a 7-day limit for legal use. If approved, this guideline would eliminate all ephedra products used for longer periods of time, including weight loss and athletic performance formulas. The FDA would not allow any ephedra product to contain caffeine or caffeine-containing herbs such as kola nut (*Cola* spp.) or guarana *(Paullinia cupana)*.

Supplement proponents are justified in asking for consistency in these regulations. Ephedra's benefit in serious health conditions such as asthma often outweighs the risks, when used judiciously. This may also be true in cases of severe obesity. However, use of ephedra by athletes is not appropriate and could lead to serious consequences, such as high blood pressure, heart-rate irregularities, and even heart attack and stroke.

In June 1998, an ephedra safety study began at Beth Israel–Deaconess Medical Center in Boston and St. Luke's–Roosevelt Hospital in New York. Researchers are monitoring changes in blood pressure, heart rate, and arrhythmia (irregular heart beat) in 150 mildly to severely overweight people taking a combination of ephedra alkaloids and caffeine. The study is sponsored by the Ephedra Research Foundation, a group of concerned members of the supplement industry. They have requested that the FDA wait to finalize rules on ephedra until these study results are complete.

SCIENTIFIC SUPPORT

All of the clinical studies on the isolated constituent ephedrine have focused on weight loss, with little research into respiratory problems such as asthma. Ephedrine may stimulate weight loss in certain overweight people, namely, those who have a physiological problem that impairs their ability to burn fat. It appears to be ineffective in more general cases of excess weight, as illustrated by the first study in the Specific Studies section. Unfortunately, no scientific studies have tested ephedra's long-term safety. In addition, the studies use an isolated or synthetic constituent from ephedra rather than the whole plant, and no study has tested ephedra in combination with herbs that could lessen its common side effects.

It is interesting to note that clinical studies combine ephedrine with a low-calorie diet, but none considers the effects of exercise. Ironically, the participants in several studies are described as "sedentary." In the search for a magic weight loss pill, it's easy to forget that exercise has a scientifically proven effect on stimulating metabolism. By now, it is a well-known fact that extremely low-calorie diets ultimately fail because they push the body into "survival" mode, actually lowering the metabolic rate. A 1997 study in the *American Journal of Physiology* found that exercise effectively reverses the well-known drop in metabolism that accompanies low-calorie dieting. Researchers found that 45 minutes of exercise three times a week stabilized the dieters' ability to burn fat and their overall metabolic rates, compared with the group who dieted without exercising.[1] Exercise may stimulate metabolism as effectively or better than ephedra, without causing negative side effects. Physical activity may also be more appropriate for dieters than ephedra in terms of mood. For example, one study linked exercise to improvements in depression associated with low-calorie dieting. In this study, those who cut calories without exercising experienced no improvements in mood.[2] On the other hand, using ephedra may actually worsen a dieter's mood because ephedra stimulates adrenaline secretion, which can lead to a "stressed-out" syndrome that eventually weakens adrenal gland function. Exercise actually helps counteract excessive adrenaline production, making it a better choice than ephedra for most dieters.[3] Regular

physical activity also has an advantage over ephedra in reducing the likelihood of developing hypertension and diabetes, both of which are more common in overweight people. Although ephedra may be of short-term help for certain people, it is no substitute for exercise, nutrition, and a positive self-image.

SPECIFIC STUDIES

Weight Loss: Clinical Study (1985)

Researchers found that ephedrine had no advantage over placebo in stimulating weight loss in a double-blind, placebo-controlled study of 46 obese people. They concluded that ephedrine is not effective in "unselected simple obesity," the type of obesity that is not linked to sluggish metabolism. During the 3-month study, the participants took either 25 or 50 mg of ephedrine three times daily or placebo. All subjects followed a low-calorie diet consisting of 1,000 calories a day for women and 1,200 calories a day for men. Those in the group taking 150 mg of ephedrine daily had significantly more side effects than the lower-dose ephedrine and placebo groups, although the symptoms tended to disappear after 3 months of treatment. Side effects included agitation, insomnia, headache, weakness, heart palpitations, giddiness, euphoria, tremors, and constipation. Despite ephedrine's tendency to raise blood pressure, blood pressure actually decreased in all three groups in this study, probably due to the low-calorie diet.[4]

Weight Loss: Clinical Study (1987)

In a very small study, researchers found that the synthetic constituent ephedrine hydrochloride (50 mg three times daily) led to a statistically significant decrease in weight in five people with low basal metabolic rates, compared with five people taking placebo. All of the study participants, with the exception of one woman, were sedentary and all had failed to lose weight with previous diets. Participants followed a strict dieting regimen (1,000 to 1,400 calories a day) and took either placebo or ephedrine for 2 months before crossing over to the opposite treatment group. Those in the ephedrine group reported mild side effects such as agitation, insomnia, heart palpitations, and giddiness.[5]

HOW IT WORKS

Whole Plant Versus Isolated Constituents

When ephedra is taken in its whole-plant form, the powerful alkaloids are absorbed more slowly and have more long-lasting effects than the isolated constituents.[6] In addition, whole plant formulas contain both of the two major alkaloids, ephedrine and pseudoephedrine, which have opposite effects on the body that help balance each other. Whereas ephedrine raises the heart rate and the blood pressure, pseudoephedrine actually lowers them. The rich tannin content of the whole plant also helps prevent constriction in blood vessels (which can lead to high blood pressure) by inhibiting angiotensin II production. Although pseudoephedrine has bronchodilating effects, it is much less stimulating to the nervous system than ephedrine, which helps lessen the plant's impact on the adrenal glands.[7]

All of this suggests that whole ephedra may have fewer side effects than its isolated constituents.

Effects on the Respiratory System

In the early 1900s, doctors gave fairly toxic adrenaline injections to people suffering from asthma attacks. Although ephedrine is similar to adrenaline in action, it is far safer, can be given orally, and has a much longer effect. Ephedrine makes breathing easier by dilating the bronchioles (small air-conveying tubes in the lungs). Although the effects are milder than those of adrenaline, they are relatively long-lasting; the peak effects occur within 1 hour and generally last for 6 hours. Ephedrine relaxes smooth muscle and is especially effective when there are spasms in the lungs.[8]

Laboratory studies show that ephedrine and pseudoephedrine also help counteract inflammation and edema (swelling), two symptoms commonly involved in asthma.

By interfering with the body's production of the PGE$_2$ series of prostaglandins, the two plant constituents inhibit the early stages of inflammation.[7] Ephedrine and pseudoephedrine prevent edema caused by substances such as histamine, serotonin, bradykin, and prostaglandin E$_1$ (PGE$_1$). The constituent pseudoephedrine also reduces edema by dilating the blood vessels of the kidneys and stimulating the flow of urine.[8]

Stimulating Effects

Ephedra's stimulant activity is often compared with that of amphetamines, though it is only one-fifth as strong.[9] The constituent ephedrine stimulates the release of noradrenaline from the sympathetic nervous system, forcing more blood to the brain and limbs.[8,10]

Unfortunately, the same constituents that stimulate the body and relieve congestion and bronchoconstriction also cause negative side effects. Ephedrine causes constriction in the veins, which raises blood pressure. The systolic blood pressure is usually elevated more than the diastolic pressure. Ephedrine also increases cardiac output and heart rate for up to 10 times longer than adrenaline.[7] A recent clinical study showed that ma-haung (ephedra) capsules caused a significant rise in heart rate in at least half of subjects, while the effects on blood pressure were more variable, depending on the individual.[11] As blood flow increases to the heart, brain, and muscle, the blood flow to the kidneys and intestines is compromised, an effect that can interfere with digestion.[7]

Weight Loss

Clinical studies show that ephedrine increases the metabolic rate by stimulating the release of noradrenaline from the sympathetic nervous system.[10] Whereas thin people experience up to a 40 percent increase in thermogenesis (heat production) after eating a meal, overweight individuals may only have an increase of 10 percent or less. This means more food is stored as fat rather than converted to energy (heat). People taking ephedrine have experienced a 10 percent increase in thermogenesis compared with control groups.[12] Researchers now believe that ephedrine increases thermogenesis primarily in skeletal muscle rather than in brown adipose (fat) tissue.[10] Ephedrine may also help suppress the appetite because blood is diverted away from the digestive tract to the limbs.[13]

Note: Although some research suggests that ephedra's effects on metabolism are heightened by combining it with caffeine or aspirin, these combinations could have serious long-term side effects and are not recommended.

MAJOR CONSTITUENTS

Alkaloids (ephedrine and pseudoephedrine)

SAFETY

Ephedra should not be used in excessive doses or for a long period of time. Many restrictions on its use apply.[14,15]

• **Side effects:** High blood pressure, heart-rate irregularities, insomnia, irritability, tremors, epigastric pain, glaucoma, nausea and vomiting, headaches, urinary disturbances, overall weakness, heavy sweating that may ultimately weaken the body, and possible dependence when used in larger amounts. More serious reactions include seizures, heart attacks, and strokes.[15]

• **Contraindications:** Ephedra should not be taken during states of anxiety and restlessness, or if you have high blood pressure, glaucoma, impaired circulation to the brain, problems of the prostate or urinary tract (such as benign prostatic hyperplasia), thrombosis or other clotting disorders, digestive problems, anorexia or bulimia, food allergies, chronic constipation or diarrhea, gastric ulcer, colitis, insomnia, cardiac asthma, thyroid disease, or diabetes. Ephedra is not appropriate for pregnant or nursing women. It should not be used by children younger than 6 years.[14,15]

• **Drug interactions:** Do not combine ephedra with cardiac glycosides or halothane, guanethidine, monoamine oxidase (MAO) inhibitors, or secale alkaloid derivatives/oxytocin. Ephedra may not be appropriate for use with St. John's wort in weight loss formulas, because the combination may compound the herbs' effects.[9]

Note: Preliminary evidence suggests that ephedra root, a part of the plant not normally used by Westerners, may actually counteract some of the common side effects of ephedra. The root does not contain any of the powerful alkaloids found in the stems, and may help lower blood pressure due to its content of ephedradine and other constituents. Unlike ephedra stems, the root of the plant is used to stop rather than to stimulate profuse sweating.[7,8,16] This may be of interest to manufacturers in search of a more balanced ephedra formulation.

DOSAGE

Because of the wide range of individual reactions to ephedra, consult a nutritionally aware health practitioner before using the plant. In order to avoid side effects, ephedra should be used in appropriate situations, in small amounts, and for short periods of time. Take ephedra on an empty stomach to avoid indigestion.

The active constituents (alkaloids) are readily absorbed by the body in tincture, capsule, tablet, or tea form. However, it is very difficult to estimate the total amount of alkaloids contained in a dose of an unstandardized ephedra product. For this reason, standardized ephedra products that disclose the amount of alkaloids per dose may be preferable, in order to stay within recommended levels.

- **Standardized extract:** 12 to 25 mg total alkaloids (calculated as ephedrine) two to three times a day
- **Capsules/tablets:** 500 to 1,000 mg of ephedra, two to three times a day[17] (This dosage is based on the crude herb, rather than a standardized preparation.)
- **Tincture:** 15 to 30 drops in water, up to three times a day[18]

STANDARDIZATION

Standardized ephedra formulations generally contain 6 percent ephedrine and pseudoephedrine.

REFERENCES

1. Nicklas BJ, Rogus EM, Goldberg AP. Exercise blunts declines in lipolysis and fat oxidation after dietary-induced weight loss in obese older women. *American Journal of Physiology* 1997; 273: E149–E155.
2. Koeppl PM, Heller J, Bleeker ER, et al. The influence of weight reduction and exercise regimes upon the personality profiles of overweight males. *Journal of Clinical Psychology* 1992; 48(4): 463–471.
3. Horowitz S. Using the body to heal the body: exercise and disease intervention. *Alternative and Complementary Therapies* June 1998: 169–172.
4. Pasquali R, Baraldi G, Cesari MP, et al. A controlled trial using ephedrine in the treatment of obesity. *International Journal of Obesity* 1985; 9: 93–98.
5. Pasquali R, Cesari MP, Melchionda N, et al. Does ephedrine promote weight loss in low-energy-adapted obese women? *International Journal of Obesity* 1987; 11: 163–168.
6. Harada M, Nishimura M. Contribution of alkaloid fraction to pressor and hyperglycemic effect of crude *Ephedra* extract in dogs. *Journal of Pharmacobiodynamics* 1981; 4(9): 691–699.
7. Robson T. *Ephedra sinica* et spp. *Australian Journal of Medical Herbalism* 1993; 7(3): 64–68.
8. Bensky D, Gamble A, Kaptchuk T, trans. *Chinese Herbal Medicine Materia Medica.* Seattle, WA: Eastland Press, 1986: 32–34; 562–563.
9. Bergner P. FDA warns against drug promotion of "herbal fen-phen." *Medical Herbalism* 1997; 9(3): 20.
10. Liu YL, Toubro S, Astrup A, et al. Contribution of ß3-adrenoceptor activation to ephedrine-induced thermogenesis in humans. *International Journal of Obesity* 1995; 19: 678–685.
11. White LM, Gardner SF, Gurley BJ, et al. Pharmacokinetics and cardiovascular effects of ma-huang (*Ephedra sinica*) in normotensive adults. *Journal of Clinical Pharmacology* 1997; 37: 116–122.

12. Astrup A, Madsen J, Holst JJ, et al. The effect of chronic ephedrine treatment on substrate utilization, the sympathoadrenal activity, and energy expenditure during glucose-induced thermogenesis in man. *Metabolism* 1986; 35(3): 260–265.

13. Pedersen M. *Nutritional Herbology: A Reference Guide to Herbs.* Warsaw, IN: Wendell W. Whitman Company, 1994.

14. McGuffin M, Hobbs C, Upton R, Goldberg A, eds. *American Herbal Products Association Botanical Safety Handbook.* Boca Raton and New York: CRC Press LLC, 1997.

15. Blumenthal M, Busse W, Goldberg A, eds. *The Complete German Commission E Monographs.* Austin, TX: American Botanical Council; Boston: Integrative Medical Communications, 1998.

16. Pizzorno JE, Murray MT. *A Textbook of Natural Medicine.* Seattle, WA: Bastyr College Publications, 1993.

17. Werbach MR, Murray MT. *Botanical Influences on Illness: A sourcebook of clinical research.* Tarzana, CA: Third Line Press, 1994.

18. Foster S. *101 Medicinal Herbs.* Loveland, CO: Interweave Press, 1998.

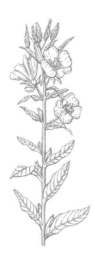

Evening Primrose

OENOTHERA BIENNIS
ONAGRACEAE

State of Knowledge: Five-Star Rating System

Clinical (human) research	✳✳
Laboratory research	✳✳
History of use/traditional use	✳
Safety record	✳✳
International acceptance	✳✳

PART USED: *Seed*

PRIMARY USES

- *Diabetic neuropathy (nerve damage) (experimental)*
- *Breast pain or tenderness (experimental)*
- *Chronic eczema (experimental)*
- *Premenstrual syndrome (experimental)*

Over the past decade, evening primrose oil (EPO) has become one of the most popular supplements on the American and European markets. Although often promoted as a virtual cure-all for a myriad of health conditions, it may actually have just a few specific uses. Research suggests that evening primrose oil may be especially valuable for treating diabetic neuropathy (nerve damage), eczema, and breast pain or tenderness. It may also be useful for some women with premenstrual syndrome (PMS), although research is still inconclusive.

Evening primrose oil is a rich source of omega-6 essential fatty acids (EFAs), which are also widely found in vegetable oils, nuts, and seeds. Essential fatty acids are "essential" to good health because they help reduce inflammation and ensure the health of cell membranes. EFAs must be consumed as part of the diet because our bodies cannot manufacture them.

What makes EPO different from vegetable oils such as safflower or olive oil? Evening primrose oil offers an added benefit: a direct, easily absorbed source of gamma-linolenic acid (GLA), a fairly unusual constituent present in only a few plants that serves as a building block for anti-inflammatory prostaglandins (hormone-like compounds). Most evening primrose supplements are composed of 7 to 10 percent GLA.[1] Oils from the seeds of black currant *(Ribes nigrum)* and borage *(Borago officinalis)* generally provide higher amounts of GLA at a lower cost, although scientific research is lacking on these two plants. Black currant oil contains 14 to 19 percent GLA, and borage seed between 20 and 26 percent GLA.[1,2]

Despite all the enthusiasm about GLA, evening primrose oil is probably not a necessary supplement for everyone. Healthy bodies easily convert omega-6 EFAs in nuts, seeds, and vegetable oils into GLA. Supplementation with evening primrose oil may be necessary only when this conversion process becomes impaired due to disease, as in the case of diabetes. Preliminary clinical research shows that EPO supplementation can significantly improve symptoms of nerve damage caused by diabetes (technically known as *diabetic neuropathy*). This could be a remarkable breakthrough for the estimated one-third of people with diabetes who are affected by this complication, which may lead to serious nerve problems in the arms and legs. Researchers do not yet know how many other health conditions may be related to impaired metabolism of GLA.

Evening Primrose Oil: The Inflammatory Debate

Some researchers are concerned that taking evening primrose oil may actually cause *increased* inflammation in the body over time. A certain amount of EPO is broken down in the body into arachidonic acid (AA), an inflammatory fatty acid commonly found in meat and dairy products. Evening primrose oil is also very rich in omega-6 fatty acids. Although necessary to good health, omega-6 oils are already abundant—perhaps even too abundant—in most people's diets. Excessive intake makes it difficult for our bodies to metabolize the more rare omega-3 oils, found mainly in flaxseed and cold-water fish. Researchers on this side of the debate believe that flax oil is a more important supplement than EPO for the majority of Americans. It is also important to achieve the right balance between omega-6 and omega-3 oils. The ideal ratio is 4 times as much omega-6 as omega-3, although most of us are currently getting 20 times more omega-6 than omega-3![1]

Other scientists maintain that evening primrose oil poses no health concerns when taken in moderation for specific conditions. Dr. David Horrobin, a leading EPO researcher, states that humans (unlike most animals) have the unique ability to convert much of this harmful AA into an anti-inflammatory substance called *prostacyclin,* so the potential for increased inflammation may not be an issue.[3] It may be years before scientists fully understand the complex role of fats in the body and the optimal balance of different types of fatty acids. For more information, see "Flax."

HISTORY

Evening primrose is native to North America and was important to many Native American tribes as a food and medicine. In Utah and Nevada, indigenous peoples consumed the seeds and young leaves of evening primrose as a food. Different parts of the plant were used medicinally by other groups. The Cherokee brewed a tea made from evening primrose flowers and leaves as a weight loss aid. The Ojibwa applied the whole plant externally to reduce the swelling and inflammation associated with bruises. The root was also taken internally for coughs and hemorrhoids, and applied externally in the belief that it helped build muscles.

Native Americans taught the early European settlers to apply evening primrose leaves to wounds. During the seventeenth century, settlers introduced the plant to England, where it became a common plant in backyard gardens. The Shakers later used a tea made from the seeds for soothing stomachaches and coating sore throats. Evening primrose roots were also boiled and eaten for their nutty flavor, and the seeds were used in breads as a substitute for poppy seeds. The use of evening primrose oil is a more modern development; its cultivation is now a huge industry.

INTERNATIONAL STATUS

Evening primrose oil is approved for the treatment of atopic eczema (a hereditary, allergy-based skin disease) in Germany, Denmark, Ireland, Spain, Greece, South Africa, Australia, and New Zealand. In the United Kingdom, it is approved for atopic eczema, as well as for PMS-related mastalgia (breast pain) and breast pain not associated with the menstrual cycle. The Canadian government permits the use of EPO for treating essential fatty acid deficiencies.

BOTANY

Evening primrose opens its beautiful, bright yellow flowers each day at dusk during its flowering season between June and October. Another common name for the plant is "evening star" because the lovely blossoms open after dark and close before sunrise. Evening primrose reaches heights of up to 8 feet tall, producing numerous four-petaled flowers during its second year of growth. It is a member of the evening primrose family (Onagraceae), which also includes fireweed and fuchsia. The name "primrose" is somewhat misleading because the plant is unrelated to true primroses, which belong to the Primulaceae family.

Native to North America, evening primrose is found growing like a weed in backyards, fields, waste places, and on roadsides throughout the United States. The plant can also be found in western Europe, Africa, China, Australia, and many other parts of the world. Even in arid and semiarid regions, evening primrose thrives and flowers voluptuously with minimal watering.

Evening primrose oil is derived from the fruit of the plant, which contains a multitude of seeds. It takes as many as 5,000 of these tiny seeds to produce just one capsule of oil. During the manufacturing process, the seeds are cleaned and cracked to expose the oil. Solvents, such as hexane, are applied before pressing the seeds, in order to extract the oil quickly and inexpensively. The oil is then separated from the solvent and encapsulated.

Today, most commercially grown evening primrose comes from Canada and the United States. Most of the large commercial farms are also equipped with processing facilities to ensure fast processing and an optimal final product. Growers cross-breed evening primrose to guarantee a product that is consistently high in GLA.

BENEFITS

- Improves some cases of diabetic neuropathy by providing a direct source of GLA, which increases nerve impulse transmission and the flow of blood and oxygen
- May help relieve breast pain by reducing the sensitivity of breast cells to estrogen
- May help relieve chronic eczema in children and adults by reducing inflammatory prostaglandins and the dilation of capillaries in the skin
- May be helpful for cases of PMS associated with abnormal essential fatty acid profiles

SCIENTIFIC SUPPORT

Researchers have built the strongest case for using evening primrose oil for diabetic neuropathy, a long-term complication of diabetes that causes nerve damage in the arms, legs, hands, and feet. At least one-third of people with either type I (insulin-dependent) or type II diabetes (non-insulin-dependent, or diabetes mellitus) eventually develop symptoms of nerve damage.[4] To date, all drugs tested for treating this condition have been rejected due to serious side effects. Preliminary evidence suggests that evening primrose oil may be a promising alternative treatment. Two randomized, double-blind, placebo-controlled studies demonstrated a significant reduction in numbness, pain, weakness, burning sensations, abnormal sensations of heat and cold, neurological symptoms (as measured by sensory examination of pinprick touch and vibrations), and nerve conduction after treatment with EPO. Results were most impressive in people with diabetes who had better blood sugar control.[5,6]

Mastalgia (breast pain) is another area in which EPO shows promise. In one study, use of EPO as a primary treatment led to positive results in 58 percent of women with breast pain related to the menstrual cycle, and in 38 percent of those with noncyclical pain.[7] A larger double-blind, placebo-controlled study of 291 women with severe breast pain found EPO to be just as effective as the drug bromocriptine in relieving cyclical breast pain, without the serious side effects of drug therapy.[8]

Some researchers are also enthusiastic about EPO's potential to relieve allergic eczema in children and adults. An analysis of nine placebo-controlled studies showed statistically significant reductions in many symptoms of eczema, particularly itching.[9] Researchers noted improvements in skin redness, surface damage, capillary dilation, watery skin secretions, and in some cases, thickening of the skin. Treatment with EPO

has even enabled some individuals to decrease their use of antihistamines or topical steroids.[10,11] It is not known how many people with eczema experience a relapse following EPO treatment.

One of the most popular uses of evening primrose oil is for the treatment of PMS. Unfortunately, the results of studies in this area have been inconclusive. A research group recently conducted a literature search of clinical trials that used EPO for PMS, with the intention of performing a meta-analysis of the results. As it turned out, only five studies were properly designed, and the two best-controlled studies were negative ones, making a meta-analysis inappropriate.[2] Dr. P. O'Brien, a leading researcher on evening primrose, believes that PMS may be related to abnormal essential fatty acid profiles in some women. He suggests that future research in this area should include only women diagnosed with EFA imbalances. This would ensure that study results are not skewed by negative responses in women with PMS who have normal fatty acid metabolism.[12]

More than 75 other clinical studies have been conducted using evening primrose for a wide variety of health conditions, including rheumatoid arthritis, multiple sclerosis, ulcerative colitis, breast cysts, attention deficit disorder (ADD), dyslexia, and Crohn's disease. For the most part, this research has either been contradictory or is still in very early stages. In some cases, treatment with omega-3 oils from flax may be more appropriate.[1]

SPECIFIC STUDIES

Diabetic Neuropathy: Clinical Study (1993)

Treatment with evening primrose oil led to a statistically significant improvement in symptoms of mild diabetic neuropathy in a randomized, double-blind, placebo-controlled study of 84 patients. All subjects had diabetes mellitus and exhibited clinical evidence of neuropathy in their limbs. Symptoms included numbness, weakness, impaired reflexes, pain, tingling, or burning sensations. Over the course of 1 year, subjects took either 12 capsules of EPO (480 mg of GLA total) daily or placebo. They were evaluated after 3, 6, and 12 months of treatment. To assess the effectiveness of EPO, the researchers used neurological exams that tested muscle strength, tendon reflexes, sensation, heat and cold thresholds, and other parameters in the arms, legs, hands, and feet. Results showed that for all 16 neurological or neurophysical parameters measured, people in the EPO group experienced greater positive changes than those in the placebo group. For 13 of these parameters, the improvements were statistically significant. Four people in the EPO group and six in the placebo group reported minor side effects, including nausea or vomiting.[6]

Adult Atopic Eczema: Clinical Study (1994)

In a double-blind, placebo-controlled study of 52 adults with moderately severe eczema, evening primrose oil was significantly more effective than placebo in reducing surface skin damage and redness. Participants were divided into three groups and treated for 16 weeks. Group A included women who experienced a premenstrual exacerbation of eczema symptoms, Group B included women without exacerbation, and Group C was made up of men. Subjects took either 12 capsules of EPO (500 mg each) daily or placebo. All patients continued treatment with their usual topical steroids during the study. Researchers examined subjects five to six times during treatment, measuring the severity of surface skin damage, skin redness related to capillary dilation (erythema), and skin thickening (lichenification) on a scale of 0 to 3. Participants kept diaries in which they recorded subjective changes in their symptoms.

Results of the study showed statistically significant reductions in skin redness and surface damage, but not thickening of the skin, compared with placebo. There was no change in the amount of topical steroids used in the active treatment or placebo groups (researchers gave no further details on this issue). Women who reported a premenstrual exacerbation of eczema symptoms experienced a greater, but not statistically significant, decrease in their symptoms. Two individuals taking EPO and one taking placebo reported minor diarrhea and/or abdominal colic.[11]

HOW IT WORKS

Evening primrose oil contains a direct source of gamma-linolenic acid (GLA), an omega-6 essential fatty acid. Our bodies break GLA down into dihomogammalinolenic acid (DGLA) and ultimately into beneficial prostaglandins (PGE1) that help decrease inflammation, dilate blood vessels, and prevent abnormal blood clotting.[3]

It is known that people with diabetes have difficulty converting omega-6 oils into GLA, making supplementation important. Over time, a lack of GLA and its metabolites decreases the flow of blood and oxygen to the nerve cells, causing tissue damage. Because essential fatty acids are vital to the structure of cell membranes, a lack of GLA affects the ability of nerve cell membranes to regulate the flow of substances in and out of the cells. Essential fatty acids are also required for normal conduction of electrical impulses. Researchers believe that people with diabetes have abnormally low levels of the enzyme delta-6-desaturase, which controls the conversion of omega-6 to GLA. Evening primrose oil has been shown to counteract nerve damage in people with diabetes without affecting blood sugar levels.[4,13]

GLA may help relieve breast pain by altering the essential fatty acid content of cell membranes and hormone receptors in the breasts. Some researchers believe that breast pain is caused by excessive levels of saturated fat in these cells. Higher levels of saturated fat may make the breast tissue overly sensitive to normal levels of circulating estrogen, causing pain. Treatment with EPO appears to restore the balance of fatty acids in breast cells and hormone receptors, making them less sensitive to estrogen.[13]

Preliminary research suggests that people with eczema may have difficulty converting omega-6 oils into GLA and its metabolites. This has been noted both in individuals with eczema and in infants born into families with a genetic history of eczema.[3] Treatment with EPO raises levels of fatty acids and helps relieve symptoms of eczema. Researchers believe this is due in part to a reduction of inflammatory prostaglandins (PGE2). EPO may also strengthen ceramides, components in the epidermal layer of skin that prevent excessive loss of water and drying of the skin.[9] There is also some evidence that EPO reduces the dilation of capillaries in the skin and has a strengthening effect on the immune system.[10]

Preliminary research has also shown that certain women with PMS may have difficulty converting omega-6 oils into GLA, leading to abnormal production of prostaglandins that cause pain and other unpleasant symptoms. Fatty acid imbalances may also exaggerate the effects of circulating hormones on cell receptors, which may contribute to the symptoms of PMS.[12]

MAJOR CONSTITUENTS

Gamma-linolenic acid (GLA)

SAFETY

Evening primrose herb and seed oil are considered safe when used appropriately.[14]

- **Side effects:** In some clinical studies, a small percentage of people experienced minor stomach upset, nausea, or headache after taking high doses of EPO. This may be avoided by lowering the overall dosage or by dividing the dose into smaller amounts taken several times during the day.
- **Contraindications:** None known.
- **Drug interactions:** Taking evening primrose oil with phenothiazine epileptogenic drugs for schizophrenia may increase the risk of temporal lobe epilepsy.[15]

DOSAGE

The following dosages were used in clinical studies with positive results. Take EPO capsules with food to ensure proper absorption. For best results, decrease your intake of saturated fats and trans-fatty acids, found in products such as margarine and shortening, because these harmful fats compete with essential fatty acids for absorption in the body. It may take several months to see noticeable improvement with evening primrose oil supplements.

- **Diabetic neuropathy:** 8 to 12 capsules a day (containing 320 to 480 mg of total GLA)
- **Breast pain:** 6 capsules a day (containing 240 mg of total GLA)
- **Chronic eczema:** 6 capsules a day
- **PMS:** 6 capsules a day

STANDARDIZATION

Evening primrose oil supplements typically contain 7 to 10 percent GLA.

REFERENCES

1. Murray M. *Encyclopedia of Nutritional Supplements.* Rocklin, CA: Prima Publishing, 1996.
2. Robbers JE, Tyler VE. *Tyler's Herbs of Choice.* New York and London: The Haworth Herbal Press, 1999.
3. Horrobin DF. Medical roles of metabolites of precursor EFA. *Inform* 1995; 6(4): 428–435.

4. Reichert R. Evening primrose oil and diabetic neuropathy. *Quarterly Review of Natural Medicine* Summer 1995:129–133.

5. Jamal GA, Charmichael H. The effect of gamma-linolenic acid on human diabetic peripheral neuropathy: a double-blind placebo-controlled trial. *Diabetic Medicine* 1990; 7: 319–323.

6. Keen H, Payan J, Allawi J, et al. Treatment of diabetic neuropathy with gamma-linolenic acid. *Diabetes Care* 1993; 16(1): 8–15.

7. Holland PA, Gately CA. Drug therapy of mastalgia: what are the options? *Drugs* 1994; 48(5): 709–716.

8. Pye JK, Mansel RE, Hughes LE. Clinical experience of drug treatments for mastalgia. *Lancet* 1985; 2: 373–377.

9. Burton JL. Essential fatty acids in atopic eczema: clinical studies. In: Horrobin DF, ed. *Omega-6 Essential Fatty Acids: Pathophysiology and Roles in Clinical Medicine.* New York: Wiley-Liss, 1990.

10. Fiocchi A, Sala M, Signoroni P, et al. The efficacy and safety of gamma-linolenic acid in the treatment of infantile atopic dermatitis. *The Journal of International Medical Research* 1994; 22: 24–32.

11. Humphreys F, Symons JA, Brown HK, et al. The effects of gamolenic acid on adult atopic eczema and premenstrual exacerbation of eczema. *European Journal of Dermatology* 1994; 4: 598–603.

12. O'Brien PMS, Massil H. Premenstrual syndrome: clinical studies on essential fatty acids. In: Horrobin DF, ed. *Omega-6 Essential Fatty Acids: Pathophysiology and Roles in Clinical Medicine.* New York: Wiley-Liss, 1990.

13. Horrobin DF. The effects of gamma-linolenic acid on breast pain and diabetic neuropathy: possible non-eicosanoid mechanisms. *Prostaglandins, Leukotrienes, and Essential Fatty Acids* 1993; 48: 101–104.

14. McGuffin M, Hobbs C, Upton R, et al., eds. *American Herbal Products Association Botanical Safety Handbook.* Boca Raton, FL: CRC Press, 1997.

15. Foster S, Tyler VE. *Tyler's Honest Herbal.* New York and London: The Haworth Herbal Press, 1999.

Feverfew

TANACETUM PARTHENIUM
ASTERACEAE

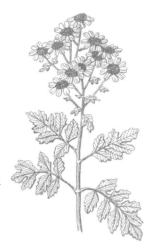

State of Knowledge: Five-Star Rating System

Clinical (human) research	✶✶
Laboratory research	✶✶✶
History of use/traditional use	✶✶✶
Safety record	✶✶✶
International acceptance	✶✶✶

PART USED: *Leaf*

PRIMARY USES

- *Migraine headaches*
- *Fever (traditional)*
- *Menstrual cramps (traditional)*
- *Arthritis (traditional)*

Sometimes called the "aspirin of the eighteenth century," feverfew has been rediscovered by modern people with migraine. During the 1970s, a research group in England advertised in a local newspaper, seeking people who had used feverfew to prevent migraine headaches. They received more than 25,000 enthusiastic responses. This spurred the first scientific studies at the London Migraine Clinic, which confirmed the plant's effectiveness.

Although feverfew is far safer than aspirin and prescription migraine drugs, it is important to remember that it may only offer symptomatic relief without addressing the underlying causes of migraines. Unfortunately, these causes still are not completely understood by doctors and researchers. A few factors that may play a role include allergies to foods and food additives, changing hormonal levels in women, and spinal problems that can be corrected by a chiropractor or osteopath. Ideally, feverfew should be used as part of a truly holistic program for heading off the deeper causes of migraines.

The High Cost of Migraines

Recent statistics from the National Headache Foundation show that migraines cost more than peace of mind. In the United States, businesses lose approximately $50 billion each year in sick-day compensation and medical bills because of employees who suffer from chronic migraine headaches.

HISTORY

Physicians have recommended feverfew as a headache remedy since the first century. In 1633, the British herbalist Gerard wrote, in the typical language of the day, that "It is good for them that are giddie in the head." During the 1700s, Culpeper instructed his migraine patients to apply bruised feverfew leaves to the crown of the head. Physician John Hill also sang the praises of feverfew: "In the worst headache this herb exceeds whatever else is known."

Traditionally, feverfew was identified as a woman's herb, due to its value in relieving menstrual cramps and problems during labor. The common names "mother herb" in Germany, "woman's plant" in Wales, and "Santa Maria" (the Blessed Virgin) in Latin America may also refer to the plant's use in treating migraine headaches, which are three times more common in women than men. Other early uses for feverfew included arthritis, psoriasis, stomachache, toothache, and respiratory problems such as asthma and bronchitis. As

the name suggests, feverfew's cooling property was also used to help break high fevers.

When the English colonists brought feverfew to America, they discovered another use for the plant: as an insect repellent. It has been cultivated as a protective border around vegetable gardens, used as a natural insect repellent on the skin, and placed in closets to discourage moths. In South America, feverfew is used for colic, stomachache, morning sickness, digestive problems, menstrual disorders, and kidney stones. In China, several related species are used for headaches and other "hot" illnesses.

INTERNATIONAL STATUS

Feverfew is approved in the United Kingdom and France for the treatment of migraine headaches and arthritis.

BOTANY

As a member of the largest family of flowering plants (Asteraceae), feverfew has many common relatives, including chrysanthemum, black-eyed susan, chamomile, sunflower, echinacea, calendula, and burdock. Feverfew grows 1 to 3 feet tall and blooms from July to October. The blossoms have white outer ray petals and a bright yellow center composed of multiple disk flowers. Native to central and southern Europe, feverfew was introduced to England and is now naturalized in most of the temperate zone, including North America. The plant is easy to grow as an ornamental or for medicinal purposes. Commonly found in poor soils, feverfew thrives in sunlight but also tolerates shade. As Gerard noted in the seventeenth century, "It joyeth to grow among rubbish."

BENEFITS

- Prevents and treats migraine headaches by decreasing platelet aggregation (the tendency of the blood platelets to clump) and by preventing the release of serotonin
- May help treat arthritis, psoriasis, and other inflammatory problems by preventing the release of inflammatory substances

SCIENTIFIC SUPPORT

Several well-controlled studies show that feverfew dramatically reduces migraine frequency, pain intensity, and accompanying nausea and vomiting in people who have chronic migraines. The duration of migraine attacks does not appear to be significantly affected. Used as a preventive, feverfew generally produces results within 1 month of regular use, with even greater benefits evident after 2 months. In fact, in one study, people who had successfully treated themselves with raw feverfew leaves for several years experienced a recurrence of incapacitating migraine after abruptly discontinuing the treatment. The same study showed that raw feverfew leaves were just as effective as freeze-dried feverfew powder in reducing migraine symptoms.[1]

To date, only one scientific study has tested feverfew in subjects with rheumatoid arthritis. Although the study found no significant effects, the participants had also been unresponsive to conventional therapies. More research is needed in this area.

SPECIFIC STUDIES

Migraine Prevention: Clinical Study (1997)

Feverfew was associated with a statistically significant reduction in migraine pain intensity, vomiting, and sensitivity to noise in a double-blind, placebo-controlled, crossover study of 57 subjects. All of the people included in the study had severe migraines, and 43 percent suffered more than 10 attacks per month. During phase 1 of the study, participants took either 2 capsules of feverfew (100 mg total) or placebo daily for 2 months. During phases 2 and 3, one group continued to receive feverfew for an additional 30 days, followed by placebo for 30 more days. The second group took placebo for 30 days followed by feverfew for an additional month. The results of phases 2 and 3 showed that the feverfew treatment continued to reduce pain intensity, whereas the placebo treatment was associated with an increase in pain. The feverfew group saw a marked improvement in their symptoms within the first 2 months of treatment.[2]

Migraine Prevention: Clinical Study (1988)

Feverfew treatment led to a statistically significant 24 percent reduction in the number and severity of migraine attacks, along with improvement in symptoms such as nausea and vomiting, in a randomized, double-blind, placebo-controlled, crossover study of 59 people. Almost half (47 percent) of the subjects had previously tried standard migraine drugs with little success. During the first 4 months of the study, participants took either 1 capsule of dried feverfew leaves (82 mg, parthenolide content 0.66 percent; equivalent to roughly two fresh feverfew leaves) daily or placebo. The two groups then switched treatments for an additional 4 months. During the placebo phase, the severity of migraine attacks increased significantly. There were no side effects with feverfew treatment.[3]

HOW IT WORKS

Although the deeper causes of migraine headaches are not fully understood, researchers now have a better understanding of what happens physiologically during an attack. Initially, blood vessels in the head constrict, reducing the flow of blood and oxygen to the brain. As the migraine progresses, blood vessels gradually dilate (widen) and become inflamed, stimulating pain receptors. Researchers now believe that platelets, a part of the blood involved in clotting, play a major role in migraines. During an attack, platelets tend to aggregate (stick together) and to release inflammatory prostaglandins and thromboxanes. The platelets also secrete serotonin, a neurotransmitter that increases blood vessel constriction.[4]

Research shows that feverfew and one of its main constituents, parthenolide, decrease platelet aggregation and inhibit enzymes that turn into inflammatory prostaglandins and thromboxanes. In addition, feverfew helps prevent the release of serotonin from platelets, an effect similar to many standard antimigraine drugs, such as methysergide. The plant may also work by restoring normal calcium mobilization in cells with defective calcium channels. This is a factor in several types of migraine, including a rare form called familial hemiplegic migraine.[5]

A fourth mode of action may account for feverfew's traditional use in treating arthritis, psoriasis, and other inflammatory problems. Studies show that feverfew discourages the release of inflammatory substances from cells known as polymorphonuclear leukocytes (PMNs) in inflamed joints. These substances are known to be a major cause of inflammation and cellular damage in rheumatoid arthritis.[5]

Parthenolide is still considered to be a major constituent in feverfew extracts. However, a 1996 clinical study suggests that it is not the only one. In this study, researchers found that an alcohol extract of feverfew had no benefits in relieving migraines, even though it had been standardized for parthenolide content.[6] These results conflict with previous studies that demonstrated positive effects using a dried whole-plant capsule standardized for parthenolide. Researchers now believe that one or more essential constituents were missing from the extract used in the 1996 study. An important constituent may be chrysanthenyl acetate, an essential oil that inhibits prostaglandin synthesis.[3] Feverfew also contains significant levels of melatonin, a hormone that acts as an antioxidant and regulates sleep. This is interesting, in light of research linking chronic migraine headaches to lower circulating levels of melatonin.[7]

Dennis Awang, Ph.D., an authority on the chemistry of feverfew, has pointed out the need for future studies that compare various cultivars of parthenolide-rich feverfew to parthenolide-free varieties and placebo. This will help researchers better understand which constituents are involved in feverfew's complex antimigraine effects.[8]

MAIN CONSTITUENTS

Parthenolide and other sesquiterpene lactones

SAFETY

Clinical studies show that feverfew is reasonably safe when used appropriately.

- **Side effects:** Side effects are uncommon but can include mild stomach upset in a small percentage of people.[9] Those who chew fresh feverfew leaves experience minor mouth ulcerations occasionally, an effect that has not been seen in capsule users.
- **Contraindications:** Do not use feverfew during pregnancy or nursing without the advice of a health-care practitioner.[9]
- **Drug interactions:** None known. If you are already taking a prescription medication for migraines, check with a health-care practitioner before using feverfew.

DOSAGE

Feverfew is most effective against migraines when used as a preventive for at least 2 to 3 months. Some health practitioners also recommend using the plant to head off acute migraine attacks. For these situations, try a dose of feverfew every 15 minutes for a maximum of four doses, until the symptoms improve.

Levels of important constituents can vary widely depending on where the plant was grown, when it was harvested, and how the preparation was manufactured. In general, it is best to eat fresh feverfew leaves or to take a standardized product made from whole dried leaves. Teas are less useful because many of the plant's active constituents are not water soluble. Be sure to store all feverfew products in a cool, dark cupboard to protect them from heat and light, which lower parthenolide levels rapidly.[5]

- **Standardized extract:** 275 mg a day
- **Capsules/tablets:** 300 to 400 mg capsules, taken up to 3 times a day[10]
- **Tincture:** 15 to 30 drops a day[10]
- **Fresh leaves:** 2 large or 4 small leaves a day (eaten raw or mixed into food)

STANDARDIZATION

Feverfew is typically standardized to contain between 0.2 and 0.7 percent parthenolide.

REFERENCES

1. Johnson ES, Kadam NP, Hylands DM, et al. Efficacy of feverfew as a prophylactic treatment of migraine. *British Medical Journal* 1985; 291: 569–573.
2. Palevitch D, Earon G, Carasso R. Feverfew *(Tanacetum parthenium)* as a prophylactic treatment for migraine: a double-blind placebo-controlled study. *Phytotherapy Research* 1997; 2: 508–11.
3. Murphy JJ, Heptinstall S, Mitchell JRA. Randomised double-blind placebo-controlled trial of feverfew in migraine prevention. *The Lancet* July 23, 1988; 189–92.
4. Robbers JE, Tyler VE. *Tyler's Herbs of Choice.* New York and London: The Haworth Press, Inc., 1999.
5. Heptinstall S, Awang DVC. Feverfew: a review of its history, its biological and medicinal properties, and the status of commercial preparations of the herb. In: Lawson L, Bauer R, eds. *Phytomedicines of Europe: Chemistry and Biological Activity.* Washington, DC: American Chemical Society, 1998; 158—175.
6. de Weerdt CJ, Bootsma HPR, Hendriks H. Herbal medicines in migraine prevention: randomized double-blind placebo controlled crossover trial of a feverfew preparation. *Phytomedicine* 1996; 3(3): 225–230.
7. Murch SJ, Simmons CB, Saxena PK. Melatonin in feverfew and other medicinal plants. *The Lancet* 1997; 350: 1598–1599.
8. Awang DVC. Feverfew trials: the promise of—and the problem with—standardized botanical extracts. *HerbalGram* 1997; 41: 16–17.
9. McGuffin M, Hobbs C, Upton R, et al., eds. *American Herbal Products Association Botanical Safety Handbook.* Boca Raton and New York: CRC Press LLC, 1997.
10. Foster S. *101 Medicinal Herbs.* Loveland, CO: Interweave Press, 1998.

Flax

LINUM USITATISSIMUM
LINACEAE

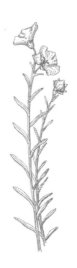

State of Knowledge: Five-Star Rating System

Clinical (human) research	✳✳
Laboratory research	✳✳✳
History of use/traditional use	✳✳✳✳
Safety record	✳✳✳✳
International acceptance	✳✳✳

PART USED: *Seed*

PRIMARY USES

- *Overall good health*
- *High cholesterol*
- *Inflammatory conditions, including arthritis, psoriasis, and ulcerative colitis (experimental)*
- *Autoimmune diseases such as cancer, lupus, and multiple sclerosis (experimental)*
- *Allergies (experimental)*
- *Chronic constipation (whole seed)*

In recent years, America seems to have developed a "fat phobia." A trip to the supermarket reveals a mind-boggling assortment of fat-free and low-fat foods, from potato chips to ice cream. Yet Americans still have one of the highest rates of heart disease and cancer in the world. Many researchers now tell us that merely reducing our fat intake to less than 30 percent of calories may not be enough to ensure good health. The answer seems to lie not simply in how much fat we consume, but in what type of fats we consume.

In the quest to avoid fat, many people neglect to provide the body with a healthful supply of essential fatty acids (EFAs), "good fats," that may actually help protect against degenerative diseases. EFAs are the beneficial components of polyunsaturated fats and are critical in building healthy cells. They

163

cannot be manufactured by the body and must be supplied through the diet. Of all the EFAs, omega-3 (also called *alpha-linolenic acid,* or ALA), found in flaxseed, is emerging as the most important for maintaining health. Americans had a much higher intake of omega-3 EFAs before the age of industrialization, hydrogenated fat, and refined vegetable oils. Currently, researchers estimate that at least 80 percent of Americans are deficient in this beneficial oil.[1]

The type of fat we eat greatly influences how well our bodies function. People who consume too many meat and dairy products get more than just a large dose of saturated fat. They also take in high levels of arachidonic fatty acids, which contribute to inflammation and heart problems because they are converted to a harmful type of prostaglandin (a hormone-like substance) in the body. Some researchers think this may explain, in part, the explosion of allergies and autoimmune diseases over the past 50 years.

Those who eat a more plant-based diet, including flaxseed or flax oil, consume larger amounts of healthful omega-3 EFAs. Our bodies convert omega-3 EFAs into beneficial prostaglandins that actually help counteract inflammation and support heart health. Current research suggests that lignans, another compound in flax, may also have powerful effects against many types of cancer, especially breast cancer. Flaxseed contains over 100 times the amount of lignans found in any other food.[2]

Balancing Act: Omega-6 Versus Omega-3 EFAs

With all this talk of omega-3 EFAs, you may be wondering about omega-6 fatty acids. Also essential to health, omega-6 EFAs are widely found in whole grains, nuts, seeds, and especially vegetable oils. However, many researchers believe that Americans already consume too many omega-6 EFAs, in the form of vegetable oils and as "hidden fats" in a variety of prepared foods. In a world of perfect fat balance, we would consume a 4:1 ratio of omega-6 to omega-3 oils, meaning four times as much omega-6 as omega-3. Most of us are currently taking in 20 times as much omega-6 as omega-3! When we eat too many omega-6 oils and hydrogenated fats, we can't properly metabolize the more precious omega-3s. Numerous clinical studies show that adding flax to the diet provided much less benefit when people failed to also lower their intake of saturated fats, hydrogenated oils, and omega-6 oils.[3]

HISTORY

With a history more than 5,000 years long, flax has earned its Latin name *usitatissimum* (meaning "useful") many times over. Flax is one of the oldest cultivated plants; its use has been traced back to cloth made during the Stone Age in what is now Switzerland. Before the invention of the cotton gin in 1794, everything from linen clothing to lamp wicks, ship sails, and wrappings for Egyptian mummies was made from flax fiber. People living in warmer climates traditionally favored linen garments over wool because of their breathability and ease of care. In an age of infrequent bathing, Charlemagne ordered his subjects to cultivate flax for clothing because of its "sanitary" nature. Flax oil (also called *linseed oil*) readily absorbs oxygen, making it perishable as a food but valuable as a pliant yet protective polish for furniture, leather shoes, and wooden tools. After pressing out the oil, people often fed the remaining linseed cakes to animals or used them as a rich "green manure," or fertilizer.[4]

Native Americans sometimes harvested wild species of flax, but the plant was not cultivated in America until the seventeenth century. During colonial times, cloth was considered so essential to survival that every household was required by law to produce a certain amount of flax or woolen cloth each year. When adventurous settlers moved west, they immediately planted flax alongside corn, wheat, and other crops. In 1809, an enterprising American invented flax-based oilcloth, which was turned into rain gear, tablecloths, and other useful household items. Fifty years later, linoleum made from linseed oil and cork was patented and soon decorated floors throughout America.[4]

Flax was also a traditional food and medicine in many countries. Because of its soothing, mucilaginous quality, ground flaxseed was used for coughs, sore throats, irritable digestive disorders, and gravel or burning in the urinary tract. Sometimes it was prepared as a tea with honey and lemon juice. Ground seeds were also mixed with honey, oil, or mashed figs and applied externally as a poultice for skin inflammation, irritation, boils, abscesses, and sunburn. The seeds have a long history of use in chronic constipation due to their gentle bulking and lubricating effects. From 1820 to 1947, flax was listed in *The United States Pharmacopoeia* for many of these uses. The plant also has a long history of use in both Chinese and Ayurvedic medicine.[4]

INTERNATIONAL STATUS

Flaxseed is approved by Germany's Commission E to treat chronic constipation, irritable colon, diverticulitis (inflammation of the small pockets in the colon wall), gastritis (inflammation of the stomach lining), and enteritis (inflammation of the small intestine); to soothe colons damaged by laxative abuse; and as a poultice (external treatment) for local inflammation. Flax is also approved for such use in France and Belgium. These uses of flax relate to its fiber and mucilage content, however, and not to EFAs.

BOTANY

In spite of their small size, it would be difficult to miss flax's delicate, blue flowers. Botanist

William Weber describes their color as "one of the truest blues found in nature." Common flax *(L. usitatissimum)* has linear green leaves and slender stems that reach up to 4 feet tall. The five-petaled blue flowers bloom from June to August, turning into autumn fruits that each hold 8 to 10 polished seeds.

Flax has been cultivated in so many parts of the world for so long that its exact origin has been lost. The plant easily escapes cultivation and has returned to a semiwild state in temperate and semitropical places around the globe. Nearly 100 different species of flax are found worldwide, including mountain flax *(L. catharticum),* a white-flowered species that is widely distributed in Europe, and prairie flax *(L. lewisii),* which is commonly found growing in the United States. Today, at least 35 percent of the commercial flaxseed crop comes from Canada, and most of the remainder from North Africa, Turkey, and Argentina. Flax is still cultivated for its fiber in Russia, China, Egypt, and parts of Europe. Growers in Maine and the Willamette Valley of Oregon are currently attempting to resurrect the flax fiber industry in the United States.

BENEFITS

- Supports overall good health by providing omega-3 EFAs, eicosapentaenoic acid (EPA), and docosahexaenoic acid (DHA), which compose the membranes of every cell in the body, including the nerves, retina of the eye, and brain
- Helps reduce inflammation by lowering arachidonic acid levels and encouraging production of "good" (series 1 and 3) prostaglandins
- Helps lower cholesterol due to its omega-3 EFAs, lignan, and fiber content
- May protect against cancer by boosting immune system function and blocking excessive levels of harmful estrogens (experimental)

SCIENTIFIC SUPPORT

Unfortunately, the studies investigating the effects of omega-3 oils on heart health have tested fish oil more often than flax oil. However, many researchers believe that flax is just as effective as fish oil, since the body readily converts linolenic acid in flax into the eicosapentaenoic acid (EPA) that occurs naturally in fish oil. EPA is important because it is converted into prostaglandins that support heart health. Flax also contains fiber and lignans, which have additional cardiovascular benefits. Though research is still preliminary, top flax researcher Stephen Cunnane, Ph.D., believes that linolenic acid also offers benefits all its own.[3]

At least four clinical trials using flax confirm its cardiovascular benefits. Several studies show that flaxseed significantly lowers total cholesterol and low-density lipoprotein

(LDL) cholesterol levels. Another study found that flax lowered levels of lipoprotein(a), a more recently discovered risk factor for heart disease. Levels of healthful high-density lipoprotein (HDL) cholesterol do not appear to be significantly affected.[5,6] Flax oil also considerably improves arterial compliance, a measure of the elasticity of arteries that is an indicator of risk for heart disease and stroke.[7]

In a 5-year French study known as the Lyon Diet Heart Study, flax helped patients who had suffered a heart attack in the previous 6 months to avoid a second heart attack. Participants were asked to substitute a flax-based spread for butter and cream and to consume a Mediterranean-style diet high in bread, fruit, vegetables, and fish. After only 2 years, researchers were so impressed by the results that they ended the study early. At that time, deaths due to heart attack were already 76 percent lower and overall mortality was 70 percent lower than in an untreated control group. Success was attributed to the threefold increase in omega-3 intake, combined with a decrease in saturated fat, cholesterol, and omega-6 EFAs.[8]

In 1990, the U.S. National Cancer Institute (NCI) launched a 5-year, $20 million program to learn more about flax and other plants that might prevent cancer. Although preliminary results with flax were extremely promising, especially against breast cancer, the NCI abruptly cancelled the project. The current evidence on flax's cancer-protective effects is encouraging, although limited primarily to laboratory and cross-cultural population studies.

Some researchers have suggested a possible link between consumption of linolenic acid and an increased risk for prostate cancer, but this evidence has largely been discredited. Studies were criticized because male patients obtained large amounts of linolenic acid from red meat, in addition to flax. There is a much stronger possibility that saturated fat and other harmful constituents in the red meat were responsible for the increased cancer risk than that linolenic acid was the cause.[3]

Several studies using flax oil in rheumatoid arthritis also had disappointing results. However, in this case, researchers noted that participants had not modified their intake of omega-6 oils to ensure proper absorption of omega-3 EFAs from flax. In addition, many subjects were diagnosed with an underlying zinc deficiency, a common problem in rheumatoid arthritis that is known to prevent conversion of omega-3 to the good prostaglandins that fight inflammation.[9] (See Balancing Act: Omega-6 Versus Omega-3 EFAs for more in-depth information about this issue.)

Researchers are currently studying flax as a possible treatment for malaria, chronic renal (kidney) transplant rejection, and systemic lupus erythematosus (SLE or lupus, an autoimmune disease involving inflamed blood vessels, kidney failure, and heart problems).

SPECIFIC STUDIES

Breast Cancer:
Case-Control Study (1997)

A case-control study conducted in Australia found that breast cancer risk was substantially reduced among women with a higher intake of phytoestrogens, including lignans from flax. Researchers compared 144 women with newly diagnosed early breast cancer (before treatment) to 144 women without breast cancer who were matched for age and area of residence. Results were measured by means of questionnaires and urine samples, which were tested for levels of the isoflavones daidzein and equol, and the lignans enterodiol, enterolactone, and matairesinol. Unfortunately, researchers were not able to measure urinary levels of genistein, which is thought to be a particularly important type of isoflavone. Risk factors were tabulated after adjusting for age at first menstruation, number of pregnancies, alcohol intake, and total fat intake. Researchers found that cancer risk was most reduced by a high intake of the isoflavone equol (formed during the metabolism of the soy isoflavone daidzein) and by enterolactone (formed during intestinal breakdown of a lignan in flax). Although the other phytoestrogens were also associated with a risk reduction, this association did not reach statistical significance.[10]

Cholesterol: Clinical Study (1998)

Researchers found that whole flaxseed and sunflower seed were equally effective in lowering total cholesterol levels (6.9 percent and 5.5 percent, respectively) in 38 postmenopausal women with mildly, moderately, or severely elevated cholesterol levels. However, only flaxseed was found to significantly lower levels of harmful LDL cholesterol (14.7 percent) and lipoprotein(a) (7.4 percent). Levels of healthful HDL cholesterol and triglycerides were unaffected by either treatment. During the double-blind crossover study, participants were randomly assigned to receive either 38 grams of flaxseed or sunflower seed daily, in the form of breads and muffins, over a 6-week period. This was followed by a 2-week wash-out period, and then another 6 weeks in which subjects switched treatment groups. Researchers attributed the superiority of flaxseed to its high linolenic acid and lignan content. Despite the higher intake of calories during both treatments, the participants did not gain weight. This may have been because they also had a higher intake of dietary fiber.[5]

HOW IT WORKS

One way to measure health is by the vitality of each individual cell in the body. Adequate levels of alpha-linolenic acid from flax are necessary for the formation of cell membranes in every part of the body. ALA is broken down into eicosapentaenoic (EPA) and docosahexaenoic acids (DHA), two substances that are vital for the health of nerves, the retina of the eye, and brain cells. These substances are also present in fish oils. Studies in humans show that EPA levels rise six- to eightfold after consuming ALA from flax, whereas increases in DHA are more unpredictable.[3] From there, our bodies convert EPA and DHA into good (series 1 and 3) prostaglandins, which regulate many important physiological processes.

One-quarter cup of whole flaxseed also contains roughly 20 grams of fiber, well over half the daily recommended dose for optimal health. Inadequate fiber intake has been linked to constipation, diverticulitis, hemorrhoids, poor blood sugar metabolism, high blood pressure and cholesterol levels, and some cancers.[11] Flax's lignan content is also considered highly protective against a number of diseases.

Inflammation

The omega-3 fatty acids in flax are converted into "good" (series 1 and 3) prostaglandins that may help reduce inflammation, pain, and allergic response in a number of conditions. In a study of patients with eczema (chronic, itchy inflamed skin), researchers found deficient levels of omega-3 EFAs, EPA, and DHA in body tissues, combined with excessive levels of omega-6 EFAs. This study demonstrates the importance of higher omega-3 intake, as well as the need to achieve the correct balance between omega-3 and omega-6 (see the previous discussion about fatty acid balance).[12]

Heart Health

Clinical studies suggest that at least three components in flaxseed are involved in its ability to lower cholesterol levels: ALA, lignans, and fiber. The conversion of ALA into beneficial prostaglandins helps support heart health by improving blood flow and decreasing platelet aggregation. When blood platelets aggregate (stick together), they release potent substances that encourage the formation of plaque in the arteries, as well as abnormal blood clots that can cause heart attacks and strokes. Flax also lowers levels of lipoprotein(a), a risk factor for heart disease that often responds to estrogen therapy but not to exercise, reduction of fat intake, or standard drugs. Researchers attribute this reduction to mild estrogenic effects produced by flax lignans.[5]

Cancer

Researchers don't completely understand how ALA might work in helping to fight cancer, but have proposed several theories. Eating a diet rich in ALA not only encourages production of "good" prostaglandins, it also decreases production of "bad" (series 2) prostaglandins, which suppress immune function.[13] Darshan Kelley, Ph.D., a top flax researcher, suggests that ALA may also work by altering the fatty acid composition of immune cells or by changing the fatty acid composition of platelets that secrete substances that affect immune cell activity.[14] Clearly, more research is needed in this area.

Breast Cancer

Flaxseed is rich in lignans, which are thought to exert protective effects against many kinds of cancer, especially breast cancer. Lignans (particularly secoisolariciresinol diglucoside, or SDG) are converted by intestinal bacteria into two active forms known as enterodiol and enterolactone.[2] *In vitro* studies suggest that lignans have mild antiestrogenic effects that enable them to compete with harmful forms of estrogen at receptor cites. Lignans may also help reduce excessive levels of circulating estrogens by stimulating sex hormone–binding globulin in the liver and by inhibiting an enzyme called aromatase.[10,15]

Research has shown that consuming flaxseed (10 grams daily for 3 months) lengthens the menstrual cycle so that a complete cycle lasts longer than 28 days, which may reduce a woman's lifetime exposure to high levels of estrogens that can increase cancer risk.[16] This study is supported by population studies which show that Japanese women who excrete higher levels of phytoestrogens, including lignans, also tend to have longer menstrual cycles than Western women.[17] A recent laboratory study provided further support for this theory by showing that flaxseed and isolated lignans (such as SDG) included as 10 percent of the diet lengthened the menstrual cycle of rats. Flax's effects in this study were comparable with the drug tamoxifen, an antiestrogenic drug used in treating breast cancer.

Several other laboratory studies demonstrated that ground flaxseed and SDG significantly reduced the number and size of breast tumors in mice after 2 to 3 months of treatment.[18,19]

Colon Cancer

Because lignans are primarily broken down in the colon through conversion by intestinal bacteria, they may also offer some protection against colon cancer. Laboratory studies have shown that lignans reduce early risk factors and have a long-term protective effect against the multiplication of aberrant crypts (atypical pitlike depressions in the colon wall), an important predictor of colon cancer. Researchers believe lignans may act as antioxidants and may also exert antiestrogenic effects on estrogen receptors in the colon. Another possibility is that lignans reduce harmful levels of reabsorbed and circulating estrogens by stimulating excretion in the feces.[13] They may also affect the breakdown of cholesterol and the production of secondary bile acids in the colon, substances that have been associated with promotion of cancer.

Land or Sea: Is Fish Oil Better than Flax Oil?

Some researchers argue that fish oil is superior to flax oil because it provides a direct source of EPA that does not need to be converted in the body. To get the benefits of flax, our bodies have to change linolenic acid in flax oil into EPA. However, the issue is more complicated than this. Although clinical studies show that fish oil is effective in improving heart health, in some cases as many as 25 to 100 capsules had to be taken daily to produce these results.[1] Studies also indicate that fish oil contains large amounts of harmful lipid peroxides (free radicals), which deplete the body's store of antioxidants.[20]

Flax appears to be just as effective as fish oil at lowering cholesterol levels, with the additional advantages of being safer and less expensive. A well-conducted study showed that flax increases levels of EPA in the tissues and lowers levels of damaging arachidonic acids just as well as fish oil—as long as levels of omega-6 oils in the diet are not too high.[21] Flax contains more than twice as much omega-3 EFA as fish oil, in addition to disease-fighting constituents such as lignans and fiber. Needless to say, you don't need to be "landlocked" in order to stay healthy. Although many health practitioners do not recommend fish oils, they do favor moderate intake of cold-water fish, such as salmon, mackerel, and herring.

MAJOR CONSTITUENTS

Alpha-linolenic acid (ALA), lignans (especially secoisolariciresinol diglucoside, or SDG), fiber

SAFETY

Flaxseed has a long history of consumption as food and is considered quite safe.[22,23]

- **Side effects:** None known.
- **Contraindications:** Flaxseed should not be used when there is bowel obstruction.[22,23] In cases of bowel inflammation, the seeds should be presoaked in water before eating.[23] Flax oil is not contraindicated in either of these situations.
- **Drug interactions:** As with any high-fiber food, flaxseed may reduce the absorption of other drugs.[22,23]

DOSAGE

To prepare whole flaxseed, use a mini food processor, food mill, or coffee grinder to break the hard outer coating of the seed. Ground flax should be taken with at least 6 ounces of water. Plan to eat it within 15

minutes of grinding in order to prevent rancidity. In cases of stomach or throat inflammation, it is best to soak whole flaxseed in 1
cup of room-temperature water for 20 to 30
minutes before consuming. The omega-3 oil
in whole flaxseed maintains its potency for
at least 1 year and is just as bioavailable in
the body as flaxseed oil.[3]

Look for certified organic flaxseed oil in
opaque polyethylene bottles that are refrigerated and dated for freshness. The best
brands provide lignans as well as omega-3
oils. To prevent rancidity, keep bottles of flax
oil tightly sealed and refrigerated. Never
cook with flax oil, because heat destroys the
valuable compounds. Flax oil and ground
seeds can be added, uncooked, to salads, ce-
real, and other dishes, as long as they are
consumed immediately.

- **Oil:** 1 to 2 tablespoons a day
- **Seed (ground):** 2 1/2 teaspoons two
  to three times a day

Note: Adequate levels of zinc and friendly
intestinal bacteria (acidophilus and others)
are needed to properly metabolize flaxseed
and flax oil.

STANDARDIZATION

Some flax supplements are standardized to
58 percent alpha-linolenic acid.

REFERENCES

1. Murray MT. *Encyclopedia of Nutritional Supplements.* Rocklin, CA: Prima Publishing,
   1996.
2. Knight DC, Eden JA. A review of the clinical effects of phytoestrogens. *Obstetrics and
   Gynecology* 1996; 87(5): 897–90.
3. Cunnane SC. Metabolism and function of
   alpha-linolenic acid in humans. In: Cunnane
   S, Thompson LU, eds. *Flaxseed in Human
   Nutrition.* Champaign, IL: AOCS Press,
   1995.
4. Haggerty WJ. Flax: ancient herb and modern medicine. *HerbalGram* 1999; 45: 51–57.
5. Arjmandi BH, Khan DA, Juma S, et al.
   Whole flaxseed consumption lowers serum
   LDL-cholesterol and lipoprotein(a) concentrations in postmenopausal women. *Nutrition Research* 1998; 18(7): 1203–1214.
6. Bierenbaum ML, Reichstein R, Watkins
   TR. Reducing atherogenic risk in hyper-
   lipemic humans with flax seed supplementation: a preliminary report. *Journal of the
   American College of Nutrition* 1993; 12(5):
   501–504.
7. Nestel PJ, Pomeroy SE, Sasahara T, et al.
   Arterial compliance in obese subjects is
   improved with dietary plant n-3 fatty acid
   from flaxseed oil despite increased LDL
   oxidizability. *Arteriosclerosis, Thrombosis, and
   Vascular Biology* 1997; 17: 1163–1170.
8. de Lorgeril M, Renaud S, Mamelle N,
   et al. Mediterranean alpha-linolenic
   acid-rich diet in secondary prevention of
   coronary heart disease. *Lancet* 1994; 343:
   1454–1459.

9. Nordstrom DCE, Honkanen VEA, Nasu Y, et al. Alpha-linolenic acid in the treatment of rheumatoid arthritis. A double-blind, placebo-controlled and randomized study: flaxseed vs. safflower seed. *Rheumatology International* 1995; 14: 231–234.

10. Ingram D, Sanders K, Kolybaba M, et al. Case-control study of phytoestrogens and breast cancer. *Lancet* 1997; 350: 990–994.

11. Whitaker J. Add flax to your diet for overall health. *Dr. Julian Whitaker's Health and Healing* 1996; 6(7): 6–7.

12. Sasaki K. Fatty acid compositions of plasma lipids in atopic dermatitis/asthma patients. *Japanese Journal of Allergies* 1994; 43(1): 37–43.

13. Jenab M, Thompson LU. The influence of flaxseed and lignans on colon carcinogenesis and ß-glucuronidase activity. *Carcinogenesis* 1996; 17(6): 1343–1348.

14. Kelley DS. Immunomodulatory effects of flaxseed and other oils rich in alpha-linolenic acid. In: Cunnane and Thompson, eds. *Flaxseed in Human Nutrition.* Champaign, IL: AOCS Press, 1995.

15. Adlercreutz H, Bannwart C, Wahala K, et al. Inhibition of human aromatase by mammalian lignans and isoflavonoid phytoestrogens. *Journal of Steroid Biochemistry and Molecular Biology* 1993; 44(2): 147–153.

16. Phipps WR, Martini MC, Lampe JW, et al. Effect of flaxseed ingestion on the menstrual cycle. *Journal of Clinical Endocrinology and Metabolism* 1993; 77(5): 1215–1219.

17. Orcheson LJ, Rickard SE, Seidl MM, et al. Flaxseed and its mammalian lignan precursor cause a lengthening or cessation of estrous cycling in rats. *Cancer Letters* 1998; 125: 69–76.

18. Serraino M, Thompson LU. Flaxseed supplementation and early markers of colon carcinogenesis. *Cancer Letters* 1992; 63: 159–165.

19. Serraino M, Thompson LU. The effect of flaxseed supplementation on the initiation and promotional stages of mammary tumorigenesis. *Nutrition and Cancer* 1992; 17: 153–159.

20. Shukla VKS, Perkins EG. The presence of oxidative polymeric materials in encapsulated fish oils. *Lipids* 1991; 26: 23–26.

21. Mantzioris E, James MJ, Gibson RA, et al. Dietary substitution with an alpha-linolenic acid-rich vegetable oil increases eicosapentaenoic acid concentrations in tissues. *American Journal of Clinical Nutrition* 1994; 59: 1304–1309.

22. Blumenthal M, Busse W, Goldberg A, eds. *The Complete German Commission E Monographs.* Austin, TX: American Botanical Council; Boston: Integrative Medical Communications, 1998.

23. McGuffin M, Hobbs C, Upton R, et al., eds. *American Herbal Products Association Botanical Safety Handbook.* Boca Raton, FL: CRC Press, 1997.

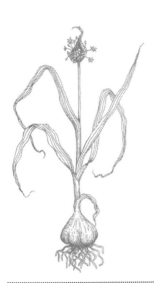

Garlic

ALLIUM SATIVUM
LILIACEAE

State of Knowledge: Five-Star Rating System

Clinical (human) research	✳ ✳ ✳
Laboratory research	✳ ✳ ✳ ✳
History of use / traditional use	✳ ✳ ✳ ✳ ✳
Safety record	✳ ✳ ✳ ✳
International acceptance	✳ ✳ ✳ ✳

PART USED: *Root (bulb)*

PRIMARY USES

- *Overall cardiovascular health*
- *High cholesterol*
- *High blood pressure*
- *Cancer protection*
- *Infections*
- *Colds and flu (traditional)*
- *Diabetes (experimental)*
- *Antioxidant*

Perhaps the world's best example of a medicinal food, garlic is also one of the most intensively studied herbs in natural medicine today. Impressive results from both clinical and laboratory studies point out the protective value of garlic against the leading diseases of the modern world, including heart disease, cancer, and infectious diseases. Although it is still unclear exactly how garlic works, few herbs—or foods—appear to fit so well into an overall lifestyle strategy for health promotion. Consumer enthusiasm for garlic's health-protective potential is reflected in sales of garlic supplements, which are the best-selling nonprescription phytomedicines in Germany and, as of 1997, the second best-selling herbal supplements in the United States.

Garlic offers a wealth of cardiovascular benefits that can help lower the risk of *atherosclerosis,* a hardening and narrowing of the arteries that can lead to heart attack, stroke, and other heart problems. Numerous clinical studies have suggested that various forms of garlic can lower cholesterol levels and improve ratios of healthful high-density lipoprotein (HDL) cholesterol to harmful low-density lipoprotein (LDL) cholesterol. Garlic has also been shown to lower blood pressure, inhibit platelet aggregation (the tendency of blood platelets to clump together), improve circulation, and protect the coronary arteries against age-related stiffening, an important indicator of cardiovascular health.

Garlic may also help protect against cancer. Compelling results from large population studies suggest that people who consume garlic regularly lower their risks of developing a number of different types of cancer, particularly cancers of the gastrointestinal tract. Garlic is strongly antimicrobial and has been used for centuries in treating infections. In addition, the herb has demonstrated potent antioxidant properties, which may contribute to its effects in a number of areas.

Not all garlic research has yielded positive results, particularly in the area of lowering cholesterol, and researchers have offered various explanations for the inconsistencies. One important issue has been variations in the type and quality of garlic products used in the clinical studies. Another complicating factor is possible problems with the quality and design of some studies. Overall, however, results of research on garlic's protective benefits against heart disease and cancer have been positive.

Much current research is aimed at determining exactly which forms of garlic and which active compounds are most important to garlic's therapeutic and health-protective benefits, and a certain amount of controversy exists. The fact is that since the 1960s, research has shown that virtually every form of garlic provides some type of health benefit—from dietary garlic eaten raw or cooked to dried garlic tablets, aged garlic supplements, enteric coated capsules, and garlic oil "perles" (or softgel capsules). In addition, numerous different garlic compounds have demonstrated a variety of health effects.

It is unlikely that any one "active ingredient" will be identified in garlic, but future research may shed new light on which forms of garlic are most appropriate for specific uses. In the meantime, it is safe to say that regular use of garlic—in food or as a dietary supplement—is a wise move for those concerned with improving overall health and longevity. *Bon appétit!*

HISTORY

Garlic's history of medicinal use spans at least 5,000 years, so a detailed account would require many pages. People from nearly every culture in the world have taken garlic both to treat disease and to enhance general health and longevity, from the ancient Chinese to early Europeans to colonial Americans. The many recorded uses of garlic are remarkably consistent from culture to culture, and garlic is still used today for many of the same purposes in traditional medicine systems around the world.

The earliest written records of the medicinal uses of garlic come from ancient India and Mesopotamia. Garlic is also included in the ancient Egyptian medical text now known as the *Ebers Codex*, which dates from about 1550 B.C.[1] According to historical records, large quantities of garlic and onions were supplied as rations to help ensure the health of the Egyptian workers who built the Great Pyramids. In traditional Chinese medicine, some of the many applications of garlic have included the treatment of colds, bronchitis, intestinal parasites, tuberculosis, diarrhea and dysentery, and a variety of skin problems. Indian Ayurvedic healers used it for many of the same purposes, and also for ear problems, heart disease, and as a general circulatory system tonic.[1] The Greek physician Hippocrates prescribed garlic for infections, pneumonia, cancer, and digestive problems, and Dioscorides recommended it for "clearing the arteries" and for treating coughs, infections, and leprosy.

Obviously, garlic was prized for its antimicrobial effects long before microbes were even discovered. French priests of the Middle Ages used garlic to protect themselves against bubonic plague, now known to be a bacterial infection. One fascinating historical account holds that during a plague epidemic in the 1700s, four convicted French prisoners were given the task of collecting and burying the bodies of the dead—an assignment that seemed tantamount to a death sentence. Much to everyone's surprise, the four prisoners proved immune to the disease. They claimed that their secret was a concoction of garlic and other herbs soaked in vinegar, which they drank and splashed on their faces and clothes. This mixture, known as *vinaigre des quatres voleurs* (four thieves' vinegar) can still be purchased in France today.[1]

During the First World War, European soldiers prevented infection by putting garlic directly on their wounds, and it was so widely used this way by Russians during the Second World War that it acquired the nickname "Russian penicillin."[1] Throughout history, some of the most popular traditional uses of garlic have been for treating colds, coughs, flu, and other infections; earaches; skin infections, ulcers, and other skin problems; intestinal parasites; digestive problems; vaginal yeast infections; and high blood pressure. Garlic was listed in *The United States Pharmacopoeia* until 1900.[1] Today, garlic is one of the best-selling preventive medicines in Europe, where it is accepted as safe and effective by both medical authorities and government officials.

INTERNATIONAL STATUS

Garlic is listed as an approved herb in the *German Commission E Monographs,* in which it is recommended as a supportive treatment for improving blood cholesterol levels and helping to prevent age-related cardiovascular changes. In the United Kingdom and France, it is approved for use in lowering cholesterol and high blood pressure and for helping to prevent the development of atherosclerosis.

BOTANY

Garlic has been cultivated for so long that it is difficult to know exactly where the plant came from, although botanists believe it originated in central Asia. Today, some 700 *Allium* species are distributed around the world, occurring in North America, Europe, North Africa, and Asia. *Allium sativum* is now unknown in the wild, but wild garlic species do exist, including *Allium ursinum.* Garlic is also closely related to onion *(Allium cepa),* which studies suggest may confer some of the same health-protective benefits as garlic. The spicy garlic "bulb" that is used as food and medicine is the root of the plant. However, all parts of the garlic plant are edible, including the flowers. Garlic, onions, leeks, chives, and other *Allium* vegetables are all members of the lily family (Liliaceae).

Large-scale commercial garlic production exists in many countries, including Egypt, China, India, South Korea, and Argentina; European nations such as France, Germany, Spain, and Hungary; and the United States. About 90 percent of the garlic grown in the United States comes from Gilroy, California, the self-proclaimed "Garlic Capital of the World."[2] Freshly harvested garlic is a special treat, and garlic is an easy plant to grow in your own garden. Plant in fall or early spring in a sunny spot in rich, moist, sandy soil, and harvest the bulbs when the leaves begin to wither.

The name *garlic* is believed to be derived from the old Anglo-Saxon words *gar* (meaning spear) and *lac* (plant), a reference to the spearlike shape of the leaves. The name *Allium* is believed to come from the Celtic word *all,* which means smarting or burning. The species name, *sativum,* means "cultivated."

BENEFITS

- Lowers serum cholesterol and triglyceride levels
- Improves the ratio of HDL (beneficial) to LDL (harmful) cholesterol
- Protects against oxidation of LDL
- Inhibits platelet aggregation
- Increases fibrinolysis
- Lowers blood pressure
- Improves peripheral circulation

- Acts as an antibacterial, antifungal, and antiviral agent
- Inhibits tumor formation (experimental)
- May protect many different organ systems against damage from toxins (experimental)
- Lowers blood sugar levels (experimental)

SCIENTIFIC SUPPORT

Garlic is one of the most extensively researched of all herbs. Modern garlic research has focused on four main areas: heart disease, cancer, infectious disease, and antioxidant effects. As of 1997, there were more than 1,200 published pharmacological studies (over 200 of these in humans) and 650 chemical studies on garlic. At least 40 countries have contributed to the body of research on garlic, with Germany, the United States, and India leading the way.[3]

Heart Health

The effects of garlic on cardiovascular health are the best known and have been studied for more than 30 years. In clinical studies, garlic reduced cholesterol levels, raised levels of healthful high-density lipoproteins (HDL cholesterol), and demonstrated antiplatelet or blood-thinning effects—all extremely important factors in preventing atherosclerosis, high blood pressure, heart attack, and stroke. Most of the best-designed research in this area—both positive and negative—used a daily dosage of 600 to 900 mg of a powdered garlic product standardized to alliin content.

HUMAN RESEARCH

A meta-analysis of clinical studies showed that consumption of the equivalent of $1/2$ to 1 clove of fresh garlic per day for time periods ranging from 2 to 4 months lowered cholesterol levels by 12 percent. The meta-analysis reviewed five well-designed placebo-controlled trials involving 365 adults with elevated cholesterol. Four of the studies in the meta-analysis used dried garlic powder tablets or spray-dried powder, and one used aged garlic.[4] Another meta-analysis, which evaluated results from 16 controlled trials involving a total of 952 subjects, also reported a 12 percent reduction in total cholesterol after at least 4 weeks of treatment with 600 to 900 mg a day of dried garlic powder (see Specific Studies).[5]

Other clinical studies showed that garlic improved circulation to the extremities both in healthy people[6] and in people with peripheral arterial disease.[7,8] In a placebo-controlled study of people with coronary artery disease, a solvent-extracted garlic oil preparation inhibited platelet aggregation (clumping), significantly lowered serum cholesterol and triglycerides, and significantly increased HDL and fibrinolysis (inactivation of a blood-clotting substance).[9]

In a cross-sectional study of elderly people, long-term garlic consumption was associated with prolonged elasticity of the aorta, the largest artery in the human body. Aortic stiffening has been linked to aging as well as to high blood pressure and cholesterol, and aortic elasticity is an important measure of the overall health of the cardiovascular system (see Specific Studies).[10] Clinical studies have also shown that garlic can help lower elevated blood pressure, particularly in mild cases.[11-14]

ANIMAL AND LABORATORY RESEARCH

The clinical results of the previously mentioned trials are well supported by animal and laboratory studies. In numerous studies, garlic powder and aged garlic supplements as well as fresh garlic have demonstrated an ability to lower cholesterol and blood pressure, reduce platelet aggregation (clumping), and inhibit the effects of fibrinogen (a protein involved in blood clotting). A certain amount of both platelet aggregation and fibrinogen are necessary for proper blood clotting, but too much can lead to atherosclerosis. All of garlic's effects in this area are important indicators of its ability to prevent the development of atherosclerosis at many different points in the process.[15-17] In addition, garlic has demonstrated an ability to protect against experimentally induced arrhythmias (abnormal heart beats) in animal studies.[18,19]

Antioxidant Effects

Because garlic is an antioxidant, it helps to prevent the oxidation of blood fats, another major contributor to the development of atherosclerosis and other forms of heart disease. Studies indicate that both dried garlic powder and aged garlic reduce the susceptibility of lipoproteins (blood fats) to oxidation.[16,20-22] In a placebo-controlled crossover study in 10 healthy volunteers, daily doses of garlic powder tablets (600 mg) taken for 2 weeks reduced the susceptibility of blood fats to oxidation by 34 percent.[21] Aged garlic extract and four of its constituents were effective in reducing oxidation of LDL in a laboratory study.[22] In another laboratory study, aged garlic and its constituent S-allyl-cysteine protected blood vessel cells from damage by oxidized LDL.[23]

Cancer

One of the most exciting areas in garlic research involves its potential cancer-preventive properties. A number of large epidemiological (population) studies have shown an association between consumption of garlic, onions, and other *Allium* vegetables and a lowered risk of certain cancers, particularly cancers of the gastrointestinal tract.[24] A Chinese population study drew a direct correlation between consumption of garlic and other *Allium* vegetables (such as onions) and a decreased risk for stomach cancer. In this study, people consuming the greatest amount of garlic and onions had only 40 percent the risk of stomach cancer of those consuming the lowest amount.[25] A 1994 study of 41,000 American women showed that one or more servings of garlic a week was associated with a 35 percent decrease in risk of colon cancer—the most significant reduction seen with any of the 127 foods studied.[26]

On the other hand, other studies detected no protective effects against breast, colon, stomach, or lung cancers.[19] Population studies like these have limitations, because even if they are very well controlled, factors other than the ones under investigation may confound the results. For example, results can be influenced by the subjects' inaccurate recall or reporting of their dietary habits.

Garlic has also demonstrated direct anticancer effects in experiments. In animal studies, garlic and a variety of garlic constituents interfered with the development of a number of different types of tumor cells, including colon, stomach, breast, prostate, esophageal, skin, and brain cancer cells.[16,19,27–31]

Antimicrobial Effects

Laboratory experiments have demonstrated that garlic has powerful effects against various disease-causing microbes, including bacteria, viruses, and fungi. These microbes include antibiotic-resistant strains of bacteria such as *Staphylococcus, Escherichia, Proteus,* and *Pseudomonas* as well as the herpes simplex virus and *Candida albicans* (the fungus that causes yeast infections).[32–35] In addition, more recent studies indicate that garlic has the ability to inhibit the growth of *Helicobacter pylori*, a bacterium associated with the development of stomach ulcers and gastric cancer.[36,37] Although laboratory results do not always translate directly into clinical benefits, these "test tube" results offer theoretical support for garlic's traditional reputation as an infection fighter and could help explain why people who consume large amounts of garlic may have a lower risk of stomach cancer.[36]

Other Actions

Based on evidence from laboratory studies, garlic also appears to have detoxifying, immune-stimulating, and liver-protective benefits, although these effects have not yet been as well studied.[16,38,39] Because some laboratory studies have suggested that garlic can lower blood sugar, the herb is under investigation for its potential in the treatment of diabetes.[16] In other studies, garlic and garlic constituents protected the liver against damage from free radicals and other toxins.[38] In addition, in a study designed to evaluate the tonic effects of garlic against physical and psychological stress, aged garlic appeared to be effective in delaying fatigue in mice undergoing different exercise tests.[40] In other preliminary research with mice, aged garlic helped prevent age-related brain changes, including atrophy and learning impairment.[41]

SPECIFIC STUDIES

Cholesterol: Meta-analysis (1994)

This analysis of clinical trials showed that treatment with garlic lowered total cholesterol levels by 12 percent after 1 to 3 months of treatment. Sixteen studies involving a total of 952 subjects were selected for inclusion in the meta-analysis. To be included, the trials had to be formally randomized and controlled, include at least two treatment groups, and be at least 4 weeks in duration. Only five of the trials were specifically designed to include people with elevated cholesterol; other trials included healthy volunteers or people with high blood pressure, existing coronary artery disease, diabetes, or increased spontaneous platelet aggregation. Eleven of the studies used standardized dried garlic powder in daily doses ranging from 600 mg to 900 mg. The other five used either fresh garlic, garlic extract, or garlic oil at various dosages.

The authors reported that many of the studies had methodological shortcomings. In the highest-quality trial, garlic lowered cholesterol as effectively as the drug bezafibrate. In addition, in the eight trials that provided data on these parameters, there was a 13 percent reduction in triglycerides and a slight, nonsignificant increase in HDL ("good" cholesterol) in subjects who took garlic powder. The rate of side effects in the trials was low, with the most frequently reported being garlic odor. The authors concluded that, "The currently available data support the likelihood of garlic therapy being beneficial, at least over a few months." However, they also emphasized the need for better designed, more rigorously controlled, and longer-lasting studies.[5]

Blood Pressure: Meta-analysis (1994)

Conducted by the same authors who performed the cholesterol meta-analysis summarized earlier, this meta-analysis suggested that standardized dried garlic may be an appropriate treatment for people with mild hypertension (high blood pressure). Here, the authors selected eight randomized, controlled, published or unpublished studies involving a total of 415 subjects. Only studies that were at least 4 weeks long, had a minimum of two treatment groups, and utilized a formal randomization method were considered for inclusion in the meta-analysis. Unfortunately, only three of the studies were specifically designed to include people with high blood pressure.

Of the six studies that compared garlic treatment with placebo, three demonstrated a significant reduction in systolic blood pressure, and four showed a significant reduction in diastolic blood pressure. Dosages used in the trials ranged from 600 mg to 900 mg a day of dried garlic standardized to 1.3 percent alliin content. Garlic odor was the most frequent side effect reported. According to the authors, "The results suggest that this garlic powder preparation may be of some clinical use in subjects with mild hypertension."

As with the previously described meta-analysis, the investigators noted that a number of the studies in the analysis had methodological shortcomings and that in their opinion, the clinical evidence on garlic's blood pressure-lowering effects remained inconclusive. They concluded that "more rigorously designed and analyzed trials are needed."[12]

Aortic Elasticity: Observational Study (1997)

In this cross-sectional observational study of 202 elderly people, researchers concluded that long-term consumption of garlic helped protect the elasticity of the aorta. Specifically, garlic consumption was associated with slowing the development of age-related aortic rigidity. The aorta is essential to the healthy function of the whole cardiovascular system, and aortic stiffening is linked with high blood pressure and elevated cholesterol as well as with aging. The study compared two equal-sized groups of healthy adults. One group had been taking standardized garlic powder supplements daily for at least 2 years in doses ranging from 300 mg to 900 mg a day, and the other reported no garlic supplementation. The subjects were also subdivided into three groups based on their level of reported garlic intake, in order to see if different dosages had any effect on improvements in aortic elasticity.

Aortic elasticity was assessed with measurements of cardiovascular function known as pulse wave velocity (PWV) and elastic vascular resistance (EVR). Both tests demonstrated a clear association between long-term garlic intake and decreased PWV and EVR, indicating greater aortic elasticity. The degree of improvement was about the same in all three dosage groups, but the differences in PWV between the garlic and control groups were more pronounced in older subjects. The investigators concluded, "These data strongly support the hypothesis that garlic intake had a protective effect on the elastic properties of the aorta related to aging in humans."[10]

HOW IT WORKS

Garlic has many actions and an extremely complex chemistry made up of hundreds of compounds. Researchers are still hard at work trying to determine which garlic constituents are responsible for its wide range of therapeutic effects.

In clinical studies, both raw and cooked garlic have demonstrated health effects, although cooking destroys the ability of garlic to produce *allicin,* a sulfur compound that many researchers believe is the most important contributor to garlic's health benefits. Technically, allicin is not present in whole garlic cloves, but is produced after the clove is crushed or chopped when an enzyme called *alliinase* interacts with alliin contained in garlic cells. In turn, allicin is the precursor to a number of other important garlic constituents, including ajoene, diallyl sulfide, and many other sulfur-containing compounds.

Studies point to allicin as the major source of garlic's antimicrobial action, and many garlic experts also consider allicin the key to garlic's cardiovascular benefits. (The characteristic strong odor of fresh garlic also comes from allicin.) However, other evidence suggests that allicin is not the only contributor to garlic's therapeutic effectiveness. For example, aged garlic (which yields little or no allicin) and cooked garlic have both demonstrated activity in clinical and pharmacological studies.

Different garlic-processing methods yield products with distinctly different chemical compositions, including variations in the amount of alliin or allicin potential. Because allicin is an unstable compound that begins to degrade shortly after it is produced, some manufacturers of garlic supplements have developed processing methods designed to stabilize or guarantee the allicin yield of the final product when it is consumed. This is what it means when you see the terms "allicin yield" or "allicin potential" on the labels of some standardized garlic products. Fresh raw garlic and products made from dried garlic powder contain the highest levels of allicin. Products made from distilled garlic oil, on the other hand, yield no allicin, but are good sources of the sulfur-containing breakdown products of allicin, such as diallyl sulfide. Products made by macerating (soaking) crushed garlic in vegetable oil yield high levels of ajoene and vinyldithiins. Aged garlic, while containing little or no alliin, contains the sulfur compounds S-allyl-cysteine and S-allyl-mercaptocysteine.

Some researchers believe that in order to provide the same benefits as fresh garlic, garlic tablets should be enteric coated so that important compounds are not destroyed by stomach acids.[3]

Cholesterol-Lowering Effects

Garlic appears to directly inhibit production of cholesterol by the liver and to enhance the excretion of cholesterol. In a laboratory study using cultured human and rat liver cells, low doses of garlic inhibited the effects of an enzyme called hydroxy-methylglutaryl-coenzyme A reductase (HMG-CoA reductase), which is important in the early stages of cholesterol synthesis. Higher doses of garlic hindered cholesterol production both at early and later stages.[42] Garlic may also enhance excretion of sterols and bile acids, as was demonstrated in an animal study comparing the cholesterol-lowering effects of S-allyl-cysteine with guggulipid.[43] Allicin, ajoene, adenosine, and a number of other compounds are believed to be important in garlic's lipid-lowering action.[3,15,41]

Effects on Blood Pressure

Garlic's precise mode of action in lowering blood pressure is not clear. However, in a laboratory study, garlic juice prepared from fresh garlic had a direct relaxant effect on cardiac and smooth muscles, which the investigators offered as an explanation for garlic's hypotensive (blood pressure–lowering) action.[44]

Antiplatelet and Antithrombotic Effects

Garlic and garlic constituents may reduce platelet aggregation by inhibiting synthesis of thromboxanes (substances that promote blood clotting) or by changing properties of the platelet membrane, or both.[45] Garlic also stimulates production of prostacyclin, which hinders the activity of thromboxane A2.[16] In one placebo-controlled clinical study, solvent-extracted garlic oil and the constituents diallyl disulfide and diallyl trisulfide inhibited the formation of thromboxanes and reduced platelet aggregation. The garlic oil preparation also increased fibrinolytic activity (the breakdown of fibrin, a blood-clotting protein derived from fibrinogen).[9]

Another group of researchers proposed that garlic's antiplatelet activity and other cardiovascular effects may be due to activation of nitric oxide synthase (NOS) and subsequent production of nitric oxide. The correlation between low levels of nitric oxide and high blood pressure has been known since 1991, and this research correlated the effect of garlic extract on NOS and platelet aggregation.[46] Raw, dried, aged, and macerated garlic as well as garlic oil have all demonstrated antiplatelet effects. Ajoene may be one of the most potent antiplatelet compounds in garlic.[19]

Studies have suggested that garlic can both increase fibrinolytic activity and lower fibrinogen levels.[45] In an *in vitro* study using an experimental model of blood vessel wall injury, the constituent ajoene prevented the formation of thrombi (blood clots) at the site of blood vessel injury. The investigators suggested that this effect is related to its ability to inhibit fibrinogen binding, that is, the adhesion of platelets to fibrinogen.[47] Aged garlic extract also interfered with platelet adhesion to fibrinogen in people with elevated cholesterol,[20] and garlic oil reduced platelet adhesiveness in rabbits with high cholesterol.[16] Researchers have shown that both fresh and dried garlic enhance fibrinolysis,[19] and studies suggest that in high doses, cooked garlic can also increase fibrinolysis and inhibit thrombus formation.[3,16,45]

Atherosclerosis Prevention

Garlic's protective actions against the development of atherosclerosis are due in part to its antiplatelet effects as well as to its ability to inhibit oxidation of LDL. In addition, studies have suggested that garlic exerts direct antiatherosclerotic effects on arterial cells.[15,17] In a laboratory study utilizing smooth muscle cells derived from human atherosclerotic plaques, treatment with garlic reduced the tendency of the cells to retain cholesterol and cholesteryl esters and inhibited plaque cell proliferation. In the same study, garlic reduced cholesterol accumulation and cell proliferation in four volunteers with atherosclerosis.[15] Part of garlic's protective effect against atherosclerosis may stem from its ability to inhibit the production of eicosanoids (such as leukotrienes) involved in inflammation, because inflammation is a factor in early-stage development of atherosclerosis.[9]

Anticancer Effects

Current anticancer research is focused on a number of different sulfur-containing compounds, including diallyl sulfide, S-allyl-mercaptocysteine, S-allyl-cysteine, and ajoene. In laboratory and animal studies, these constituents inhibited the growth of tumors at different stages in cancer development.[19,27–31,48] Researchers theorize that garlic's sulfur compounds may exert anticancer effects by affecting the activity of enzymes involved in carcinogenesis, such as cytochrome P-450 and glutathione S-transferases.[27,49]

Antimicrobial Effects

Although allicin is widely believed to be the most important antimicrobial compound in garlic, other constituents are important contributors. Ajoene in particular has demonstrated effects against a number of different bacterial and fungal disease-causing organisms.[19,50]

"Garlic Breath" and Other Respiratory Effects

The unmistakable odor known as "garlic breath" is a well-known consequence of eating fresh garlic. For about the first hour after consumption, garlic odor on the breath is caused by excretion of allyl mercaptan from the throat. After that, however, the smell can be largely attributed to excretion of allyl methyl sulfide through the lungs, which lasts for about 24 hours.[3]

Traditional herbalists believe that in the presence of respiratory tract infection, the excretion of garlic compounds through the lungs brings some of garlic's antimicrobial properties into direct contact with the site of infection. This is one possible explanation for garlic's reputation for effectiveness in the treatment of colds, flu, and other respiratory tract infections.

MAJOR CONSTITUENTS

Alliin, alliinase (depending on preparation, breakdown products include allicin and other thiosulfinates, diallyl sulfide and other allyl sulfides, ajoene, vinyldithiins, S-allyl-cysteine, S-allyl-mercaptocysteine, and many other sulfur-containing compounds); amino acids; glycosides; vitamins; minerals; trace elements, including selenium and germanium

SAFETY

Garlic has a long history of safe use as a food. Garlic supplements have an excellent safety record and are well tolerated by most people.

- **Side effects:** There is no known toxicity, although garlic can cause mild stomach upset or irritation in sensitive individuals.[51] Taking garlic supplements with food may reduce the chance of stomach irritation. Fresh garlic or garlic oil applied externally may burn the skin.[1]
- **Contraindications:** Consumption of garlic as a food during pregnancy has a long history of safe use. However, some experts recommend that concentrated garlic products be used with caution during pregnancy and nursing. Garlic excreted in breast milk could cause colic in sensitive infants. In addition, garlic may flavor breast milk, although some babies are reported to like the taste.[3] If you have a blood-clotting disorder, talk to your doctor before using concentrated garlic products.

- **Drug interactions:** None known. However, because of garlic's blood-thinning effects, avoid taking concentrated garlic products in combination with prescription anticoagulant medications or other medications with blood-thinning effects, such as aspirin. By the same token, if you are scheduled to have surgery, it is a good idea to discontinue garlic supplements beforehand to reduce the risk of excessive postoperative bleeding. Consult your doctor.

DOSAGE

Because of the telltale odor garlic leaves on the breath when eaten as a food, many people prefer to take garlic in the convenient forms of concentrated supplements, including tablets, capsules, and softgel "perles" of garlic oil.

Garlic supplements vary considerably in strength. Some manufacturers make specific claims about the allicin yield or the allicin-releasing potential of their extracts. If in doubt, ask the manufacturer for substantiation of the benefits of the dosage they recommend for their product.

The health benefits of garlic are associated with regular and long-term use. All of the dosages listed here are based on effective dosages used in clinical studies with various product forms.

- **Garlic powder tablets/capsules:** 600 to 900 mg per day

- **Aged garlic extract:** 4 ml a day
- **Garlic oil "perles":** 10 mg a day
- **Fresh garlic:** One moderate-size fresh clove a day (3 to 4 grams)

STANDARDIZATION

Garlic is often standardized to "allicin yield" or "allicin potential." For example, garlic may be standardized to contain 1.3 percent alliin, corresponding to an allicin release of 0.6 percent.

REFERENCES

1. Bergner P. *The Healing Power of Garlic.* Rocklin, CA: Prima Publishing, 1995.
2. Hahn G. Botanical characterization and cultivation of garlic. In: Koch HP, Lawson LD, eds. *Garlic: The Science and Therapeutic Application of Allium sativum L. and Related Species.* Baltimore: Williams & Wilkins, 1996.
3. Lawson LD. Garlic: a review of its medicinal effects and indicated active compounds. In: Lawson LD, Bauer R, eds. *Phytomedicines of Europe.* Washington, DC: American Chemical Society, 1998.
4. Warshafsky S, Kamer RS, Sivak SL. Effect of garlic on total serum cholesterol. A meta-analysis. *Annals of Internal Medicine* 1993; 119: 599–605.
5. Silagy C, Neil A. Garlic as a lipid-lowering agent—a meta-analysis. *The Journal of the Royal College of Physicians* 1994; 28(1): 39–45.
6. Okuhara T. A clinical study of garlic extract on peripheral circulation. *Japanese Pharmacology and Therapeutics* 1994; 22(8): 3695–3701.
7. Kiesewetter H, Jung F, Jung EM, et al. Effects of garlic coated tablets in peripheral arterial occlusive disease. *The Clinical Investigator* 1993; 71: 383–386.
8. Kiesewetter H, Jung F, Pindur G, et al. Effect of garlic on thrombocyte aggregation, microcirculation, and other risk factors. *International Journal of Clinical Pharmacology, Therapy, and Toxicology* 1991; 29(4): 151–155.
9. Bordia A, Verma SK, Srivastava KC. Effect of garlic *(Allium sativum)* on blood lipids, blood sugar, fibrinogen and fibrinolytic activity in patients with coronary artery disease. *Prostaglandins, Leukotrienes and Essential Fatty Acids* 1998; 58(4): 257–263.
10. Breithaupt-Grögler K, Ling M, Boudoulas J, et al. Protective effect of chronic garlic intake on elastic properties of aorta in the elderly. *Circulation* 1997; 96(8): 2649–2655.
11. Auer W, Eiber A, Hertkorn E, et al. Hypertension and hyperlipidaemia: garlic helps in mild cases. *The British Journal of Clinical Practice* 1990; 44(8)(suppl 69): 3–6.
12. Silagy CA, Neil HAW. A meta-analysis of the effect of garlic on blood pressure. *Journal of Hypertension* 1994; 12(4): 14–18.
13. McMahon FG, Vargas R. Can garlic lower blood pressure? A pilot study. *Pharmacotherapy* 1993; 13(4): 406–407.
14. Barrie SA, Wright JV, Pizzorno JE. Effects of garlic oil on platelet aggregation, serum lipids and blood pressure in humans.

Journal of Orthomolecular Medicine 1987; 2(1): 15–21.

15. Orekhov AN, Tertov VV, Sobenin IA, et al. Direct anti-atherosclerosis-related effects of garlic. *Annals of Medicine* 1995; 27: 63–65.

16. Reuter HD. *Allium sativum* and *Allium ursinum:* part 2. Pharmacology and Medicinal Application. *Phytomedicine* 1995; 2(1): 73–91.

17. Efendy JL, Simmons DL, Campbell GR, et al. The effect of the aged garlic extract, 'Kyolic,' on the development of experimental atherosclerosis. *Atherosclerosis* 1997; 132: 37–42.

18. Martin N, Bardisa L, Pantoja C, et al. Anti-arrhythmic profile of a garlic dialysate assayed in dogs and isolated atrial preparations. *Journal of Ethnopharmacology* 1994; 43: 1–8.

19. Nagourney RA. Garlic: medicinal food or nutritious medicine? *Journal of Medicinal Food* 1998; 1(1): 13–27.

20. Steiner M, Lin RS. Changes in platelet function and susceptibility of lipoproteins to oxidation associated with administration of aged garlic extract. *Journal of Cardiovascular Pharmacology* 1998; 31(6): 904–908.

21. Phelps S, Harris WS. Garlic supplementation and lipoprotein oxidation susceptibility. *Lipids* 1993; 28(5): 475–477.

22. Ide N, Nelson AB. Aged garlic extract and its constituents inhibit $Cu2+$-induced oxidative modification of low density lipoprotein. *Planta Medica* 1997; 63: 263–264.

23. Ide N, Lau BHS. Garlic compounds protect vascular endothelial cells from oxidized low density lipoprotein-induced injury. *Journal of Pharmacy and Pharmacology* 1997; 49: 908–911.

24. Ernst E. Can Allium vegetables prevent cancer? *Phytomedicine* 1997; 4(1): 79–83.

25. You W-C, Blot WJ, Chang Y-S, et al. Allium vegetables and reduced risk of stomach cancer. *Journal of the National Cancer Institute* 1989; 81: 162–164.

26. Steinmetz KA, Kushi LH, Bostick RM, et al. Vegetables, fruit, and colon cancer in the Iowa women's health study. *American Journal of Epidemiology* 1994; 139(1): 1–15.

27. Sigounas G, Hooker J, Anagnostou A, et al. S-Allylmercaptocysteine inhibits cell proliferation and reduces the viability of erythroleukemia, breast, and prostate cancer cell lines. *Nutrition and Cancer* 1997; 27(2): 186–191.

28. Pinto JT, Qiao C, Xing J, et al. Effects of garlic thioallyl derivatives on growth, glutathione concentration, and polyamine formation of human prostate carcinoma cells in culture. *American Journal of Clinical Nutrition* 1997; 66: 398–405.

29. Dorant E, van den Brandt PA, Goldbohm RA, et al. Garlic and its significance for the prevention of cancer in humans: a critical view. *British Journal of Cancer* 1993; 67: 424–429.

30. Welch C, Wuarin L, Sidell N. Antiproliferative effect of the garlic compound S-allyl cysteine on human neuroblastoma cells in vitro. *Cancer Letters* 1992; 63: 211–219.

31. Wargovich MJ. Diallyl sulfide, a flavor component of garlic *(Allium sativum),* inhibits dimethylhydrazine-induced colon cancer. *Carcinogenesis* 1987; 8(3): 487–489.

32. Ashan M, Islam SN. Garlic: a broad spectrum antibacterial agent effective against common pathogenic bacteria. *Fitoterapia* 1996; 67(4): 374–376.

33. Singh KV, Shukla NP. Activity on multiple resistant bacteria of garlic *(Allium sativum)* extract. *Fitoterapia* 1984; 55(5): 313–315.

34. Weber ND, Andersen DO, North JA, et al. In vitro virucidal effects of *Allium sativum* (garlic) extract and compounds. *Planta Medica* 1992; 58: 417–423.

35. Adetumbi M, Javor GT, Lau BHS. Allium sativum (garlic) inhibits lipid synthesis by *Candida albicans. Antimicrobial Agents and Chemotherapy* 1986; 30(3): 499–501.

36. Sivam GP, Lampe JW, Ulness B, et al. *Helicobacter pylori*—in vitro susceptibility to garlic *(Allium sativum)* extract. *Nutrition and Cancer* 1997; 27(2): 118–121.

37. Cellini L, Di Campli E, Masulli M, et al. Inhibition of *Helicobacter pylori* by garlic extract *(Allium sativum). FEMS Immunology and Medical Microbiology* 1996; 13: 273–277.

38. Nakagawa S, Kasuga S, Matsuura H. Prevention of liver damage by aged garlic extract and its components in mice. *Phytotherapy Research* 1989; 3(2): 50–53.

39. Lau BHS. Detoxifying, radioprotective, and phagocyte-enhancing effects of garlic. *International Clinical Nutrition Review* 1989; 9(1): 27–31.

40. Ushijima M, Sumioka I, Kakimoto M, et al. Effect of garlic and garlic preparations on physiological and psychological stress in mice. *Phytotherapy Research* 1997; 2: 226–230.

41. Moriguchi T, Saito J, Nishiyama N. Anti-ageing effect of aged garlic extract in the inbred brain atrophy mouse model. *Clinical and Experimental Pharmacology and Physiology* 1997; 24: 235–242.

42. Gebhardt R. Multiple inhibitory effects of garlic extracts on cholesterol biosynthesis in hepatocytes. *Lipids* 1993; 28(7): 613–619.

43. Sheela CG, Augusti KT. Effects of S-allyl cysteine sulfoxide isolated from *Allium sativum* Linn and gugulipid on some enzymes and fecal excretions of bile acids and sterols in cholesterol fed rats. *Indian Journal of Experimental Biology* 1995; 33: 749–751.

44. Aqel MB, Gharaibah MN, Salhab AS. Direct relaxant effects of garlic juice on smooth and cardiac muscles. *Journal of Ethnopharmacology* 1991; 33: 13–19.

45. Neil A, Silagy C. Garlic: its cardioprotective properties. *Current Opinion in Lipidology* 1994; 5: 6–10.

46. Das I, Khan NS, Sooranna SR. Potent activation of nitric oxide synthase by garlic: a basis for its therapeutic applications. *Current Medical Research and Opinion* 1995; 13(5): 257–263.

47. Apitz-Castro R, Badimon JJ, Badimon L. Effect of ajoene, the major antiplatelet compound from garlic, on platelet thrombus formation. *Thrombosis Research* 1992; 68(2): 145–155.

48. Scharfenberg K, Ryll T, Wagner R, et al. Injuries to cultivated BJA-B cells by ajoene, a garlic-derived natural compound: cell viability, glutathione metabolism, and pools of acidic amino acids. *Journal of Cellular Physiology* 1994; 158: 55–60.

49. Lee ES, Steiner M, Lin R. Thioallyl compounds: potent inhibitors of cell prolifera-

tion. *Biochimica et Biophysica Acta* 1994; 1221: 73–77.

50. Yoshida S, Kasuga S, Hayashi N, et al. Antifungal activity of ajoene derived from garlic. *Applied and Environmental Microbiology* 1987; 53(3): 615–617.

51. McGuffin M, Hobbs C, Upton R, et al., eds. *American Herbal Products Association Botanical Safety Handbook*. Boca Raton, FL: CRC Press, 1997.

Ginger

ZINGIBER OFFICINALE
ZINGIBERACEAE

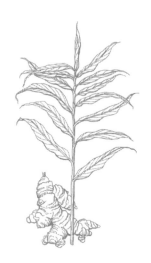

PART USED: *Rhizome*

PRIMARY USES

- *Motion sickness*
- *Nausea and vomiting*
- *Appetite and digestion*
- *Heart health*
- *Pain and inflammation of arthritis (traditional/experimental)*
- *Migraine (traditional)*
- *Antioxidant*

Pungent, aromatic ginger is one of the best-known folk remedies for settling upset stomachs. But what some may not realize is that this remarkable "kitchen medicine" is a veritable treasure-chest of health benefits. While the most extensively researched medicinal uses of ginger are for alleviating nausea and vomiting, preventing motion sickness, and aiding digestive function, research continues to confirm other traditional uses and reveal potential new ones. Some of the most promising research suggests that ginger may have value in the prevention of heart disease. Other preliminary studies offer scientific support for ginger's traditional use for arthritis in the Ayurvedic healing tradition.

Numerous cultures throughout the ages have appreciated ginger's warming, soothing effects on the digestive tract. The herb also has a long history of use worldwide for improving appetite and promoting healthy digestion. Now scientists know that ginger contains digestion-enhancing enzymes very similar to those found in papaya fruit, another well-known digestive aid.

In laboratory studies, ginger has demonstrated antioxidant activity and the ability to kill many different types of bacteria and fungi. In hot tropical countries where ginger is a daily food staple, these antioxidant and antimicrobial properties serve as preservatives to help keep food from spoiling.

Ginger offers important benefits for the circulatory system, too. As with herbs like garlic, ginkgo, and turmeric, ginger inhibits platelet-activating factor (PAF), a naturally occurring substance in the body that is essential to blood clotting and inflammatory processes. While adequate levels of PAF are needed to maintain proper body function, excess PAF has been implicated in the development of many conditions, including heart disease, allergies, asthma, and inflammatory disorders such as psoriasis.

HISTORY

Possibly one of the first plants to be cultivated by humankind, ginger has been employed and valued by nearly every major culture in the world. Ginger has been in continuous use as food and medicine in Asia for at least 5,000 years, and to this day the herb remains a key remedy in both traditional Chinese medicine and Indian Ayurvedic

medicine. Ancient Indians called ginger *vishwabhesaj*, meaning "the universal medicine."

One of the most important traditional Ayurvedic uses of ginger is for reducing the pain and inflammation of arthritis. It is sometimes applied externally, as a paste, to painful joints. Ayurvedic healers also consider ginger a treatment for neurological disorders (including migraine), digestive problems, fever, asthma, gout, and coughs. In traditional Chinese medicine, ginger has been used to treat ulcers, colds, hemorrhage, stomachache, diarrhea, and nausea, and as an external remedy for wounds and burns.

In the Western world, herbalists from the Greek Dioscorides to the American Eclectic physicians (an important group of doctors who practiced during the late nineteenth and early twentieth centuries) have regarded ginger as a premier digestive remedy. Ginger has a strong traditional reputation for settling digestive upsets of all kinds and for helping to dispel flatulence and relieve gastrointestinal spasms. In numerous cultures, ginger is a staple remedy for colds and is brewed into a soothing expectorant tea for relieving coughs. The herb has also been used to expel parasites, to warm the body and enhance circulation, and to promote diaphoresis (perspiration) in order to cool the body during fever.

INTERNATIONAL STATUS

Today, ginger is sold as an approved over-the-counter remedy for nausea and motion sickness in a number of European countries, including Germany, Belgium, and the United Kingdom. It is listed in the *German Commission E Monographs* as an approved herb for treating dyspepsia (indigestion) and preventing motion sickness.[1] In the United Kingdom, ginger is also sold as an antimigraine preparation.

BOTANY

Ginger (*Zingiber officinale*) is a member of the tropical plant family Zingiberaceae, a group of important spice-producing plants that also includes turmeric, cardamom, and galanga. Although many people think of the medicinal part of ginger as a root, it is actually a *rhizome,* which is a kind of creeping, underground stem. The knotty, irregularly shaped fresh ginger rhizomes sold in grocery stores are known in the botanical trade as "hands." Both fresh and dried ginger are used medicinally. The botanical name *Zingiber* comes from the original Sanskrit word for ginger, *singabera,* meaning "shaped like a horn."

Believed to have originated in southern Asia, ginger is now widely cultivated in tropical regions around the globe for the spice and medicinal plant trade. Among the most important ginger-producing nations in the world are Indonesia, Jamaica, China, Australia, India, and a number of African countries. A multitude of different varieties are grown, each possessing subtle variations in aroma, flavor, and pungency. Ginger is reported to be virtually unknown in the wild today.

BENEFITS

- Enhances peristalsis (gastrointestinal motility)
- Reduces gastrointestinal spasms
- Promotes secretion of digestive juices, including bile
- May help lower cholesterol
- Inhibits platelet-activating factor and prostaglandins

SCIENTIFIC SUPPORT

A number of well-controlled clinical studies have demonstrated ginger's effectiveness in preventing motion sickness.[2–4] Ginger does not work for everyone, but in some of the clinical trials, it was as effective or more effective than the commonly used motion sickness medicines against which it was tested, including Dramamine. In the studies, ginger alleviated or reduced the intensity of all symptoms related to the motion sickness syndrome, including nausea, vomiting, dizziness, and cold sweating. Ginger has a major advantage over synthetic motion sickness drugs in that it has a much better safety record. Motion sickness drugs can cause side effects such as drowsiness and visual disturbances, a potentially serious risk in drivers, pilots, and others who need to stay alert. Two motion sickness studies reported negative findings for the efficacy of ginger.

According to other studies, ginger may help with some of the most troubling causes of stomach upset, including postoperative nausea and vomiting,[5,6] chemotherapy,[7] and *hyperemesis gravidarum,* an extremely severe, sometimes life-threatening form of morning sickness.[8] Once again, ginger's excellent safety profile gives it an edge over conventional antinausea drugs, which cause side effects that can be especially problematic during pregnancy or recovery from anesthesia.

A limited amount of research in humans has shown that ginger may be helpful in the treatment of arthritis and migraine, two traditional uses of ginger in Ayurvedic medicine. One paper reported on 56 case studies of patients with rheumatic and musculoskeletal disorders who treated themselves with ginger for time periods ranging from 3 months to 2.5 years. Twenty-eight of these patients had rheumatoid arthritis, 18 osteoarthritis, and 10 muscular discomfort. More than 75 percent of the people with arthritis reported relief of pain and inflammation, and all of the people with muscular discomfort noted a marked reduction in pain.[9] This was not a controlled study, but the results are encouraging. Future research should shed more light on ginger's role in the treatment of these common and crippling disorders.

Preliminary research suggests that ginger may help protect against the development of stomach ulcers, lower cholesterol by stimulating the production of bile, protect the liver from toxins, tone the heart muscle, and regulate blood pressure.[10] Although more research is needed before these results can be directly applied to humans, it seems safe to conclude that regular ginger use can be a valuable addition to an overall strategy for maintaining wellness.

SPECIFIC STUDIES

Motion Sickness: Clinical Study (1994)

This large-scale study showed that ginger was just as effective as a variety of synthetic motion sickness drugs for preventing typical symptoms, including malaise, nausea, vomiting, and cold sweating. The randomized double-blind study involved 1,741 tourists participating in a Norwegian whale-watching safari, a 6-hour trip on high seas. According to the tour company, when no motion sickness prophylaxis (prevention) was taken, the trip usually resulted in seasickness for about 80 percent of passengers.

The study compared the effects of ginger against seven commonly used motion sickness medicines (cinnarizine, cinnarizine with domperidone, cyclizine, dimenhydrinate with caffeine, meclizine with caffeine, and scopolamine). The volunteers took either ginger or one of the test medications 2 hours before boarding the boat and recorded their symptoms on questionnaires, which were collected at the end of the trip. Overall, 82 to 85.5 percent of the volunteers reported feeling well or very well during the trip. Although none of the test medications protected every one of the study volunteers against seasickness, ginger proved to be "as potent an agent as the others." People taking scopolamine experienced more illness and a greater number of adverse effects than those using other substances. The dose of ginger used in the study was 250 mg.[3]

Postoperative Nausea and Vomiting: Clinical Study (1990)

In a double-blind, placebo-controlled study of 60 women undergoing major gynecological surgery, ginger performed significantly better than placebo and was as effective as the injectable antinausea drug metoclopramide in preventing the nausea and vomiting caused by anesthesia. The women in the study were randomized into three study groups of 20 each. One group received treatment with a ginger capsule plus a placebo injection, one with a placebo capsule and an injection of metoclopramide, and the third with a placebo capsule and a placebo injection.

Compared with placebo, there were significantly fewer incidences of nausea and vomiting among women who took ginger. The rate of nausea and vomiting was similar among patients who received ginger or the synthetic drug (specifically, 28 percent, 30 percent, and 51 percent in the ginger, metoclopramide, and placebo groups, respectively). The researchers concluded, "Ginger has the major advantage over other substances in that it does not have any recorded side effects." The dose of ginger used in the study was 1 gram.[5]

Morning Sickness: Clinical Study (1990)

This double-blind crossover study showed ginger to be significantly better than placebo in alleviating the nausea and vomiting of hyperemesis gravidarum, a particularly severe form of morning sickness. Thirty pregnant women underwent 4 days of treatment with either placebo or powdered ginger capsules at a dosage of 250 mg given four times a day (a total daily dose of 1 gram of ginger). Next, the two treatment groups were switched so that the women who had been taking placebo took ginger, and vice versa. (Three patients were excluded from the study before the end of the treatment period, two because they did not take the required number of ginger capsules, and one because she was diagnosed with a gallstone during the trial.)

At the end of the study, 70 percent of the women stated that they had greater relief of morning sickness symptoms during the time they were taking ginger. Objective assessment of relief scores by the investigators confirmed that ginger provided significantly greater symptom relief. One woman in the study had a miscarriage at 12 weeks, but the investigators did not feel that this was related to treatment with ginger. The other women had normal deliveries of healthy infants. No side effects were reported.[8]

HOW IT WORKS

The pungent principles (the ingredients responsible for ginger's fragrance), especially gingerol and shogaol, are believed responsible for most of ginger's therapeutic effects.

Antinausea, Digestive, and Cholesterol Lowering Effects

Researchers currently believe that ginger's effectiveness against motion sickness is due to direct action on the digestive system. Synthetic motion sickness drugs, on the other hand, prevent nausea and vomiting by acting on the central nervous system, often causing side effects such as drowsiness and visual disturbances.

Laboratory studies show that ginger improves gastrointestinal motility (peristalsis), reduces spasms, and absorbs and neutralizes toxins in the gastrointestinal tract. Ginger also increases the secretion of digestive juices, including saliva and bile. Ginger's ef-

fect on cholesterol appears to be twofold. In studies, ginger both inhibited the absorption of cholesterol by the body and enhanced its excretion by encouraging the conversion of cholesterol to bile acids.[10]

Anti-Inflammatory Effects

Ginger shares two important actions with the nonsteroidal anti-inflammatory drugs (NSAIDs) commonly used to treat arthritis and other painful conditions. Like NSAIDs, ginger inhibits the synthesis of prostaglandins and leukotrienes, substances that play a key role in pain, inflammation, and fever. However, unlike NSAIDs, ginger selectively blocks only certain prostaglandins, leaving levels of beneficial prostaglandins unaffected.

Antiplatelet Activity

The other action that ginger shares with NSAIDs is its effect on platelet aggregation. Ginger exerts powerful antiplatelet effects, meaning that it helps prevent blood platelets from adhering to one another and forming clumps. This antiplatelet action supports the healthy function of the circulatory system, helping to keep blood flowing smoothly to all parts of the body and preventing the development of atherosclerotic plaques in the blood vessels.

Aspirin also has antiplatelet effects, which is why doctors recommend it in small daily doses to help protect against heart disease.

However, unlike aspirin and other NSAIDs, therapeutic doses of ginger inhibit platelet aggregation without affecting the ability of the blood to coagulate. In one study in healthy volunteers, 2 grams of dried ginger had no effect on the results of bleeding time tests, which are used to assess the ability of the blood to coagulate. The dose of ginger used in this study was twice as high as that used in most clinical studies.[11]

Ginger inhibits platelet-activating factor by hindering the formation of thromboxanes, substances that promote blood clotting, while encouraging the synthesis of prostacyclin, an inhibitor of platelet aggregation. In one comparative experiment, ginger had a more potent antiplatelet effect than garlic and onion, two plants well known for their blood-thinning actions.[12]

Pain Relief

Like capsaicin from cayenne peppers, ginger may help to relieve pain when used externally by blocking the effects of a neurotransmitter called *substance P,* which is responsible for transmitting pain impulses in nerve endings.[10]

MAJOR CONSTITUENTS

Pungent principles (gingerol, shogaol, zingerone), volatile oils (bisabolene, zingiberene, zingiberol), proteolytic enzymes

SAFETY

Fresh ginger root is considered safe for consumption when used appropriately. Any contraindications for dried ginger are based on medicinal use, not on consumption in small doses as a spice.[13]

- **Side effects:** Rare reports of heartburn.
- **Contraindications:** People with gallstones should consult a physician before using dried ginger root in therapeutic doses.[1] The *German Commission E Monographs* recommends against the use of ginger in pregnancy (see Ginger and Pregnancy: A Continuing Debate).[1]
- **Drug interactions:** None known.[1,13] Theoretically, because of its antiplatelet (blood-thinning) effects, therapeutic doses of ginger might enhance the effects of other blood-thinning medications. However, one study showed that ginger at a dose of 2 grams had no effect on bleeding times in normal volunteers.[11]

Ginger and Pregnancy: A Continuing Debate

The German Commission E recommends against the use of ginger by pregnant women. However, an editor's note in the English translation of the *Monographs* states,

"A review of clinical literature could not justify this caution. There is no evidence that ginger causes harm to the mother or fetus."[1] Some experts feel that the caution is based not on direct evidence of harm but on reluctance to recommend any substance that has not been fully studied for use in pregnancy. There are no reports in the scientific literature of miscarriage or birth defects related to the use of ginger during pregnancy.[14]

As a food, ginger has been consumed by millions of pregnant women throughout history, without any evidence of adverse effects. The FDA considers doses of ginger up to 5 grams to be safe for consumption as a food.[14] The dose of ginger used in the hyperemesis gravidarum study described earlier was 1 gram a day, which, in the study authors' words, "did not exceed amounts prescribed in recipes for cakes or tarts."[8]

DOSAGE

Most clinical studies investigating ginger's effects in motion sickness and nausea used a dosage of 1 gram per day of powdered dried ginger taken as capsules. To prevent motion sickness, ginger is best taken at least one-half hour before beginning travel. (If you are already feeling sick, it is probably too late for ginger!)

- **Dried ginger capsules:** 1 gram (1,000 mg) a day

STANDARDIZATION

Some ginger products are standardized to 0.8% essential oils or 4% volatile oils.

REFERENCES

1. Blumenthal M, Busse W, Goldberg A, et al., eds. *The Complete German Commission E Monographs.* Austin, TX: The American Botanical Council; Boston: Integrative Medical Communications, 1998.

2. Mowrey DB, Clayson DE. Motion sickness, ginger, and psychophysics. *The Lancet* 1982; March 20: 655–657.

3. Schmid R, Schick T, Steffen R, et al. Comparison of seven commonly used agents for prophylaxis of seasickness. *Journal of Travel Medicine* 1994; 1(4): 203–206.

4. Grøntved A, Brask T, Kambskard J, et al. Ginger root against seasickness. *Acta Otolaryngology* 1988; 105: 45–49.

5. Bone ME, Wilkinson DJ, Young JR, et al. Ginger root—a new antiemetic. *Anaesthesia* 1990; 45(8): 669–672.

6. Phillips S, Ruggier R, Hutchinson SE. *Zingiber officinale* (ginger)—an antiemetic for day case surgery. *Anaesthesia* 1993; 48: 715–717.

7. Meyer K, Schwartz J, Crater D, et al. *Zingiber officinale* (ginger) used to prevent 8-MOP associated nausea. *Dermatology Nursing* 1995; 7(4): 242–244.

8. Fischer-Rasmussen W, Kjaer SK, Dahl C, et al. Ginger treatment of hyperemesis gravidarum. *European Journal of Obstetrics & Gyne-*

cology, and Reproductive Biology 1990; 38: 19–24.

9. Srivastava KC, Mustafa T. Ginger (Zingiber officinale) in rheumatism and musculoskeletal disorders. Medical Hypotheses 1992; 39: 432–348.

10. Murray M. The Healing Power of Herbs. Rocklin, CA: Prima Publishing, 1995.

11. Lumb AB. Effect of dried ginger on human platelet function. Thrombosis and Haemostasis 1994; 71(1): 110–111.

12. Srivastava KC. Effects of aqueous extracts of onion, garlic and ginger on platelet aggregation and metabolism of arachidonic acid in the blood vascular system: in vitro study. Prostaglandins Leukotrienes and Medicine 1984; 13: 227–235.

13. McGuffin M, Hobbs C, Upton R, et al., eds. American Herbal Products Association Botanical Safety Handbook. Boca Raton, FL: CRC Press, 1997.

14. Bergner P. Is ginger safe during pregnancy? Medical Herbalism 1991; 3(3): 7.

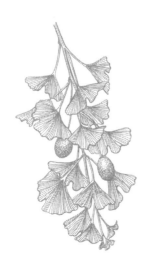

Ginkgo

GINKGO BILOBA
GINKGOACEAE

PART USED: *Leaf*

PRIMARY USES

- *Memory and brain function*
- *Circulation enhancement to the brain, heart, limbs, ears, and eyes*
- *Alzheimer's disease, cerebral insufficiency, senile dementia*
- *Peripheral artery disease*
- *Certain eye and ear disorders*
- *Cardiovascular health*
- *Antioxidant*

As one of the oldest surviving species on earth, ginkgo's reputation as an "anti-aging" herb seems especially appropriate. The remarkable effects of *Ginkgo biloba* on memory, brain function, and circulation have made this venerable tree one of the most extensively studied and widely used botanicals in the world. The herb's popularity is well deserved, because strong clinical evidence shows that it can help improve declining brain function in elderly people, even those with Alzheimer's disease.

Ginkgo has a broad range of beneficial actions that many researchers believe work synergistically to contribute to its benefits as a *neuroprotective agent*—a technical term for a substance that helps protect the brain and enhance brain function. No other known circulation enhancer, natural or synthetic, can increase blood flow not only to healthy areas of the brain but also to areas already damaged by disease or injury. Ginkgo leaf extract also improves circulation to the limbs, reducing symptoms such as coldness, numbness, and cramping, and increasing pain-free walking distance in people with peripheral artery disease.

Best known for its beneficial effects in cerebral insufficiency (impaired blood flow to the brain) and senile dementia, ginkgo is also recommended by European physicians for disorders such as peripheral artery disease, tinnitus (ringing in the ears), and dimming vision due to lack of blood flow and consequent oxygen deprivation. Not long ago, an important study published in the *Journal of the American Medical Association* confirmed that ginkgo leaf extract can be helpful in improving brain function and slowing the progression of Alzheimer's disease.[1] This is welcome news to the thousands of people whose lives are painfully affected by this devastating disorder.

Today, millions of Americans and Europeans enjoy the benefits of ginkgo for enhancing cognitive function, maintaining healthy blood flow, and treating a variety of health conditions. In addition, ginkgo's powerful antioxidant effects have earned it an international reputation among young and old alike as a longevity herb.

HISTORY

Contrary to popular belief, the use of ginkgo leaf to enhance brain function is relatively new in worldwide herbal traditions. Although ginkgo fruit and nut have been used for thousands of years as food and medicine in Asia, ginkgo leaf was not widely prescribed by traditional Chinese practitioners. The modern use of ginkgo leaf became popular in the 1950s, when German researchers began investigating its beneficial effects in improving circulation. Today, Chinese herbalists recommend ginkgo leaf for the treatment of asthma, bronchitis, and brain disorders.

INTERNATIONAL STATUS

Ginkgo is listed as an approved herb in the *German Commission E Monographs,* in which it is indicated for the treatment of organic brain syndrome manifested by symptoms such as "memory deficits, disturbances in concentration, depressive emotional condition, dizziness, tinnitus, and headache."[2]

BOTANY

Often called a "living fossil," the magnificent *Ginkgo biloba* tree is the oldest known living tree species and the last survivor of its botanical family, Ginkgoaceae. Individual ginkgo trees may live as long as 1,000 years, growing to heights of 80 feet or more. Legend has it that ginkgo was saved from extinction by ancient Chinese monks, who used it in temple plantings. Ginkgo gets its species name, *biloba,* from its graceful two-lobed leaves, which turn brilliant yellow in autumn.

Although native to Asia, ginkgo trees are commonly planted as ornamentals in North America. Today, large, stately ginkgo trees line the streets of many American cities. They are popular not only for their beauty but because they are hardy, able to withstand cold temperatures and pollution, and to resist insects, disease, and disease-causing organisms.

Although they are slow growing, ginkgo trees are not difficult to cultivate. Botanists classify ginkgo as a *dioecious* plant, meaning that individual trees possess either male- or female-type reproductive parts. Horticulturalists generally prefer to plant male ginkgo trees, because the fruit produced by female trees is considered messy and foul smelling.

BENEFITS

- Enhances microcirculation
- Improves blood flow and oxygen supply to the brain, eyes, ears, and limbs
- Protects cells from free radical damage
- Inhibits platelet-activating factor

SCIENTIFIC SUPPORT

Hundreds of published laboratory studies document the complex and varied effects of ginkgo, and at least 44 double-blind clinical studies involving 9,772 people have investigated the effects of ginkgo in a variety of different health conditions. Most clinical studies of ginkgo use a 50:1 concentrated extract standardized to contain 24 percent ginkgo flavone glycosides and 6 percent terpene lactones (ginkgolides).

In at least 10 controlled clinical studies in elderly people with declining brain function due to cerebral insufficiency, those taking ginkgo experienced significant improvements in mental performance, including short-term memory and concentration. Researchers also noted benefits to mood, attention, and sociability.

In 1997, a well-controlled clinical study showed that ginkgo was helpful in the treatment of Alzheimer's disease as well as multi-infarct dementia (a decline in brain function caused by multiple strokes). The researchers believed that the improvements seen in the participants with Alzheimer's disease were equivalent to "a six-month delay in the progression of the disease."[1] This trial supports positive results achieved in earlier trials in people with Alzheimer's disease.[3,4] The evidence is especially promising in light of the fact that no satisfactory treatments currently exist for this common and debilitating disease.

Limited but promising research suggests that ginkgo may also help maintain and improve brain function in young, healthy people. In several small studies in healthy people, short-term memory, attention, and response time were significantly improved after single doses of ginkgo extract.[5,6] These findings are supported by the results of studies testing the effects of ginkgo in young, healthy rodents. These studies used well-accepted models for testing learning and memory in animals.[7,8]

In addition, a number of clinical studies have demonstrated the effectiveness of ginkgo extract in the treatment of *intermittent claudication* (also called *peripheral artery disease*), a narrowing of the arteries in the legs that causes painful cramping. In these trials, there was a significant increase in pain-free walking distance after treatment with ginkgo extract.[9,10]

Currently, researchers are evaluating the effects of ginkgo extract in the treatment of asthma, cataracts, depression (in people unresponsive to drug treatment), hearing loss, head injuries, and a variety of other conditions. In addition, researchers observed positive results in one clinical trial investigating ginkgo's effects on altitude sickness. In this study ginkgo was significantly more effective than placebo in improving tolerance to high altitude and preventing typical symptoms of altitude sickness.[11]

SPECIFIC STUDIES

Alzheimer's Disease and Multi-Infarct Dementia: Clinical Study (1997)

In this important American study, treatment with standardized ginkgo extract helped improve or stabilize a number of daily living and cognitive functions in elderly patients with mild to severe dementia due either to Alzheimer's disease or multi-infarct dementia. The authors of the study suggested that the improvements seen in patients with Alzheimer's could be equated to a six-month delay in the disease's progression. The 309 people in the placebo-controlled double-blind study were randomized to receive 52 weeks of treatment with either placebo or ginkgo extract at a dosage of 40 mg three times a day. At the end of the treatment period, 202 subjects were included in the endpoint analysis, which was based on standard tests of cognitive impairment, daily living and social behavior, and general psychopathology. Daily living and social behavior improved in 37 percent of patients taking ginkgo, compared with 23 percent of those taking placebo. In contrast, 40 percent of the placebo group had a worsening of symptoms, compared with only 19 percent of those in the ginkgo group. Side effects with ginkgo were no different from placebo.[1]

Cerebral Insufficiency: Clinical Study (1994)

Researchers observed significant improvements in mental performance, including short-term memory and concentration, after 6 weeks of treatment with standardized ginkgo extract in this placebo-controlled, double-blind trial in 90 elderly patients with cerebral insufficiency. For 12 weeks, 45 subjects received treatment with standardized ginkgo extract at a total daily dose of 150 mg, and 45 received placebo. Of particular interest to the investigators were ginkgo's effects on long- and short-term memory, concentration, mental flexibility, stress, family problems, and general life satisfaction. Three patients (one in the ginkgo group, two in the placebo group) dropped out without giving any reasons. In assessing data from the remaining patients, researchers saw significant improvements in nearly all parameters in the group taking ginkgo. Although many benefits became evident earlier than 6 weeks into the trial, others did not appear until 6 weeks or more had passed.[12]

Short-Term Memory in Healthy Volunteers: Clinical Study (1988)

Although small, this study offers some support for the idea that ginkgo extract can help improve memory and brain function in young, healthy people. The double-blind, placebo-controlled, crossover trial compared the effects of placebo with those of varying doses of ginkgo extract in eight healthy women between the ages of 25 and 40. Results were assessed 1 hour after treatment with a battery of standard tests for short-term memory, reaction time, and sensory capability. The investigator reported that short-term memory was "very significantly

improved" after 600-mg doses of ginkgo extract, compared with placebo.[5]

Peripheral Artery Disease: Meta-analysis (1992)

Analysis of the combined results of five similar placebo-controlled trials showed that patients with peripheral arterial disease had a highly significant increase in pain-free walking distance after treatment with standardized ginkgo extract. Peripheral artery disease (intermittent claudication) is a type of circulation disorder that can cause painful cramping in the legs. The five trials assessed improvements in pain-free walking distance, using a standard treadmill test. All but one of the studies in the meta-analysis used a daily ginkgo extract dose of 160 mg.[10]

HOW IT WORKS

Researchers classify ginkgo as a *nootropic* agent, meaning that it is a substance that acts on the central nervous system but for which no single pharmacological mechanism of action is known. As with many herbs, ginkgo's neuroprotective effectiveness is likely the result of a complex interplay among many different actions.

Effects on Circulation

Among its numerous effects, ginkgo enhances *microcirculation,* meaning that it improves blood flow to tiny blood vessels called *capillaries* in the brain, eyes, ears, limbs, and other body parts. This effect is believed to be due to a combination of factors, one of which is ginkgo's antioxidant activity. The antioxidant plant compounds in ginkgo act as free radical scavengers, absorbing toxic chemicals in order to prevent oxidative cell damage (including damage related to aging). Ginkgo's antioxidant action is likely a major contributor to its "anti-aging" benefits, because the central nervous system and brain are especially susceptible to free radical damage.

Ginkgo's antioxidant properties also help strengthen blood vessel walls and improve their overall tone and elasticity. By preventing free radical damage, ginkgo appears to stabilize cell membranes and make blood vessel walls and red blood cells more flexible, improving the flow of blood and oxygen to the brain, limbs, and other areas supplied by tiny capillaries, such as the eyes and ears. By enhancing microcirculation, ginkgo can improve a variety of brain functions, including memory, concentration, and problem solving.

Another part of the story is ginkgo's ability to inhibit the effects of a substance called *platelet-activating factor* (PAF). PAF is important in blood clotting and inflammatory reactions, and some PAF is necessary for good health. However, too much PAF has been linked to the development of allergies, asthma, inflammatory disorders such as psoriasis, and cardiovascular diseases. Ginkgo's antiplatelet (or blood-thinning) action supports the healthy function of the circulatory system, helping to keep blood flowing smoothly to all parts of the body. Ginkgo's antiplatelet effect may be partly explained by the fact that the extract enhances the body's production of prostacyclin, a substance that inhibits platelet aggregation. Increased production of prostacyclin may also have a relaxing effect on blood vessels.

Herbs such as ginger, turmeric, and garlic also provide antiplatelet actions. Aspirin has antiplatelet effects, which is why many Western doctors recommend a dosage of 1 aspirin a day to help reduce risks of cardiovascular diseases such as stroke and heart attack. In theory, regular use of antiplatelet herbs might be expected to provide the same health-protective benefits.

Other Effects on the Brain

There is some evidence that ginkgo may enhance the uptake of serotonin (a neurotransmitter), increase the number of serotonin receptors in the brain,[13] and inhibit the effects of monoamine oxidase (MAO).[14] Serotonin and MAO are two substances important in the regulation of anxiety and mood.

MAJOR CONSTITUENTS

Flavonoids (ginkgo flavone glycosides) and terpenoids (ginkgolides and bilobalide)

SAFETY

Ginkgo appears to be extremely safe and is well tolerated by most people. No major adverse effects or drug interactions were noted in 44 clinical trials involving more than 9,772 participants, and side effects of any kind are rare.[15]

- **Side effects:** The most common side effects are mild gastrointestinal discomfort, headache, and rash.[2,16] However, very large doses have been reported to cause diarrhea, nausea, vomiting, and restlessness.
- **Contraindications:** None are known,[2] although caution may be advised for people with blood-clotting disorders.
- **Drug interactions:** Some experts advise that ginkgo should not be taken by those who are taking prescription antidepressant drugs known as monoamine oxidase inhibitors (MAOI),[16] because there is a theoretical possibility that the combination could result in a negative drug interaction. In addition, because ginkgo has mild blood-thinning actions, it may be best avoided by those taking prescription blood-thinning medications.

DOSAGE

Almost all of the clinical research on ginkgo leaf has been conducted with one particular form of extract, namely, a 50:1 concentrated extract standardized to contain 24 percent ginkgo flavone glycosides and 6 percent terpene lactones. In most of the clinical studies, the effective dosage of standardized extract was 40 mg three times a day, a total daily dose of 120 mg of ginkgo leaf extract.

The effects of ginkgo are not immediate. In most of the clinical studies, from 4 to 24 weeks of treatment were required before benefits were seen.

- **Standardized extract:** 40 mg three times a day

STANDARDIZATION

Standardized ginkgo leaf extract is a 50:1 concentrated extract standardized to contain 24 percent ginkgo flavone glycosides and 6 percent terpene lactones.

REFERENCES

1. LeBars PL, Katz MM, Berman N, et al. A placebo-controlled, double-blind, randomized trial of an extract of *Ginkgo biloba* for dementia. *Journal of the American Medical Association* 1997; 278: 1327–1332.
2. Blumenthal M, Busse W, Goldberg A, et al., eds. *The Complete German Commission E Monographs.* Austin, TX: The American Botanical Council; Boston: Integrative Medical Communications, 1998.

3. Hofferberth B. The efficacy of EGb 761 in patients with senile dementia of the Alzheimer type, a double-blind, placebo controlled study on different levels of investigation. *Human Psychopharmacology* 1994; 9: 215–222.

4. Kanowski S, Herrmann WM, Stephan K, et al. Proof of efficacy of the *Ginkgo biloba* extract EGb 761 in outpatients suffering from mild to moderate primary degenerative dementia of the Alzheimer type or multi-infarct dementia. *Phytomedicine* 1997; 4(1): 3–13.

5. Hindmarch I. Activity of *Ginkgo biloba* extract on short-term memory. In: Füngeld EW, ed. *Rökan* (Ginkgo biloba). *Recent Results in Pharmacology and Clinic*. Berlin, Heidelberg, and New York: Springer Verlag, 1988; 321–326.

6. Allard M. Effects of *Ginkgo biloba* extract on normal or altered memory function in man. In: Christen Y, Costentin J, Lacour M, eds. *Effects of* Ginkgo biloba *extract (EGb 761) on the Central Nervous System*. Paris: Elsevier, 1992.

7. Rapin JR, Lamproglou I, Drieu K, et al. Demonstration of the "anti-stress" activity of an extract of *Ginkgo biloba* (EGB 761) using a discrimination learning task. *General Pharmacology* 1994; 25(5): 1009–1016.

8. Winter E. Effects of an extract of *Ginkgo biloba* on learning and memory in mice. *Pharmacology, Biochemistry & Behavior* 1991; 38: 109–114.

9. Peters H, Kieser M, Hölscher U. Demonstration of the efficacy of *Ginkgo biloba* special extract EGb 761® on intermittent claudication—a placebo-controlled, double-blind multicenter trial. *Vasa* 1998; 27: 106–110.

10. Schneider B. *Ginkgo biloba* Extrakt bei peripheren arteriellen Verschlusskrankeheiten. *Arzneimittel-Forschung / Drug Research* 1992; 42(1): 428–436.

11. Roncin JP, Schwartz F, D'Arbigny P. EGb 761 in control of acute mountain sickness and vascular reactivity to cold exposure. *Aviation, Space and Environmental Medicine* 1996; 67(5): 445–452.

12. Vesper J, Hänsgen KD. Efficacy of *Ginkgo biloba* in 90 outpatients with cerebral insufficiency caused by old age. *Phytomedicine* 1994; 1: 9–16.

13. Ahlemeyer B, Krieglstein J. Neuroprotective effects of *Ginkgo biloba* extract. In: Lawson LD, Bauer R, eds. *Phytomedicines of Europe*. Washington, DC: American Chemical Society, 1998; 210–220.

14. White HL, Scates PW, Cooper BR. Extracts of *Ginkgo biloba* leaves inhibit monoamine oxidase. *Life Sciences* 1996; 58(16): 1315–1321.

15. Murray M. Intermittent claudication: Trental vs. *Ginkgo biloba* extract. *American Journal of Natural Medicine* 1995; 2(1): 10–13.

16. McGuffin M, Hobbs C, Upton R, et al., eds. *American Herbal Products Association Botanical Safety Handbook*. Boca Raton, FL: CRC Press, 1997.

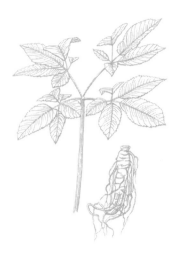

Ginseng

PANAX GINSENG
ARALIACEAE

State of Knowledge: Five-Star Rating System

Clinical (human) research	✶ ✶
Laboratory research	✶ ✶ ✶ ✶
History of use/traditional use	✶ ✶ ✶ ✶ ✶
Safety record	✶ ✶ ✶
International acceptance	✶ ✶ ✶

PART USED: *Root*

PRIMARY USES

- *Endurance*
- *Stress and fatigue*
- *Environmental stress*
- *Recovery after illness (traditional)*
- *Concentration*
- *Normalizing body functions (traditional)*
- *Overall health and vitality*

Ginseng is sometimes called the king of herbs. Perhaps the world's best-known herb, *Panax ginseng* has been used medicinally in Asia for more than 5,000 years. Especially treasured in China, at times ginseng has been valued even more highly than gold. For years, it was one of only two or three herbs known at all to American consumers. Hundreds of ginseng products have been sold worldwide, including everything from ginseng chewing gum to ginseng gin. Today, ginseng remains the fourth best-selling herb in the United States. The mystique of wild, old ginseng roots has at least partially given way to the new luster of standardized ginseng extracts backed by clinical research. Ginseng is perhaps still best known for its ancient reputation as an aphrodisiac or virility herb, an effect that lacks scientific backing. But there are tantalizing bits of support for the claim that this legendary herb may enhance your chances of a longer, healthier life.

Russian researchers introduced the term *adaptogen* to describe an herb that strengthens body functions and the immune system to help people adapt to the effects of physical stress. Ginseng was the first adaptogenic herb to be recognized, and it is still the best known. It is popularly used as a health-enhancing tonic and for increasing energy and stamina during physical activity. Even more than most herbs, ginseng has complex and varied effects. Among Western scientists, the credibility of ginseng suffers from the sheer diversity of its purported effects. The genus name *Panax* means "panacea" (cure-all), a term that is automatically discounted in modern health care. We are accustomed to thinking of a single substance having a single effect; for example, relieving pain or reducing blood pressure. Ginseng has many different effects, and sometimes even contradictory effects. For example, depending on the situation, ginseng can enhance both energy *and* quality of sleep.

Clinical studies confirm that ginseng can help enhance endurance, reduce fatigue, and improve coordination and reaction time. There is also some evidence that ginseng can boost immune function, helping the body to fight off infection during times of stress. In laboratory studies, ginseng has shown promise in protecting heart health, regulating the function of reproductive hormones, normal-izing cholesterol and blood sugar levels, and improving memory and learning. More studies in humans are needed to investigate the effectiveness of ginseng in these promising areas. There is also some research support for antitumor and cancer-protective effects, and possibly liver-protective benefits as well. The combination of potential benefits for heart health, protection against cancer, immune system support, liver health, and general balancing of body systems makes ginseng a prime candidate for more clinical research.

Different ginseng species and preparation methods provide distinctly different effects. Even within the single species *Panax ginseng,* different traditional preparation methods result in different actions. "Red" Asian ginseng, for example, is steamed and cured, resulting in a product that is considered more stimulating than the unsteamed "white" ginseng. American ginseng (*Panax quinquefolius*) is traditionally considered less stimulating, or "yang," than white ginseng. Ginseng is thought of as an energizing tonic, but has not been shown to stimulate the central nervous system the way coffee does. People taking ginseng often report feelings of improved overall well-being.

HISTORY

Ancient healers in India, Russia, China, and Japan all revered ginseng for its medicinal and health-enhancing properties. In traditional Chinese medicine (TCM), ginseng is used to normalize blood pressure and blood sugar, to strengthen overall health when the body is debilitated, and as a sexual tonic for both men and women, among other purposes.

The first written mention of ginseng dates from more than 2,000 years ago and refers to use even more ancient. Historians believe ginseng has been used continuously for at least 5,000 years. In TCM, ginseng is classified as a "superior" herb, meaning that it is considered to be among the safest and most useful herbs available. It has always been regarded as a strengthening tonic, especially helpful for the elderly, those recovering from illness, and those in weakened condition. Many notable figures in history have extolled the virtues of ginseng, including Marco Polo and Sir Richard Burton, who attributed the health and vitality of wealthy elderly Chinese people to ginseng. In 1904 it was noted that all of the 400 million people in China used ginseng to some extent. Because of its reputation for promoting virility, general health, and longevity, the Chinese considered ginseng as valuable as gold.

It is easy to see why ginseng gained a reputation as a cure-all. The herb has dozens of traditional applications. In Asian folk medicine, ginseng is used for amnesia, anemia, anorexia, asthma, atherosclerosis (hardening of the arteries), boils, bruises, cancer, convulsions, cough, debility, and diabetes; as a diuretic (an agent that promotes urination);

against dysentery, dysmenorrhea (painful menstruation), dyspepsia (indigestion), epilepsy, fatigue, fear, fever, forgetfulness, gastritis (inflammation of the stomach lining), hangover, headache, heart conditions, hemoptysis (spitting of blood from the lungs), hemorrhage, hyperglycemia (high blood sugar), hypertension (high blood pressure), hypotension (low blood pressure), impotence, insomnia, and intestinal complaints; for longevity, malaria, nausea, palpitations, polyuria (excessive urination), rhinitis (inflammation of the nasal membranes), rheumatism, and digestive distress; and as a cough remedy, nervine (a therapeutic agent for the nervous system), sedative, stimulant, and tranquilizer, among other uses.

The second best-known species of ginseng, American ginseng *(P. quinquefolius)* was widely used by some Native Americans. Whereas the Chinese believed that Asian ginseng was generally inappropriate for women, the Cherokee and Menonimi tribes used American ginseng for women's health concerns, including cramps and other menstrual problems. These and other tribes also used ginseng in ways similar to those of the Chinese: for longevity, increasing mental powers, and stimulating sexual response.

Ginseng is still a precious crop, one of the highest-priced legal herbs on the market. It is an important export crop from the United States and Canada as well as from China, Korea, Japan, and Taiwan. Because of its high value, ginseng has been overcollected from the wild everywhere it grows. In China, wild ginseng is probably extinct, and in the United States, it is threatened or endangered in most states in which it occurs naturally. Most ginseng available today is cultivated.

INTERNATIONAL STATUS

The German Commission E has approved ginseng as a tonic for fortification in times of fatigue and debility, for combating declining capacity for work and concentration, and for use during convalescence. Ginseng also appears in the Swiss, Austrian, and French pharmacopoeias, as well as those of Japan, Korea, Russia, and China.

BOTANY

Panax is a genus of the aralia family (Araliaceae) that includes six species. The botanical name *Panax* comes from the Greek word *panacea,* meaning "cure-all," in reference to the wide range of uses attributed to the herb. The Chinese name for ginseng, *ren shen*, means "man root," so called because of its characteristic shape that resembles the trunk, arms, and legs of a human being.

The ginseng plant is a small perennial herb that grows up to 25 inches tall. It has palmate (palm-like) compound leaves, usually with five leaflets, an umbel of greenish-white flowers in summer, and red berries in autumn. It grows in deep shady forests or under shadecloth when in cultivation. Under cultivation, ginseng is notoriously sensitive to diseases, especially fungal diseases.

The Asian ginseng most prized by the Chinese is *Panax ginseng*. Other Asian ginseng species include Japanese ginseng *(P. japonicus)* and sanchi or tienchi ginseng *(P. notoginseng)*. Closely related to *Panax ginseng* is wild American ginseng *(P. quinquefolius),* which was widely used by Native Americans. Unfortunately, this North American plant has become endangered in the wild due to over-collection and habitat loss. Ironically, much wild American ginseng is harvested for export to China. American ginseng is now cultivated extensively, and environmentally conscious consumers should make a special effort to purchase ginseng products made from cultivated sources.

BENEFITS

- Enhances energy metabolism during exercise
- Reduces fatigue
- Improves resistance to heat, cold, and other sources of environmental stress
- Increases well-being
- Boosts stamina and endurance
- May reduce the risk of certain cancers

SCIENTIFIC SUPPORT

Thousands of clinical, laboratory, and animal studies have been performed to investigate the actions and chemistry of ginseng. Much of this research has taken place in China, Russia, Korea, and Japan. Unfortunately, the quality of the research is quite variable and the results inconsistent. The inconsistencies may be due to differences in the ginseng sources and preparations used in the studies, problems with trial design, or deficiencies in controls. Although there are relatively few clinical studies of exemplary quality, the combination of long-term human use, clinical trials, and laboratory research adds up to a fairly impressive justification for use—and for continued and higher-quality research. Recent studies have been better designed, and the testing of standardized ginseng products is creating greater consistency in results.

The best-documented effects of ginseng in humans are improving resistance to stress and enhancing mental and physical performance. Ginseng seems to be most effective for those in a weakened condition; for those under demanding conditions such as shift work, sleep deprivation, or rigorous athletic training; and for those exposed to environmental stress, including heat and cold. For many years scientists have considered the most important chemical compounds in ginseng to be glycosides called *ginsenosides,* and numerous laboratory and clinical studies have been carried out on these constituents. Ginsenoside fractions and purified single ginsenosides have been researched for a wide variety of effects. Some have antiplatelet effects, and others affect the central nervous system, protein synthesis, immune function, and other diverse body processes.

Overall Well-Being

Ginseng's ancient reputation as an anti-aging tonic is supported by modern pharmacological research that shows that both ginseng extracts and natural compounds in ginseng roots have protective effects. Two ginsenosides have antioxidant effects, including the prevention of blood lipid oxidation, which can contribute to heart disease. Some have blood-thinning (antiplatelet) activity, some stimulate immune function, some protect the brain and nervous system against toxins and radiation, and some possess antitumor actions. In one laboratory experiment, daily oral doses of ginseng lessened age-related learning impairment in rats navigating a maze.[1] In another experiment, oral doses of ginseng extract increased the activity level in old rats, while decreasing it in young rats.[2] This is one of many studies that highlights the "adaptogenic" effects of ginseng by demonstrating how it can affect different subjects in different ways according to their needs.

There is also some clinical research in this area. A placebo-controlled, double-blind clinical trial of 49 elderly people demonstrated that 1,500 mg of red ginseng daily significantly improved reaction time and coordination, and participants reported increased energy and alertness.[3] In a clinical trial of 120 healthy individuals, ginseng extract enhanced performance, lung function, and well-being, especially in older subjects.[4] In another placebo-controlled, double-blind trial, 12 student nurses working night shifts experienced benefits in mood and performance and a reduction of fatigue after taking unstandardized ginseng extract at a daily dose of 1,200 mg.[5]

Physical Performance

Russian research, beginning in the 1950s, focused on athletic performance. Ginseng helped a group of Russian soldiers run faster in a 3-km race than a control group given placebo.[6] In a placebo-controlled, double-blind 20-week trial involving 28 male athletes between 20 and 30 years old, a daily dose of 200 mg standardized ginseng extract increased performance significantly by increasing the oxygen transport capacity of the heart and shortening reaction time to visual stimuli.[7] Animal studies have shown that mice can swim farther, and perform better in cold or hot environments, after treatment with ginseng.[8,9]

Mental Function

Ginseng also appears to stimulate mental function. Early Russian research showed that telegraph operators given ginseng showed improved speed and accuracy of performance,[6] and researchers began performing experiments to duplicate these results in animal studies.[10–12] In an animal study, ginseng increased learning and memory in rats, in contrast to caffeine and methamphetamine, which increased physical speed but slowed learning and mental performance.[13] In another study, ginsenosides appeared to increase nerve-fiber growth and prevented nerve damage from irradiation.[14] Ginseng may also improve sleep: One test in rats showed that it could increase slow-wave sleep, the deepest sleep cycles, which are most important to physical renewal. The authors of this study speculated that some of the well-known health-improving effects of ginseng may be due, as least in part, to enhancement of sleep.[15]

Fatigue

In one clinical study, ginseng provided impressive relief in people suffering from long-term fatigue. Using a detailed questionnaire to record typical symptoms of fatigue, both patients and their doctors reported that ginseng outperformed placebo in combating symptoms.[16] In another clinical trial, subjects reported overall improvements in quality of life, especially in mood, vitality, and alertness (see Specific Studies).[17]

Anxiety

Anxiety is one of the items typically tracked on the quality-of-life questionnaires used in clinical studies. Laboratory research in rats and mice indicated that white and red ginseng had antianxiety effects comparable with those achieved with injections of diazepam (Valium). In this study, ginseng powder was given orally at doses of 20 or 50 mg/kg of body weight and compared with diazepam injected at a dose of 1 mg/kg. Researchers measured the results according to behavioral tests (maze performance and conflict behavior) and monoamine oxidase (MAO) activity in the brain, an indicator of anxiety reactions.[18]

Anticancer Effects

Another intriguing potential action of ginseng is a protective effect against cancer. In a large case-control study involving 905 pairs of cases and controls, those taking ginseng extract or powder had a significantly decreased cancer risk. The study was controlled for age, sex, and date of admission to a cancer treatment hospital in Korea. Researchers took into account a multitude of factors to eliminate differences due to marital status, education, religion, economic status, occupation, and other factors. Those taking ginseng had about half the cancer risk of those who did not. Ginseng extract and powder appeared to be more effective than fresh ginseng root or ginseng tea.[19]

Other Actions

Although the results of research to date have been inconclusive, ginseng has demonstrated some promise in diabetes. Daily doses of 200 mg ginseng were associated with improved mood, psychophysical performance (the ability to mentally perceive physical stimuli), and glucose (blood sugar) balance in a placebo-controlled, double-blind 8-week trial in 36 people with non-insulin-dependent diabetes.[20] Furthermore, when given by injection, some ginsenosides demonstrated hypoglycemic (blood sugar–lowering) effects in animals. However, more research is needed in this area.

SPECIFIC STUDIES

Fatigue: Clinical Study (1996)

People suffering from functional fatigue improved significantly after taking a combination of standardized ginseng and other nutrients, compared with placebo, in this 42-day double-blind clinical trial of 232 subjects aged 25 to 60 years. Functional fatigue was defined as long-term fatigue (lasting longer than 15 years) without a known underlying physical disorder. Participants took multivitamin/multimineral capsules with 40 mg concentrated and standardized ginseng or placebo twice a day. On the 1st, 21st, and 42nd days of the study, subjects recorded changes on a questionnaire, describing their symptoms from a list of 20 common complaints related to fatigue (for example, "difficulty in getting up in the morning," "feeling exhausted," and "lack of motivation").

By the end of the trial, there was a statistically significant improvement in the total "fatigue score" in the test group compared with the placebo group, with 5.7 percent in the ginseng group reporting fatigue symptoms compared with 15.2 percent in the placebo group. Both patients and their physicians judged the efficacy of ginseng as better than placebo. Side effects were rare, the most frequently reported being nausea.[15]

Quality of Life: Clinical Study (1994)

In a placebo-controlled, double-blind study, 205 people using ginseng in combination with vitamins, minerals, and trace elements experienced increased alertness, relaxation, appetite, and improvements in total quality-of-life score compared with 185 people taking placebo. The test substance, which was taken twice daily, included 40 mg concentrated ginseng extract plus nutrients. Quality of life (QOL) was measured using an index of 22 items describing anxiety, depression, well-being, self-control, health, and vitality; a sleep dysfunction scale was also used. Those who started the trial with the lowest QOL scores experienced the most improvement. The most significant benefits were in depressed mood, vitality, and alertness. There was no significant difference in sleep dysfunction between the groups.[17]

Well-Being and Performance: Clinical Study (1981)

In a placebo-controlled, double-blind 12-week trial involving 60 men and 60 women, daily doses of 200 mg of standardized ginseng improved reaction times, pulmonary function, and self-assessments of general well-being. Researchers gave subjects 100 mg of standardized ginseng extract (equivalent to 500 mg of ginseng root) or placebo twice daily. Participants completed tests at the beginning of the study and after 3, 6, and 12 weeks of treatment. The investigators tested the participants using an automated reaction-time tester for both visual and acoustic stimuli, spirometry (a device for analyzing pulmonary function), and measurement of sex hormones (testosterone for men, estradiol for women) and gonadotropic hormones (luteinizing hormone and follicle-stimulating hormone). Participants made self-assessments using a questionnaire that covered sleep quality, concentration, vitality, and mood.

Reaction times were significantly better in older subjects (aged 40 to 60) taking ginseng compared with placebo, but not in younger subjects. Pulmonary function was also significantly improved only in older subjects. All subjects except young men (aged 30 to 39) reported significant improvements in all 10 criteria measured by the questionnaire. There was no significant effect on hormone levels.[4]

HOW IT WORKS

Through the years, there have been a number of theories about how ginseng works. Most ginseng researchers have assumed a hormonal action because of the wide range of effects on diverse body systems, all of which are under hormonal control.

The body reacts to many types of stress, including environmental factors such as heat and cold, and environmental toxins; emotional factors such as fear, grief, and anger; and mental stresses like worry, anxiety, and time pressures. Our coping mechanisms involve an extremely complex interplay of neurochemicals, hormones, and immunological factors. As a survival technique, animals developed a powerful rapid-response ability called the "fight or flight" reflex. This is mediated by adrenaline and diverts many of the body's resources in times of crisis into peak physical and mental performance. A key part of this process is called the alarm phase, which involves adrenal hormones such as glucocorticoids, which are used to measure physiological stress. Ginseng strengthens our ability to cope with stress by helping to moderate and mediate hormonal reactions.

Counteraction of Stress Effects

The effect on the hypothalamic-pituitary-adrenal axis is the most often postulated mechanism of action, and there is some experimental support for this hypothesis. For example, ginseng counteracted the effect of cold on body temperature in rats. Scientists confirmed that ginseng stimulated adrenal function because it increased the size of one part of the adrenal gland (the zona fasciculata) in the animals.[6] In animals that had their adrenal glands removed, ginseng had no effect, also clear evidence that ginseng's effect on the adrenals is responsible for its action against this form of environmental stress.

In another study, ginseng saponins exerted their effects on rats with intact pituitary glands, but not on those that had the gland removed. In the normal rats, ginseng stimulated the hypothalamus and pituitary to secrete adrenocorticotropic hormone (ACTH) which, in turn, stimulated the adrenal cortex. The study also showed that the drug dexamethazone reversed ginseng's effects by acting directly on the hypothalamus and pituitary.

Researchers point out that ginseng's antifatigue effects are different from those of standard stimulants, such as coffee. Whereas ordinary stimulants exert their effects under most circumstances, ginseng does so only under conditions of stress. And unlike corticoids, ginseng does not cause the adrenals to shrink, but actually strengthens their function.[6]

Ginseng stimulates the pituitary-adrenocortical system, speeding the recovery of glucocorticoid levels to normal after stress and reducing glucocorticoid production during prolonged stress. (Glucocorticoids are measures of physiological stress.) It also increases adrenal capacity and raises the level of ACTH and cortisone in the blood of nonstressed subjects.

In terms of physical performance, ginseng improves oxygen utilization at a cellular level. When muscle cells are deprived of oxygen, they deplete glycogen, a chemical used to store energy. Depletion of glycogen in the muscles and the accumulation of lactic acid are associated with fatigue and muscle soreness. Ginseng is said to have a "glycogen-sparing effect," shifting energy production away from glycogen and toward fatty acids, which reduces fatigue and enhances physical performance.[21]

Other Effects

Research shows that the isolated ginsenosides Rg3 and Rh2, polyacetylenes, and polysaccharides possess antitumor activity.[22–26] The polysaccharides possess cytoprotective (cell-protecting) effects.[27] Ginseng increases the general activity of the immune system, including natural killer-cell activity; production of immune system compounds, including interferon and interleukins; and the speed of development and activity level of white blood cells.[28]

Several preliminary studies demonstrate the ability of ginseng saponins to lower blood cholesterol, low-density lipoprotein (LDL) cholesterol, and triglyceride levels in rats and rabbits eating a high-cholesterol diet. In some studies, ginseng also significantly raised healthful levels of high-density lipoprotein (HDL) cholesterol. Ginseng also stimulated the conversion of cholesterol into bile acids, in addition to speeding up its excretion from the body.[6]

Ginseng's antioxidant effects may be related to enhancement of nitric oxide synthesis in the endothelial cells in the lungs, heart, and kidneys. This effect could increase vasodilation (widening of blood vessels) and blood flow, and may even contribute to an aphrodisiac action. Endothelial cells, which line the walls of the vascular system, are an early target of harmful free radicals. *In vitro* ginsenosides protect vascular cells from the effects of free radicals and increase the cells' production of nitric oxide, causing vasorelaxation and reducing the pulmonary edema (swelling) associated with free radical damage.[29]

MAJOR CONSTITUENTS

Ginsenosides (at least 31 have been identified, classified as triterpene saponins), sesquiterpenes, polyacetylenes, and polysaccharides

SAFETY

At recommended doses, ginseng is well tolerated by most people. However, taking large doses of ginseng in combination with stimulants, including caffeine, is not recommended.[30] Some researchers recommend that ginseng not be used continuously for longer than 3 months. The *British Herbal Compendium* recommends occasional use or use for a period of 1 month followed by a rest period of 2 months. Others recommend taking ginseng for periods ranging from 3 weeks to 3 months.[30]

- **Side effects:** There have been rare reports of sleeplessness, nervousness, and diarrhea in people taking large doses of ginseng.
- **Contraindications:** Ginseng is best avoided by those with high blood pressure. Some authors recommend against its use during pregnancy, but data to support this warning are lacking.[30]
- **Drug interactions:** Taking large doses of ginseng in combination with stimulants, including caffeine, is not recommended.[30]

DOSAGE

Recent clinical studies on ginseng have used ginseng extract standardized to 4 percent ginsenosides at a dosage of 200 mg to 500 mg a day. In other clinical studies, nonstandardized extracts were used at dosages ranging from 0.5 to 8 grams daily. Korean, Chinese, and Russian research used unextracted ginseng at dosages of 1 to 2 grams of root daily and higher. The dosage approved by the German Commission E is 1 to 2 grams of root or equivalent preparations.

- **Standardized extract:** 200 to 500 mg a day
- **Capsules:** 200 to 500 mg of extract or 1 to 4 grams of powdered root a day
- **Tincture:** 1 to 2 ml a day of 1:1 extract (equivalent to 1 to 2 grams ginseng root)

STANDARDIZATION

Ginseng extracts are often standardized to 4 to 5 percent ginsenosides. The Swiss pharmacopoeia requires ginseng roots to contain at least 2.0 percent total ginsenosides, whereas the German standard requires 1.5 percent or more.[31]

REFERENCES

1. Nitta H, Matsumoto K, Shimizu M, et al. *Panax ginseng* extract improves the performance of aged Fischer 344 rats in radial maze task but not in operant brightness discrimination task. *Biological and Pharmaceutical Bulletin* 1995; 18(9): 1286–1288.
2. Watanabe H, Ohta H, Imamura L, et al. Effect of *Panax ginseng* on age-related changes in the spontaneous motor activity and dopaminergic nervous system in the rat. *Japanese Journal of Pharmacology* 1991; 55(1): 51–56.

3. Fulder S, Kataria M, Gethyn-Smith B. A double-blind clinical trial of *Panax ginseng* in aged subjects. Presented at the Fourth International Ginseng Symposium, Daejeon, Korea, 18–20 September, 1984.

4. Forgo I, Kayesseh L, Staub JJ. Effect of a standardized ginseng extract on general well-being, reaction capacity, pulmonary function and gonadal hormones [in German]. *Medizinische Welt* 1981; 32(19): 751–756.

5. Hallstrom C, Fulder S, Carruthers M. Effects of ginseng on the performance of nurses on night duty. *Comparative Medicine East and West* 1982; 6(4): 277–282.

6. Shibata S, Tanaka O, Shoji J, et al. Chemistry and pharmacology of *Panax*. In: Wagner H, Hikino H, Farnsworth NR, eds. *Economic and Medicinal Plant Research*. Vol 1. London: Academic Press, 1985.

7. Forgo I, Schimert G. The duration of effect of the standardized ginseng extract G115® in healthy competitive athletes [in German]. *Notobene Medici* 1985; 15(9): 636–640.

8. Ramachandran U, Divekar HM, Grover SK. New experimental model for the evaluation of adaptogenic products. *Journal of Ethnopharmacology* 1990; 29: 275–281.

9. Yuan W-X, Wu X-J, Yang F-X, et al. Effects of ginseng root saponins on brain monoamines and serum corticosterone in heat-stressed mice. *Acta Pharmaologica Sinica* 1989; 10(6): 492–496.

10. Brekhman II, Dardymov IV. New substances of plant origin which increase nonspecific resistance. *Annual Review of Pharmacology* 1969; 9: 419–430.

11. Brekhman II, Dardymov IV. Pharmacological investigation of glycosides from ginseng and eleutherococcus. *Lloydia* 1969; 32(1): 46–51.

12. Petkov W. *Panax ginseng*—ein Reaktivitätsregler [in German]. *Pharmaceutische Zeitung* 1968; 113(35): 1281–1286.

13. Saito H, Tsuchiya M, Naka S, et al. Effects of *Panax ginseng* root on conditioned avoidance response in rats. *Japanese Journal of Pharmacology* 1977; 27: 509–516.

14. Saito H, Lee Y-M, Handa S. The activity of tyrosine hydroxylase in superior cervical ganglion and sub-maxillary gland of senescent and irradiated mice. In: Usdin E, Kvetnansky R, Kopin IJ, eds. *Catecholamines and Stress: Recent Advances*. New York: Elsevier North-Holland, 1980: 371–374.

15. Rhee YH, Lee SP, Honda K, et al. Panax ginseng extract modulates sleep in unrestrained rats. *Psychopharmacology* 1990; 101 (4): 486–488.

16. Le Gal M, Cathebras P, Strüby K. Pharmaton capsules in the treatment of functional fatigue: a double-blind study versus placebo evaluated by a new methodology. *Phytotherapy Research* 1996; 10: 49–53.

17. Wiklund I, Karlberg J, Lund B. A double-blind comparison of the effect on quality of life of a combination of vital substances including standardized ginseng G115 and placebo. *Current Therapeutic Research* 1994; 55(1): 32–42.

18. Bhattacharya SK, Mitra SK. Anxiolytic activity of *Panax ginseng* roots: an experimental study. *Journal of Ethnopharmacology* 1991; 34: 87–92.

19. Yun T-K, Choi SY. A case-control study of ginseng intake and cancer. *International Journal of Epidemiology* 1990; 19(4): 871–876.

20. Sotaniemi EA, Haapakoski E, Rautio A. Ginseng therapy in non-insulin-dependent diabetic patients. *Diabetes Care* 1995; 18 (10): 1373–1375.

21. Avakian EV, Evonuk E. Effects of *Panax ginseng* extract on tissue glycogen depletion and adrenal cholesterol depletion during prolonged exercise. *Planta Medica* 1979; 36: 43–48.

22. Ahn B-Z, Kim S-I. Relation between structure and cytotoxic activity of panaxydol analogs against L1210 cells [in German]. *Archiv der Pharmazie* 1988; 321: 61–63.

23. Matsunaga H, Katano M, Yamamoto H, et al. Studies on the panaxytriol of *Panax ginseng* CA Meyer: isolation, determination and antitumor activity. *Chemical and Pharmaceutical Bulletin* 1989; 37(5): 1279–1281.

24. Matsunaga H, Katano M, Yamamoto H, et al. Cytotoxic activity of polyacetylene compounds in *Panax ginseng* CA Meyer. *Chemical and Pharmaceutical Bulletin* 1990; 38(12): 3480–3482.

25. Matsunaga H, Saita T, Nagumo R, et al. A possible mechanism for the cytotoxicity of a polyacetylenic alcohol, panaxytriol: inhibition of mitochondrial respiration. *Cancer Chemotherapy and Pharmacology* 1995; 35; 291–296.

26. Mochizuki M, Yoo YC, Matsuzawa K, et al. Inhibitory effect of tumor metastasis in mice by saponins, ginsenoside-Rb2, 20(*R*)- and 20(*S*)-ginsenoside-Rg3, of red ginseng. *Biological and Pharmaceutical Bulletin* 1995; 18(9): 1197–1202.

27. Sun X-B, Matsumoto T, Kiyohara H, et al. Cytoprotective activity of pectic polysaccharides from the root of *Panax ginseng*. *Journal of Ethnopharmacology* 1991; 31: 101–107.

28. Murray M. *The Healing Power of Herbs*. Rocklin, CA: Prima Publishing, 1995.

29. Gillis CN. *Panax ginseng* pharmacology: a nitric oxide link? *Biochemical Pharmacology* 1997; 54: 1–8.

30. McGuffin M, Hobbs C, Upton R, et al., eds. *American Herbal Products Association Botanical Safety Handbook*. Boca Raton, FL: CRC Press, 1997.

31. Sticher O. Biochemical, pharmaceutical, and medicinal perspective of ginseng. In: Lawson LD, Bauer R, eds. *Phytomedicines of Europe*. Washington, DC: American Chemical Society, 1998; 222–240.

Goldenseal

HYDRASTIS CANADENSIS
RANUNCULACEAE

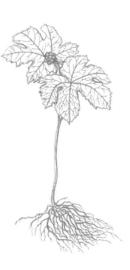

State of Knowledge: Five-Star Rating System

Clinical (human) research	✳
Laboratory research	✳
History of use/traditional use	✳✳✳
Safety record	✳✳✳
International acceptance	✳✳

PART USED: *Rhizome, root*

PRIMARY USES

- *First aid for superficial wounds (traditional)*
- *Mouthwash for canker sores and other conditions (traditional)*
- *Wash for inflamed or infected eyes (traditional)*
- *Sinus infections (traditional)*
- *Digestive problems such as peptic ulcers, colitis, and gastritis (traditional)*
- *Parasitic infections of the gastrointestinal tract (berberine)*

Do you reach for goldenseal as an "herbal antibiotic" when you feel a cold coming on? Have you heard that goldenseal can mask the presence of illegal drugs during urinalysis? Both of these common uses of goldenseal are based on myths that lack scientific support. Unfortunately, such mistaken beliefs have contributed to its over collection, helping to put goldenseal on the endangered species list in a number of its native states.

Today, people tend to characterize goldenseal either as a cure-all for everything from colds to cancer or as an herb with few legitimate uses. In reality, the truth lies somewhere in between these two opposing views. Despite the immense popularity of echinacea-goldenseal combinations for cold and flu, goldenseal was not traditionally employed this way by Native Americans or by early American herbalists. Known as the "king of the mucous membranes," by the Eclectic physicians (a group of prominent American physicians who used natural remedies around the turn of the century), goldenseal has several limited and very specific applications, all of which center around its ability to act as a stimulant, antiseptic, astringent, and anti-inflammatory in the mouth, sinuses, throat, lungs, eyes, digestive tract, and on the skin. As a consumer, the most important step you can take to help ensure the future survival of this plant is to educate yourself and others about the rational uses of goldenseal.

HISTORY

Cherokees traditionally used goldenseal for indigestion, poor appetite, as a general tonic, and as a wash for local inflammatory conditions and skin cancer. The Iroquois used the roots for diarrhea, whooping cough, liver troubles, fever, sour stomach and gas, tuberculosis, pneumonia, "rundown" systems, heart troubles, and as drops for earaches and sore eyes. The bright yellow root was also a popular source of natural dye for clothing.

After learning about goldenseal from Native Americans, the early pioneers came to consider it a virtual cure-all. By the early 1800s, the Eclectic physicians were relying on goldenseal heavily, mainly as a mucous membrane tonic. They used it for liver congestion, stomach and intestinal complaints, chronic diarrhea, coughs, nasal mucus, sinusitis, tonsillitis, as a bitter tonic, and as a douche for vaginal infections. Externally, it was employed for eye inflammation and skin problems such as eczema and ringworm. The plant was listed as a remedy for inflammations of the mucous membranes in *The United States Pharmacopoeia* from 1830 to 1840 and again from 1860 to 1926. Goldenseal was a prominent ingredient in many turn-of-the-century proprietary medicines, including a product known as Dr. Pierce's Golden Medical Discovery. The myth that goldenseal masks the presence of illicit drugs in the urine dates back to a fictitious plot in a 1900 novel written by well-known plant pharmacist John Uri Lloyd. Unfortunately, this myth continues to affect the plant's threatened status.

In early twentieth-century America, the most popular use of goldenseal was as a wash for eye conditions. In fact, until the 1970s, the goldenseal constituents berberine and hydrastine were the active ingredients in many commercial eyedrops because of their antiseptic properties and ability to relieve bloodshot eyes. Although both goldenseal and berberine have virtually disappeared from mainstream American medicine, they remain as official pharmaceutical medicines in 11 countries around the world. In China and India, plants containing berberine have been utilized for centuries, primarily as a treatment for diarrhea. According to the principles of traditional Chinese medicine, these plants are bitter and cooling and have the ability to dispel heat, counteract dampness, and remove toxins from the body. Berberine-containing plants found in these countries—especially Chinese goldthread, *Coptis chinensis*—are employed for many of the same purposes as the American plant goldenseal. Currently, goldenseal is one of the few popular American herbs not commonly used in Germany, although a good deal of it is imported each year to the United Kingdom.

INTERNATIONAL STATUS

Goldenseal is approved in the United Kingdom for menorrhagia (excessively long or heavy menstrual periods), atonic dyspepsia (indigestion caused by lack of tone), gastritis (inflammation of the stomach), mucosal inflammations, and for topical use as an eyewash. Goldenseal or the constituent berberine are listed as official medicines in the pharmacopoeias of at least 11 nations.

BOTANY

Goldenseal gets its common name from its bright yellow roots, which resemble the wax seals that were once used on envelopes. The root's wrinkled, yellow appearance, distinctive odor, and bitter taste come from the constituent berberine. A member of the buttercup family (Ranunculaceae), goldenseal is native to the moist forests and damp meadows of eastern North America, from Vermont to Georgia, west to Alabama and Arkansas, and north to eastern Iowa and Minnesota. Goldenseal's love of moisture is reflected in its genus name, *Hydrastis,* which means "water." In the spring, the plant puts up one small, hairy stem with five to nine lobed, serrated leaves and a small, solitary, greenish-white or rose-colored flower. The plant is a perennial and grows 8 to 20 inches high. Its raspberrylike berries hold shiny black seeds, which are distributed in the fall by feasting birds.

A Word About Sustainability

By the late 1800s, many herb books were already referring to goldenseal as "scarce." Today, the destruction of natural habitats and renewed interest in complementary medicine have taken a greater toll on wild populations of goldenseal and other plants. In 1997, the U.S. government classified the plant as "endangered" (in danger of extinction throughout all or a portion of its range) in Connecticut, Georgia, Massachusetts, Minnesota, North Carolina, and Vermont. It is considered "imperiled" (meaning very rare, with between 6 and 20 occurrences in the state) in Alabama and New York, and "threatened" (likely to become endangered) in Maryland, Michigan, and Tennessee. In September 1997, the Convention on International Trade in Endangered Species (CITES) began to limit the number of wild-harvested goldenseal roots being exported from the United States.[1]

GOLDENSEAL CULTIVATION

Although some goldenseal cultivation has begun in Oregon, Washington, and North Carolina, success has been mixed. Large-scale operations using synthetic fertilizers are taking place in Ontario, Canada, and growers in Southern Australia have also had some luck with the plant. One problem is the difficulty of meeting the sheer demand for the plant with cultivated sources. Wildcrafters continue to dig approximately 45 to 68 *million* goldenseal plants from eastern U.S. forests each year.[1] In order to meet current requirements, approximately 500 to 1,000 acres of cultivated goldenseal would be needed. By the year 2007, this figure is expected to rise to at least 2,000 acres.[2] Currently, only 2.5 percent of goldenseal is derived from cultivated sources.[3]

On the brighter side, there are many signs that goldenseal cultivation is on the rise, according to a 1998 tonnage survey commissioned by the American Herbal Products Association (AHPA). There are currently 140 acres of goldenseal under cultivation in North America, most of which will be harvested over the next four years. This could mean that as much as 19 percent of the goldenseal supply will come from cultivated sources during the years 1999 through 2003. Based on several large-scale

agricultural plans, up to 78 percent of goldenseal may be cultivated by the year 2003.[3] Although these projections are reassuring, AHPA cautions that the information is insufficient to lift goldenseal from the "at risk" list. A second survey for 1999 (to be released in 2000) may provide additional insight, hopefully with cause for more optimism.[3]

Several experimental cultivation projects with goldenseal have been ongoing for many years. United Plant Savers (UpS), a non-profit organization that is working to protect endangered American plants, is striving to define sustainable wild-harvesting guidelines and successful cultivation techniques for goldenseal and other plants at the UpS Botanical Sanctuary in Rutland, Ohio. They are working hard to replant goldenseal in its native woodlands and to establish other plant reserves. Three responsible herb companies have also instituted "save the goldenseal" projects, including Frontier Herbs of Norway, Iowa; Ohio-based Equinox Botanicals; and the Eclectic Institute of Sandy, Oregon. These companies are cultivating goldenseal and working to educate consumers about inappropriate uses of the plant.[2]

GOLDENSEAL "ALTERNATIVES"

Although several berberine-containing herbs are often recommended as alternatives to goldenseal, many fear that over harvesting could lead these herbs to a similar fate. These substitutes include Oregon grape (*Mahonia aquifolium)*, American goldthread *(Coptis trifolia)*, and Chinese goldthread. Often called "poor man's goldenseal," Oregon grape grows slowly and usually is required in higher doses than goldenseal to achieve similar therapeutic benefits. Already, large amounts of Oregon grape root have reportedly been harvested to fulfill the moderate demand for this herb. American goldthread is also a less-than-ideal substitute for goldenseal because it has small roots and its cool, swampy habitat is rapidly disappearing. To date, it is unknown what ecological effect the large-scale harvest of Asian goldthread is having in China.[1] Although it does not contain berberine, some herbalists believe that yerba mansa *(Anemopsis californica)* has some properties in common with goldenseal. Unfortunately, much of its habitat has been polluted by agribusiness in its native California range, making safe, sustainable harvest questionable.[4] Clearly, use of these goldenseal "alternatives" is little more than a short-term solution.

How You Can Help

Fortunately, wild goldenseal is a strong, hardy plant that could survive for generations to come with a little assistance from concerned Americans. You can help by encouraging herb and pharmaceutical companies to actively support cultivation of goldenseal, rather than continuing to take it from the wild. If you are interested in growing goldenseal or other berberine-rich plants in your own garden, or would like to

know how you can support the work of United Plant Savers, please contact UpS for more information (see appendix E).

BENEFITS

- Acts as an antiseptic (skin and digestive systems)
- Has astringent properties (skin and mucous membranes)
- Works as an anti-inflammatory agent (topically and when used as an eyewash)
- Acts as a mucous membrane tonic
- Stimulates the flow of mucus
- Inhibits growth of bacterial parasites (berberine)

SCIENTIFIC SUPPORT

Because it is not widely used in Germany or other European countries, goldenseal has not been well studied. To date, not a single clinical study has been performed on goldenseal as a whole-plant remedy. There is no scientific evidence that goldenseal stimulates the function of the immune system, as echinacea does.

Goldenseal's reputation as an "herbal antibiotic" comes from *in vitro* (laboratory) studies showing that the constituent berberine was effective against a wide range of bacteria (including some strains of *Escherichia coli, Staphylococcus,* and *Streptococcus*), fungi (such as *Candida albicans*), and parasites, including some strains of *Giardia* and *Trichomonas*.[5] However, whole-plant goldenseal contains only small amounts of berberine, which is poorly absorbed when taken by mouth, making it unlikely that goldenseal itself acts as a systemic (full-body) antibiotic.[6]

In-depth data on berberine's path through the human body are lacking. Researchers do know that berberine is poorly absorbed from the small intestine,[7] and at least some berberine is excreted unchanged in the urine.[8] What this means is that goldenseal generally needs to come in direct contact with mucous membranes in order to affect them. This is possible when the plant is used as an eyewash or mouthwash, an inhalation for sinus problems, a first aid treatment for skin wounds, and as an aid for certain digestive complaints.

Since the 1970s, scientists have conducted numerous studies on isolated berberine. Clinical research suggests that berberine may have value in the treatment of diarrhea associated with cholera and other bacteria, intestinal parasites such as *Giardia,* and eye infections (especially those caused by the bacterium *Chlamydia trachomatis*). Berberine given by injection has also been studied for its possible role in treating certain heart-rhythm disturbances. It is currently being tested as a potential treatment for tumors, AIDS, and liver problems such as cirrhosis.[6] Although there have been a large number of clinical trials with berberine, very few have been placebo controlled.[8]

Several studies have laid to rest the idea that goldenseal masks the presence of illegal drugs during urinalysis.[9] Rumors that the plant can actually yield false positive results are equally unfounded. A 1993 study tested 50 different herbs—including goldenseal—and found that none produced a false positive outcome in relation to use of amphetamines, opiates, barbiturates, cocaine, methadone, or their analogs.[10]

HOW IT WORKS

Goldenseal is known as a mucous membrane "alterative" because it both increases mucus secretion and has astringent properties that help counter the flow. Depending on the situation, it either helps increase deficient mucus flow or decrease excessive flow. According to modern herbalists, one of the most common misuses of goldenseal is during the first stages of a cold. At this time, the natural flow of mucus distributes immunoglobulin A (IgA) to help destroy viral invaders, carries the remains out of the body, and creates a state of temporary inflammation that prevents the problem from spreading. Taking goldenseal at this time is inappropriate because it may overstimulate the mucus glands, leading to excessive dryness. On the other hand, when mucus production stagnates or thickens, or mucus turns a green or yellow color, taking goldenseal may be an excellent way to keep the mucus flowing and prevent bacterial infection from setting in. This situation is common during the third or fourth day of a cold or flu.[11]

Goldenseal may be helpful for treating bacterial diarrhea, because its constituent berberine has a direct effect against bacteria such as *Vibrio cholerae* and *E. coli*. Berberine also appears to prevent certain bacteria from adhering to the lining of the intestinal tract and delays small intestine transit time, through a relaxing effect on smooth muscle. In addition, it may interfere with the metabolic processes of infectious organisms and have a direct action against toxins.[5]

According to clinical studies, goldenseal's berberine content may also help prevent the growth of intestinal parasites such as *Giardia lamblia*. *Giardia* is the number one cause of intestinal disease in all 50 of the United States and a growing international problem as well.[5] Likewise, goldenseal may be an ally in treating strep throat because of berberine's ability to prevent the *Streptococcus* bacteria from adhering to host cells.[12]

MAJOR CONSTITUENTS

Alkaloids (hydrastine and berberine)

SAFETY

Goldenseal should not be taken for longer than a few days to a week.

- **Side effects:** Large doses or overreliance can cause side effects such as overly dry or irritated mucous membranes and injury to the stomach and intestines.[11] Use of goldenseal may reduce beneficial bacteria in the intestines. It is recommended that an acidophilus supplement be used after finishing a course of treatment with this herb, as is advised after taking a prescription antibiotic.[13]
- **Contraindications:** Not for use during pregnancy.[14]
- **Drug interactions:** None known.

DOSAGE

Goldenseal is generally effective in fairly small doses.

- **Capsules:** Up to four 500- to 600-mg capsules a day
- **Tincture (1:10):** 2 to 4 ml
- **Powder:** A pinch ($1/2$ to 1 gram of the powdered root), divided into three doses

STANDARDIZATION

At this time, goldenseal is not available in standardized form.

REFERENCES

1. Cech R. An ecological imperative: growing a future for native plant medicinals. *United Plant Savers Newsletter* Fall 1997; 1–5.

2. Liebmann R. Saving goldenseal: a number one concern. *United Plant Savers Newsletter* Winter 1997; 6–7.

3. McGuffin M. AHPA goldenseal survey measures increased agricultural production. *HerbalGram* 1999; 46: 66–67.

4. Moore M. *Medicinal Plants of the Pacific West.* Santa Fe, NM: Red Crane Books, 1993.

5. Birdsall TC, Kelly GS. Berberine: therapeutic potential of an alkaloid found in several medicinal plants. *Alternative Medicine Review* 1997; 2(2): 94–103.

6. O'Hara M, Kiefer D, Farrell K, et al. A review of 12 commonly used medicinal herbs. *Archives of Family Medicine* 1998; 7: 523–536.

7. Bhide MB, Chavan SR, Dutta NK. Absorption, distribution, and excretion of berberine. *Indian Journal of Medical Research* 1969; 57(11): 2128–2131.

8. Lampe KF, Keller K, Hänsel R, Chandler RF, eds. Berberine. In: DeSmet PAGM, ed. *Adverse effects of herbal drugs.* Berlin: Springer-Verlag, 1992: 97–104.

9. Foster S. Goldenseal masking of drug tests: from fiction to fallacy. *HerbalGram* 1989; 21: 7.

10. Winek CL, Elzein EO, Wahba WW, et al. Interference of herbal drinks with urinalysis for drugs of abuse. *Journal of Analytical Toxicology* 1993; 17: 246–247.

11. Bergner P. Goldenseal and the common cold: the antibiotic myth. *Medical Herbalism* 1996/1997; 8(4): 1–10.

12. Sun D, Courtney HS, Beachey EH. Berberine sulfate blocks adherence of *Streptococcus pyogenes* to epithelial cells, fibronectin, and hexadecane. *Antimicrobial Agents and Chemotherapy* September 1988; 1370–1374.

13. Tierra M. *Planetary Herbology.* Santa Fe, NM: Lotus Press, 1988.

14. McGuffin M, Hobbs C, Upton R, Goldberg A, eds. *American Herbal Products Association Botanical Safety Handbook.* Boca Raton and New York: CRC Press LLC, 1997.

Grape Seed

VITIS VINIFERA
VITACEAE

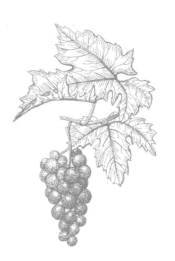

PART USED: *Seed*

PRIMARY USES

- *Antioxidant*
- *Poor vision and eye problems*
- *Varicose veins*
- *Circulatory problems*
- *Capillary fragility and easy bruising*
- *Sports injuries*
- *Heart health (experimental)*
- *Diabetes (experimental)*
- *Degenerative diseases (experimental)*

A votre santé! You now have permission to relish a glass or two of red wine, thanks to research showing that red wine (and red grape juice) can help reduce the risk of heart disease. The French have long boasted a low rate of heart disease despite their penchant for rich foods, sugar, and refined carbohydrates. Researchers believe the health benefits of red wine are one of the main explanations for this "French paradox." Red wine gets many of its health-enhancing qualities from pigment constituents in grape skins and from a flavonoid complex in the seeds known as *procyanidolic oligomers* (PCOs, or procyanidins). These antioxidant compounds are not present in white wine. Both red and green grapes are used in making white wine, but winegrowers immediately separate the juice from the skins and seeds, so that the healthful compounds from the skins and seeds do not get extracted into the juice. This is why researchers recommend red wine over white wine for health purposes.

Today you can buy superconcentrated, standardized sources of PCOs in the form of grape seed or pine bark extracts. PCOs have been shown to help protect against *free radicals,* unstable molecules that damage cells and tissues throughout the body. Researchers are now linking free radicals with premature wrinkles, sun damage, and more than 100 diseases, including cataracts, rheumatoid arthritis, heart disease, and cancer.[1] The body produces some enzymes designed to fight free radicals, but our natural defenses can easily be overwhelmed by poor diet, stress, pollution, and other modern problems. PCOs also reinforce the structure of *collagen,* the substance that makes up blood vessels and skin.

Although found in many plants, PCOs are often concentrated in barks, seeds, and other plant parts we don't usually eat. In fact, the first PCOs were isolated from the red skins of shelled peanuts. A young French Ph.D. candidate named Jacques Masquelier made this discovery during the Second World War while seeking a concentrated source of nutrition for his war-torn country. Looking for a source closer to home, Dr. Masquelier turned next to the pine forests stretching from Bordeaux to Spain, and later to grape seeds—a by-product of the French wine-making industry. When Dr. Masquelier discovered PCOs in pine bark, he originally called them "pycnogenols" as a way of distinguishing PCOs from other types of flavonoids. This term is now outdated from a scientific standpoint, but it remains in use as a trademark owned by a leading extract manufacturer. *Pinus maritima* is the species of pine found most widely in Europe and is used for the PCO-rich pine bark extracts. Despite their relatively short history in the West, grape seed and pine bark extracts have both risen to the top of the supplement charts in Europe and the United States.

HISTORY

For thousands of years, people have sipped wine, fed grapes to their lovers, and munched on raisins. Many cultures traditionally used grapes for a variety of medicinal purposes as well. Archeologists have traced wild grapes back to fossilized leaves from the Miocene and Tertiary period of ancient Europe, England, Iceland, and North America. At least 4,500 years ago, the Egyptians left behind the first detailed "manual" on wine making in the form of hieroglyphics painted on tomb walls. Grape cultivation began in the Caspian Sea region sometime before the eighteenth century B.C., gradually spreading to Greece, Italy, and France. In the United States, the first grape orchards were established on the East Coast around 1616. These were eventually abandoned because of cold temperatures and plant diseases, and California has been America's preeminent wine-making region ever since. Although the consumption and medicinal use of grapes has extended over many years, grape seed extract was patented only fairly recently, in 1970.

INTERNATIONAL STATUS

Grape seed is not officially approved for use in any European nation.

BOTANY

Wild grapes *(Vitis sylvestris)* and the first cultivated species *(Vitis vinifera)* are both native to the Caspian Sea region. The common grapevine is a perennial that climbs walls and arbors on its many tendrils. During the summer, clusters of pale green flowers perfume vineyards and backyard plots throughout the world. Grapes have green, yellow, or reddish-purple skins and two to four seeds inside the soft, pulpy flesh. Today, more than 8,000 grape cultivars exist, although only about 20 percent of these are actually grown. Most grape cultivation occurs in warm, temperate regions of the Northern Hemisphere and in cooler regions of South Africa, South America, China, Australia, and New Zealand.

BENEFITS

- Helps protect against free radical damage to cells and tissues throughout the body
- Reinforces the collagen structures of skin, blood vessels, ligaments, tendons and cartilage
- May help protect against allergies and many types of inflammation (experimental)

SCIENTIFIC SUPPORT

Since the 1970s, most of the research on procyanidins has focused on grape seed extract. (Although much of this evidence has been extrapolated to pine bark extract, not much actual research has been conducted with pine bark.) Grape seed extract demonstrated an ability to improve a number of vision problems, including computer-related fatigue and sensitivity to glare, in two double-blind, placebo-controlled clinical studies (see Specific Studies).[2,3] In another study, nearsighted patients taking grape seed extract experienced greater visual improvements than a placebo group.[4]

Grape seed extract has shown benefits in reducing capillary fragility caused by hypertension and diabetes, two conditions that are known to weaken the structure of veins and capillaries.[5] People with varicose veins have also noted improvements.[6] In a slightly more unusual study, grape seed extract helped reduce the volume and duration of postoperative edema (swelling) in women who had just had face-lifts, compared with an untreated group. In this study, women took 300 mg of grape seed extract daily for 5 days preceding surgery, and again from the second to sixth day after surgery.[7]

Grape seed's ability to protect cells and tissues from free radical damage could give it an important role to play in other health conditions as well, according to preliminary in vitro and in vivo research. One study indicated that grape seed extract may be helpful against heart disease, by protecting the heart during periods of ischemia (lack of blood and oxygen flow) and reperfusion (restoration of blood flow to the heart, which may cause oxidative damage and stress to the heart muscle).[8] In addition, researchers found that grape seed's antioxidant properties protect the lining of the gastrointestinal tract from damage, suggesting its potential benefit in conditions such as gastritis, gastric and duodenal ulcers, dyspepsia, and possibly even gastric cancer.[9]

Preliminary research suggests that grape seed extract may also offer protection to regular users of acetaminophen, an over-the-counter pain-reliever. In two studies, the extract helped protect liver and kidney cells from damage caused by a toxic dose of this common drug.[10,11]

Grape seed extract is currently being tested in the laboratory as a possible anticancer agent and as an adjunct treatment to help reduce the toxicity of chemotherapeutic drugs. The results of one study suggest that grape seed is more effective than vitamins C and E in protecting smokers against cell damage caused by tobacco-induced free radicals. This is good news, in light of the fact that roughly one-third of all cancers in the United States are tobacco-related.[12] Research also indicates that grape seed's antioxidant activity helps protect against UV damage, giving it a possible role to play in preventing skin cancer and premature aging.[13]

One of the main drawbacks of standard anticancer drugs is their negative impact on healthy cells. In an in vitro study, grape seed extract demonstrated selective toxicity toward cultured human breast, lung, and gastric cancer cells, while enhancing the growth and health of normal cells.[14] In an animal study, researchers found that the extract significantly prevented heart injury caused by doxorubicin, an important anticancer drug, when grape seed extract was given prior to drug therapy.[15] Scientists are currently testing the supplement's anticancer effects in several clinical trials at research centers in the United States.

SPECIFIC STUDIES

Computer-Related Visual Fatigue: Clinical Study (1990)

Grape seed extract relieved computer-related visual stress more effectively than bilberry *(Vaccinium myrtillus)* or placebo in a randomized, placebo-controlled, double-blind Italian study. During the 2-month study, 75 people (aged 20 to 60) who worked on computers for at least 6 hours a day were randomly assigned to one of three treatment groups. Group I took 300 mg of grape seed extract daily, group II took 300 mg bilberry daily, and group III took placebo. More than half of the subjects had an additional eye problem, and researchers distributed these subjects equally between the three groups.

By the end of the study, the grape seed group was experiencing significantly less visual stress, measured as an increase in scores at all points of a contrast sensitivity curve. The bilberry group improved at six points of the curve, and the placebo group at only two points. There was no change in visual acuity or color sense in any of the groups. Objective improvements were confirmed by reports of less visual fatigue in those taking grape seed extract, compared with little change in groups II and III. A few cases of mild stomach upset were reported, but these occurred just as frequently in the placebo group as in the active treatment groups.[2]

Sensitivity to Glare; Night Vision: Clinical Study (1988)

Grape seed extract was significantly more effective than placebo in reducing sensitivity to glare and improving night vision in a double-blind, placebo-controlled study. During the 5-week trial, 98 people were randomly assigned to take either 4 grape seed extract tablets daily (200 mg total) or placebo. Before the study, all subjects experienced prolonged visual stress from computers or strong lights and glare, or both. Those with more serious eye problems were excluded from the study. Investigators measured improvements by nycometer, scotoptometer, and ergovision. Mild side effects such as dizziness and stomach upset were reported by just two subjects taking grape seed extract.[3]

Capillary Fragility: Clinical Study (1981)

In a French study of 28 patients, grape seed extract was more effective than placebo in reducing capillary fragility caused by kidney problems, hypertension, diabetes, or obesity. During the preliminary open study, all 28 participants took 2 to 3 grape seed extract tablets daily (total 100 to 150 mg). After 3 months, 18 of 28 patients demonstrated a statistically significant increase in capillary resistance (strength of capillaries), measured by an instrument known as a capillaro-dynometer.

Researchers followed initial testing with a double-blind, placebo-controlled study in which subjects were randomly assigned to take grape seed extract or placebo for an additional 3 months. Grape seed again produced a statistically significant increase in capillary resistance, compared with insignificant improvement in the placebo group. Four people taking grape seed reported minor side effects, including stomachache and an itchy rash. Three hypertensive patients demonstrated a more positive "side effect"—a substantial drop in blood pressure.[5]

How It Works

Grape seed extract has two important properties that may give it a role to play in a variety of health conditions. The extract has demonstrated an ability to strengthen collagen, the most abundant protein in the body. Research shows that grape seed extract also neutralizes free radicals before they can cause damage to the body. Free radicals are unstable molecules that destroy tissues by oxidizing the fats that compose cell membranes and by damaging DNA, the body's genetic material.

Scientists now believe that free radicals are a common denominator in many health problems, including those related to vision, heart health, the gastrointestinal system, premature aging, and even cancer. Procyanidins (PCOs), the major constituents in grape seed and pine bark extracts, are potent antioxidants that help neutralize free radicals. According to *in vitro* research, PCOs from grape seed are more potent antioxidants than vitamins C, E, and beta-carotene.[16] Grape seed extract has also demonstrated superior antioxidant effects in living systems. In an animal experiment, the extract protected liver and brain tissues against free radical damage more effectively than any of these well-known antioxidant vitamins. For example, grape seed extract reduced free radical production by 70 percent, compared to only 47 percent, 18 percent, and 16 percent respectively for vitamins E, C, and beta-carotene. Grape seed extract reduced DNA fragmentation in liver tissue by 47 percent, compared to 36 percent, 12 percent, and 10 percent respectively for the other antioxidants. Similarly, reductions in DNA fragmentation in brain tissue were 48 percent for grape seed extract, compared to just 31 percent, 14 percent, and 11 percent for vitamins E, C, and beta-carotene. Results against lipid peroxidation (damage to the fats that compose cell membranes) in these tissues were similar.[9]

PCOs also have the remarkable ability to strengthen collagen and to prevent its destruction. The most abundant protein in the body, collagen maintains the structural integrity of the skin, blood vessels, tendons, ligaments, cartilage, and connective tissue. PCOs have been shown to reinforce collagen by binding and cross-linking to collagen fibers.[17] They also prevent the destruction of collagen by enzymes such as elastase, collagenase, hyaluronidase, and beta-glucuronidase, which are commonly released during inflammation.[18,19] In studies on vision-related problems, grape seed extract demonstrated an ability to fortify the collagen that makes up the capillaries. It also increased microcirculation to the retina of the eye.[5] In vision problems such as difficulty adjusting to glare, PCOs also appear to restore visual purple (an important protein in the rods of the eye) after damage by strong lights.[3]

Other studies suggest that PCOs may play a role in a range of inflammatory and allergic conditions by preventing the formation and release of harmful compounds such as prostaglandins, leukotrienes, serine proteases, and histamine.[17]

Some research suggests that grape seed extracts may contain a more potent form of PCOs than pine bark extract. This special form is known as gallic esters of procyanidins (especially proanthocyanidin B2-3′-O-gallate).[20] This hypothesis cannot be confirmed until more research is available on pine bark extract.

MAJOR CONSTITUENTS

Procyanidolic oligomers (PCOs) (also called oligomeric procyanidins, or OPCs)

SAFETY

Grape seed extract is considered nontoxic and has been extremely well tolerated in clinical trials.

- **Side effects:** Side effects are rare. Those reported in clinical studies included mild stomach upset, dizziness, or itchy rash.
- **Contraindications:** None known.
- **Drug interactions:** None known.

DOSAGE

- **Tablets/capsules:** For general support, 50 to 100 mg a day; for therapeutic purposes, 150 to 300 mg a day

STANDARDIZATION

Grape seed extract is typically standardized to contain 85 to 95 percent procyanidins.

REFERENCES

1. Bagchi D, Garg A, Krohn RL, et al. Protective effects of grape seed proanthocyanidins and selected antioxidants against TPA-induced hepatic and brain lipid peroxidation and DNA fragmentation, and peritoneal macrophage activation in

mice. *General Pharmacology* 1998; 30(5): 771–776.

2. Fusi L, Czimeg F, Pesce F, et al. Effects of procyanidolic oligomers from *Vitis vinifera* in subjects working at video-display units [in Italian]. *Annali di Ottalmologia e Clinica Oculista* 1990; 116: 575.

3. Corbe CH, Boissin JP, Siou A. Chromatic sense and chorioretinal circulation: a study of the effects of OPC (Endotelon) [in French]. *Journal Francais d'Ophtalmologie* 1988; 1(5): 453–460.

4. Proto F, Meucci B, Rispoli E, et al. Electrophysiological study of *Vitis vinifera* procyanoside oligomers: effects on retinal function in myopic subjects [in Italian]. *Annali di Ottalmologia e Clinica Oculista* 1988; 114: 85–93.

5. Lagrue G, Olivier-Martin F, Grillot A. A study of the effects of procyanidol oligomers on capillary resistance in hypertension and in certain nephropathies. *Semaine des Hoitaux de Paris* 1981; 57(33-36): 1399–1401.

6. Gomez Trillo JT. Varicose veins of the lower extremities: symptomatic treatment with a new vasculotrophic agent. *Prensa Medica Mexicana* 1973; 38(7-8): 293–296.

7. Baruch J. Effect of Endotelon in postoperative edema: results of a double-blind study versus placebo in 32 female patients [in French]. *Annales de Chirurgie Plastique et Esthetique* 1984; 29(4): 393–395.

8. Sato M, Maulik G, Ray P, et al. Cardioprotective effects of a novel IH636 grape seed proanthocyanidin extract. Paper presented at the IX Biennial Meeting of the International Society of Free Radical Research; September 7–11, 1998; Sao Paulo, Brazil.

9. Bagchi M, Williams CB, Milnes M, et al. Acute and chronic stress-induced gastrointestinal injury in rats, and protection by a novel IH636 grape seed proanthocyanidin extract (GSPE). *Free Radical Biology and Medicine* 1998a; 25 (suppl 1): S83.

10. Ray SD, Kumar MA, Bagchi D. *In vivo* abrogation of acetaminophen-induced hepatic genomic DNA fragmentation and apoptotic cell death by a novel grape seed proanthocyanidin extract (GSPE). *The FASEB Journal* 1998; 12(5): 3.

11. Ray SD. Effect of a novel IH636 grape seed proanthocyanidin extract on acetaminophen-induced nephrotoxicity. *Journal of the American College of Nutrition* 1998a; 17: abstract 49.

12. Bagchi M, Balmoori J, Bagchi D, et al. Protective effects of vitamins C and E, and a grape seed proanthocyanidin extract (GSPE) on smokeless tobacco-induced oxidative stress and apoptopic cell death in human oral keratinocytes. Paper presented at the Fourth Annual Meeting of the Oxygen Society; November 22, 1997; San Francisco, CA.

13. Facino RM, Carini M, Aldini G, et al. Photoprotective action of procyanidins from *Vitis vinifera* seeds on UV-induced damage: *in vitro* and *in vivo* studies. *Fitoterapia* 1998; 69(5): 39–40.

14. Joshi SS, Ye X, Liu W, et al. The cytotoxic effects of a novel grape seed proanthocyanidin extract on cultured human cancer cells. Paper presented at the 89th Annual Meeting of the American Association for

Cancer Research; March 28–April 1, 1998; New Orleans, LA.

15. Wong V, Fu K, Kohanchi B, et al. Antioxidant grape seed proanthocyanidin extract (GSPE) and a DNA repair modulator 3-aminobenzamide (3-AB) protect doxorubicin (DOX)-induced cardiotoxicity *in vivo*. Paper presented at the 38th Annual Meeting of the Society for Toxicology: March 15, 1999; New Orleans, LA.

16. Bagchi D, Krohn RL, Garg A, et al. Comparative *in vitro* and *in vivo* free radical scavenging abilities of grape seed proanthocyanidins and selected antioxidants. *The FASEB Journal* 1997a; 11(3): 4.

17. Masquelier J. Procyanidolic oligomers (leucocyanidins). *Parfums Cosmetiques Aromes* 1990; 95: 89–97.

18. Tixier JM, Godeau G, Robert AM, et al. Evidence by *in vivo* and *in vitro* studies that binding of pycnogenols to elastin affects its rate of degradation by elastases. *Biochemical Pharmacology* 1984; 33(24): 3933–3939.

19. Facino RM, Carini M, Aldini G, et al. Free radicals scavenging action and anti-enzyme activities of procyanidines from *Vitis vinifera. Arzneimittel-Forschung* 1994; 44(1): 592–601.

20. Schwitters B, Masquelier J. *OPC in Practice*. Rome: Alfa Omega Editrice, 1995.

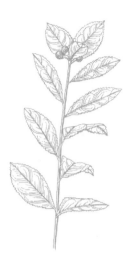

Green Tea

CAMELLIA SINENSIS
THEACEAE

State of Knowledge: Five-Star Rating System

Clinical (human) research	✳✳
Laboratory research	✳✳✳
History of use/traditional use	✳✳✳✳
Safety record	✳✳✳
International acceptance	✳✳✳✳

PART USED: *Leaf*

PRIMARY USES

- *Overall well-being*
- *Heart and liver health*
- *Cancer prevention*
- *Dental health (experimental)*

In 1992, results of a long-term study revealed that Japanese women who practiced the art of *Chanoyu* (the Japanese tea ceremony) had astonishingly low mortality rates compared with the general population of Japanese women. The good health and longevity of these women was attributed, at least in part, to their regular consumption of green tea.[1] This correlation, along with other strong scientific support, is testimony to the remarkable health benefits offered by one of the world's oldest and best-loved beverages.

Green tea is one of the most widely consumed beverages in the world, reported by one source to be second only to water.[2] An estimated 88 percent of the Chinese population drinks it daily. In many areas of Asia, such as China, India, and Japan, tea drinking is a highly evolved art. Tea ceremonies are considered sacred and are used to commemorate special events, such as marriage. Tea consumption is not limited to Asia: Americans drink more than 2 billion gallons every year, mostly iced.[3] Many Americans are familiar only with black tea, but green tea varieties are becoming increasingly popular as their impressive health benefits are brought to light.

The benefits of green tea are primarily preventive, not therapeutic. The healthful effects of green tea consumption are attributed to the presence of compounds called *polyphenols,* a type of compound called flavonoids—which are also found in many fruits, vegetables, and other herbs—that exert beneficial antioxidant properties. Oxidative damage to proteins and DNA in the body is caused by chemical reactions involving potentially harmful free radicals, which are thought to play an important role in aging and the development of many diseases. For example, cancer and heart disease both are believed to be linked to free radical damage. Green tea polyphenols are powerful antioxidants. In particular, polyphenols called *catechins* prevent these free radical reactions from happening. Some constituents in green tea even promote the activity of our own naturally occurring antioxidants.

Green, black, and oolong teas all come from the same plant, *Camellia sinensis.* The difference among the three lies in the processing method. Green tea is simply dried tea leaves, oolong tea is semifermented, and black tea is fermented, giving it the strongest flavor, darkest color, and lowest content of tannins and other polyphenols. The "fermentation" is not microbial like the fermentation of wine or yogurt. Instead, tea leaves are bruised by rolling to release enzymes that quickly convert green tea to darker forms. While the antioxidant benefits of green tea have been the most extensively studied, black tea also shows some promise in this area, although the evidence is not yet conclusive.

HISTORY

The oldest written mention of tea dates back to A.D. 780. The *Cha Ching* "tea book" relates that Chinese King Shen Nong discovered the beverage about 3,500 years earlier when some tea leaves blew into a pot of boiling water.[4] An early legend from ancient India holds that Prince Siddhartha Gautama, the founder of Buddhism, ripped off his eyelids and flung them to the ground out of frustration with his inability to stay awake during meditation while making a pilgrimage through China. A tea plant with leaves shaped like eyelids supposedly sprouted from the spot where the prince's eyelids fell.[4]

Many Eastern religious sects drank tea to stay alert during long meditations. The ancient tea ceremony of Japan has been honored for many generations and continues to play an important role in the spiritual life of many Japanese people. Many cultures believed that tea offered health benefits, including increased longevity. Today, India is the world's largest tea-producing nation, with China a close second.

Tea was introduced to Western culture in the sixth century by Turkish traders, who used it as a commodity of barter. For many years, both the Dutch and the British had strong footholds in tea-growing regions of the world. Tea arrived in America with the first settlers, but today is second in popularity to coffee and is more widely consumed as an iced, rather than hot, beverage. In American folk medicine, cooled tea bags were recommended as a poultice for puffy eyes, and cold tea as a wash for sunburn.

INTERNATIONAL STATUS

In general, green tea is considered a food. Green tea supplements are popular in Asia and are regulated as dietary supplements in the United States.

BOTANY

A member of the botanical family Theaceae, *Camellia sinensis* is a shrub native to Asia that is believed to have originated in the western Yunnan region of China, on the border between Burma and China.[5] The tea plant ranges in height from about 3 to 40 feet and has small, shiny, dark green leaves. The small, fragrant flowers have white petals, and the fruits contain one round, pale brown seed. This perennial evergreen grows in a variety of climates throughout the world, flourishing at altitudes from sea level to more than 7,000 feet. Tea does well in shade or direct sunlight, tolerates high rainfall, and prefers temperatures between 64 and 86° F.

Harvest time plays an important role in tea quality. Nearly all tea is handpicked, and only the top two leaves and the leaf bud are used to make fine tea. The first spring leaf buds, called the *first flush,* are considered the highest-quality leaves. When the first flush leaf bud is picked, another one grows, which is called the second flush, and later on, an autumn flush appears. Leaves picked farther down the stem are considered to be of poorer quality and are sometimes harvested by machine and processed into instant teas.

Tea varieties often reflect the growing region (such as Ceylon or Assam), the district (for example, Darjeeling), the form (pekoe is cut, gunpowder is rolled), and the processing method (green, black, or oolong). The plant is easily hybridized, which alters its genetic and biochemical makeup. In the future, we may see tea selectively grown to achieve a larger proportion of the constituents considered to be the most biologically active.

BENEFITS

- Contains powerful antioxidant compounds that inhibit free radical reactions
- Increases activity of certain protective antioxidant enzymes in the body

- Improves the ratio of LDL (low-density lipoprotein, or "bad" cholesterol) to HDL (high-density lipoprotein, or "good" cholesterol)
- Helps diminish the number of harmful compounds created by oxidative liver enzymes
- Encourages dental health by helping to prevent cavities

Scientific Support

In the last 15 years, green tea's cancer-preventive effects have received considerable scientific attention and support, including some noteworthy population studies. There have also been a large number of laboratory experiments demonstrating the action of antioxidants, and specifically tea polyphenols, in preventing and slowing disease. Population (epidemiological) studies have built-in limitations because even if they are very carefully controlled, factors other than the ones being studied may influence the results. For example, a review of epidemiological studies on tea consumption suggests that green tea may protect against colon cancer but not stomach cancer. It also points out that black tea consumption may be associated with increased risks for lung and colon cancers. However, inadequate controls in many of the experiments discussed could have confounded the results—that is, factors such as diet and exercise could be producing the effects researchers

observed. Nonetheless, there still is substantial evidence for the role of green tea in preventing cancer, particularly from more recent research.

Reduction of Cancer Risk

Consumption of caffeine-containing beverages, especially green tea, may alter hormone levels and reduce breast cancer risk.[6] In another study, green tea consumption appeared to decrease some of the mutagenic effects of smoking.[7] A lowered incidence of stomach cancer was observed in a case-control study of people who consumed more than 10 cups of green tea a day (actually about 40 ounces), although a later review suggests that this study may not have been properly controlled.[8] More recently, a large Chinese case-control study presented evidence suggesting that green tea might reduce the risk of colon and pancreatic cancers, with the trend appearing to be stronger in women than in men.[9] Finally, several small investigations also have offered evidence that green tea may protect against colon cancer, though this effect has not been tested in a large population study.[10]

Heart and Liver Health

Population studies also support the benefits of green tea in maintaining heart and liver health. In one investigation of Japanese people over 40, increased consumption of green tea (more than 10 cups daily) was associated with lowered levels of cholesterol and tri-glycerides. In this study, green tea was also associated with liver-protective effects, based on assessments of enzymes that indicate liver damage.[11] In another study, researchers found total cholesterol levels to be lower in individuals who consumed green tea than in those who did not, although it is possible that other Japanese dietary habits contributed to this effect.[12] Yet another study demonstrated a lowered rate of stroke in Japanese women who drank green tea frequently, compared with those who consumed less.[13] Though black tea contains many of the same constituents as green tea, at least one study was unable to show a relationship between black tea consumption and reduction of several cardiovascular disease risk factors.[14]

Laboratory studies of green tea also offer encouraging evidence with regard to heart disease. For example, researchers found that a green tea extract decreased the level of LDL cholesterol, which is associated with increased risk of cardiovascular disease.[15]

Numerous laboratory experiments underscore the power of tea polyphenols in preventing or slowing the progression of disease. In a recent study, tea polyphenols called catechins inhibited the growth of three types of human cancer cells, but not normal cells.[16] Epigallocatechin gallate, one of the major compounds in green tea, appears to exert an even stronger cancer-preventive influence when used in combination with cancer drugs such as sulindac and tamoxifen and even when combined with epicatechin, a tea polyphenol that normally does not show antioxidant activity.[17] In other laboratory studies, polyphenolic compounds from tea inhibited the growth of mouse and human cell tumors[18,19] and prevented or reduced the incidence of some tumors in rats.[20]

Dental Health

At least one laboratory study has investigated the use of green tea polyphenols in improving dental health. In this investigation, tea polyphenols prevented both the formation of certain sugars and the attachment of bacteria to dental surfaces, resulting in less tooth decay.[21] Other studies have shown reductions in tooth decay in animals.

Antioxidant Properties

Although the antioxidant benefits of green tea have been the most extensively studied, black tea has been the subject of some research in this area. Both green and black tea are rich sources of antioxidant polyphenols, though black tea has a lower concentration of polyphenols than green tea and is therefore only 20 percent as potent.[22] Evidence of black tea's anticancer potential is not conclusive, and there is even some suggestion that black tea consumption may increase the risk of certain cancers.[10]

Adding milk to tea seemed to dramatically decrease its antioxidant capabilities in some studies. Although no effects were observed when milk was added to green or black tea in *in vitro* laboratory studies, milk did inhibit the capacity of polyphenols to act *in vivo* (in the body).[22] This may be because proteins in the milk bind to the polyphenols. In another study, milk did not appear to lessen the body's ability to absorb tea catechins, although that study did not concern itself with whether the tea compounds remained active.[23] Obviously, further investigation is needed to clarify this issue.

SPECIFIC STUDIES

Cancer Prevention: Population Study (1997)

In a study of 8,552 Japanese men and women older than 40, researchers noted a lowered incidence of cancer in people who drank green tea regularly. The investigation began with a questionnaire about health history and dietary habits, including tea consumption. Researchers analyzed blood from all participants for the effects of green tea on cardiovascular and liver function; these results were reported in a separate study,[11] which is discussed later. The researchers followed the subjects to track how many cases of cancer developed over the next 9 years. They assessed the effects of tea consumption by observing the age at which cancer appeared in tea drinkers and by comparing daily tea consumption rates with cancer incidence.

The results suggested that the more tea was consumed, the later the onset of cancer. The effects of tea consumption were particularly striking for women who drank more than 10 cups of green tea daily. In that group, consumption of green tea was associated with a much later onset of cancer than is the norm. On the other hand, some men had an increased rate of cancer with green tea consumption, but this finding could be attributed to the effects of smoking and other lifestyle variables. In conclusion, daily consumption of more than 10 cups of green tea decreased the risk of cancer incidence in both men and women, but more dramatically in nonsmokers. Future studies will be directed at defining which organs benefit most from green tea's protective effects.[24]

Improved Cancer Prognosis: Population Study (1998)

Results of this 7-year study suggest that green tea consumption may help improve prognoses for patients with certain types of breast cancer. The study involved 472 women with stage I, II, or III breast cancer. The women provided an extensive health, lifestyle, and dietary history and underwent tests to determine tumor sizes, numbers of metastasized lymph nodes, and other disease markers. Increased green tea consumption was associated with decreased numbers of lymph node metastases in premenopausal women with stage I and II breast cancer, and with an increase in progesterone and estrogen receptors in postmenopausal women; all of these factors are important in determining cancer prognosis. Long-term consumption of more than 5 cups of tea daily was also significantly associated with decreased cancer recurrence in stage I and II patients who were in remission at the time of the follow-up study 6 years later. Researchers indicated that although other lifestyle changes may have influenced the improved prognosis, adjustments made when analyzing the results left green tea as the only potential predictor of decreased cancer recurrence. Green tea had no effect in stage III breast cancer patients.[25]

Cholesterol:
Population Study (1995)

In a population study of 1,371 Japanese men, researchers found that increased consumption of green tea (more than 10 cups a day, or about 40 ounces) was associated with decreased total cholesterol and blood fats. Blood samples from the subjects drinking tea showed an increase in HDL ("good") cholesterol, a decrease in LDL ("bad") cholesterol, and decreased concentrations of certain chemicals related to liver cell damage. An improved ratio of LDL to HDL cholesterol was also observed, indicating a reduced risk of arteriosclerosis. The researchers concluded that increased consumption of green tea is directly related to prevention of liver and heart disease.[11]

HOW IT WORKS

Today, researchers know that numerous diseases are associated with free radicals, highly reactive toxic chemicals that can damage DNA, proteins, and other molecules in the body. The main antioxidant compounds in green tea are its polyphenolic constituents, particularly flavonoids called catechins, which laboratory studies have identified as having the highest antioxidant activity of all tea compounds.[26]

Tea polyphenols exert their effects in several different ways. First, they may inhibit cytochrome P-450 activation of carcinogens. Cytochrome P-450 is a liver enzyme system which generally helps the body eliminate toxins and metabolize drugs, but in some cases can activate carcinogens. Second, polyphenols may also increase the antioxidant capacity of some tissues, decreasing their susceptibility to tumor formation.[26] This may be because they enhance the actions of several antioxidant enzymes that occur naturally in the body, including glutathione reductase and glutathione-S-transferase. Finally, polyphenolic flavonoids also appear to prevent the formation of certain carcinogens, including some potentially mutagenic compounds present in prepared foods.[27]

Epigallocatechin gallate, one of the major polyphenolic constituents of green tea, has been shown to prevent tumor initiation and promotion induced by various carcinogens, although the mechanism of action has not yet been fully determined.

MAJOR CONSTITUENTS

Polyphenolic flavonoids, including epicatechin, epigallocatechin, and gallate esters; quercetin, myricetein; tannins, terpenoids, and alkaloids (caffeine, theobromine, and theophylline)

SAFETY

Green tea is generally safe and nontoxic. It contains up to 50 mg of caffeine per cup, compared with 85 mg in coffee. Caffeine is a nervous system stimulant and is not recommended for long-term or excessive use.[28] Some green tea extracts are decaffeinated, which does not affect their polyphenol content.

- **Side effects:** Both green and black tea contain caffeine and, like coffee, may cause side effects, including nervousness, heart irregularities, anxiety, restlessness, insomnia, and digestive irritation.[28] The tannins may upset sensitive stomachs.

- **Contraindications:** Tea is considered nontoxic, but beverages containing caffeine should be avoided during pregnancy and by those with hypertension, other heart conditions, anxiety, eating disorders, insomnia, diabetes, and ulcers. Tea is not recommended for infants.
- **Drug interactions:** None known.[28]

DOSAGE

Between 2 and 3 cups a day is an average dose, but in some studies, subjects drank up to 10 cups (40 ounces) a day. Standardized tea extracts vary in strength, so dosages may need to be adjusted.

- **Standardized extract:** 250 to 400 mg a day of extract standardized to 90 percent polyphenols.
- **Tea:** 2 to 5 cups a day. Use 1 teaspoon of tea leaves per cup of hot water.

Tea brewing tips: For optimum brewing, green tea requires slightly cooler water temperatures and less brewing time (about 3 minutes) than other teas in order to bring out its subtle flavors. Let the boiling water cool slightly before steeping the tea. Black and oolong tea varieties require boiling water and slightly longer steeping time (3 to 5 minutes).

STANDARDIZATION

Green tea supplements are often standardized to contain up to 97 percent polyphenols, including up to 60 percent catechins.

REFERENCES

1. Sadakata S, Fukao A, Hisamichi S. Mortality among female practitioners of chanoyu (Japanese "tea-ceremony"). *Tohoku Journal of Experimental Medicine* 1992; 166: 475–477.

2. Graham HN. Green tea composition, consumption, and polyphenol chemistry. *Preventive Medicine* 1992; 21: 334–350.

3. McCord H. Tea time. *Prevention* March 2, 1999; 68–71.

4. Gutman RL, Ryu B-H. Rediscovering tea. *HerbalGram* 1996; 37: 33–40.

5. Bisset NG, ed. *Herbal Drugs and Phytopharmaceuticals.* Boca Raton, FL: CRC Press, 1994.

6. Nagata C, Kabuto M, Shimizu H. Association of coffee, green tea, and caffeine intakes with serum concentrations of estradiol and sex hormone-binding globulin in premenopausal Japanese women. *Nutrition and Cancer* 1998; 30(1): 21–24.

7. Shim JS, Kang MH, Kim YH, et al. Chemopreventive effect of green tea among cigarette smokers. *Cancer Epidemiology, Biomarkers and Prevention* 1995; 4: 387–391.

8. Kono S, Ikeda M, Tokudome S, et al. A case-control study of gastric cancer and diet in northern Kyushu, Japan. *Japanese Journal of Cancer Research* 1988; 79: 1067–1074.

9. Ji B-T, Chow W-H, Hsing AW, et al. Green tea consumption and the risk of pancreatic and colorectal cancers. *International Journal of Cancer* 1997; 70: 255–258.

10. Kohlmeier L, Weterings KGC, Steck S, et al. Tea and cancer prevention: an evaluation of the epidemiologic literature. *Nutrition and Cancer* 1997; 27(1): 1–13.

11. Imai K, Nakachi K. Cross sectional study of effects of drinking green tea on cardiovascular and liver diseases. *British Medical Journal* 1995; 310: 693–696.

12. Kono S, Shinchi K, Ikeda N, et al. Green tea consumption and serum lipid profiles: a cross-sectional study in northern Kyushu, Japan. *Preventive Medicine* 1992; 21: 526–531.

13. Sato Y, Nakatsuka H, Watanabe T, et al. Possible contribution of green tea drinking habits to the prevention of stroke. *Tohoku Journal of Experimental Medicine* 1989; 157: 337–343.

14. Bingham SA, Vorster H, Jerling JC, et al. Effect of black tea drinking on blood lipids, blood pressure and aspects of bowel habit. *British Journal of Nutrition* 1997; 78: 41–55.

15. Luo M, Kannar K, Wahlqvist M, et al. Inhibition of LDL oxidation by green tea extract (letter). *The Lancet* 1997; 349: 360–361.

16. Chen ZP, Schell JB, Ho C-T, et al. Green tea epigallocatechin gallate shows a pronounced growth inhibitory effect on cancerous cells but not on their normal counterparts. *Cancer Letters* 1998; 129: 173–179.

17. Suganuma M, Okabe S, Kai Y, et al. Synergistic effects of (–)-epigallocatechin gallate with (–)-epicatechin, sulindac, or tamoxifen on cancer-preventive activity in the human lung cancer cell line PC-9. *Cancer Research* 1999; 59: 44–47.

18. Menon LG, Kuttan R, Kuttan G. Inhibition of lung metastasis in mice induced by B16F10 melanoma cells by polyphenolic compounds. *Cancer Letters* 1995; 95: 221–225.

19. Liao S, Umekita Y, Guo J, et al. Growth inhibition and regression of human prostate and breast tumors in athymic mice by tea epigallocatechin gallate. *Cancer Letters* 1995; 96: 239–243.

20. Chen J. The effects of Chinese tea on the occurrence of esophageal tumors induced by *N*-nitrosomethylbenzylamine in rats. *Preventive Medicine* 1992; 21: 385–391.

21. Otake S, Makimura M, Kuroki T, et al. Anticaries effects of polyphenolic compounds from Japanese green tea. *Caries Research* 1991; 25: 438–443.

22. Serafini M, Ghiselli A, Ferro-Luzzi A. *In vivo* antioxidant effect of green and black tea in man. *European Journal of Clinical Nutrition* 1996; 50: 28–32.

23. van het Hof KH, Kivits GAA, Weststrate JA, et al. Bioavailability of catechins from tea: the effect of milk. *European Journal of Clinical Nutrition* 1998; 52: 356–359.

24. Imai K, Suga K, Nakachi K. Cancer-preventive effects of drinking green tea among a Japanese population. *Preventive Medicine* 1997; 26: 769–775.

25. Nakachi K, Suemasu K, Suga K, et al. Influence of drinking green tea on breast cancer malignancy among Japanese patients. *Japanese Journal of Cancer Research* 1998; 89: 254–261.

26. Agarwal R, Mukhtar H. Cancer chemoprevention by polyphenols in green tea and artichoke. In: *Dietary Pharmaceuticals in Cancer Prevention and Treatment.* Edited under the auspices of the American Institute for Cancer Research. New York: Plenum Press, 1996.

27. Stich HF. Teas and tea components as inhibitors of carcinogen formation in model systems and man. *Preventive Medicine* 1992; 21: 377–384.

28. McGuffin M, Hobbs C, Upton R, Goldberg A, eds. *American Herbal Products Association Botanical Safety Handbook.* Boca Raton and New York: CRC Press LLC, 1997.

Guggul

COMMIPHORA MUKUL
BURSERACEAE

State of Knowledge: Five-Star Rating System

Clinical (human) research	✳✳
Laboratory research	✳✳
History of use / traditional use	✳✳✳✳
Safety record	✳✳✳✳
International acceptance	✳✳

PART USED: *Resin*

PRIMARY USES

- *High cholesterol*

In 1966, inspired by an ancient Sanskrit text, a young Indian doctoral candidate named G.V. Satyavati first reported on the cholesterol-lowering action of an Ayurvedic herb called guggul. She based her work on insights provided in an obscure portion of the famous Ayurvedic treatise *Sushrutasamhita*—insights related to the treatment of obesity and associated serum lipid (blood fat) disorders with guggul. Intrigued by the similarities between the ancient concept of *medoroga* (obesity and

related blood-fat disorders) and modern understanding of the cardiovascular disease we call *atherosclerosis* (hardening and narrowing of the arteries), Satyavati and her advisor carried out the first laboratory studies of guggul. Their early work showed that guggul resin significantly lowered serum cholesterol in rabbits with high blood cholesterol while protecting the animals against atherosclerosis caused by cholesterol buildup in the blood vessels.[1]

More than three decades have passed since this groundbreaking work. Today, because of the well-established connection between elevated cholesterol levels and heart disease, the research spawned by Satyavati's insight is more important than ever. Clinical and laboratory studies have confirmed the cholesterol- and lipid-lowering effects of certain components of guggul resin.

Unprocessed guggul resin, known as gum guggul or guggulu, yields two distinct portions when extracted. One portion is toxic and is not used medicinally, but the nontoxic portion, a mixture of lipid steroids called *guggulipid,* contains compounds that have shown cholesterol-lowering and anti-inflammatory activity. The best-researched of these are steroid constituents called *guggulsterones.* Other compounds also appear to exert a synergistic effect that supports guggulipid's beneficial activity. Studies show that standardized extracts of guggulipid not only lower levels of cholesterol and other blood fats that may contribute to the development of heart disease, but also increase levels of high-density lipoprotein cholesterol (HDL, or "good" cholesterol).

In 1986, guggulipid was approved for sale in India as a cholesterol-reducing agent. Although its acceptance in India is widespread, guggul is catching on slowly in the Western world. With its cholesterol-lowering power and good safety record, backed both by centuries of traditional medical wisdom and by modern clinical trials, guggul's popularity in the West is likely to expand.

HISTORY

Guggul's history of use in Ayurvedic medicine extends over many centuries, with references dating as far back as 600 B.C. The best-known Ayurvedic applications of the herb are for the treatment of various forms of arthritis, obesity, diabetes, and gout. Ancient Ayurvedic texts stress the importance of using older samples of gum guggul in the effective treatment of obesity and inflammatory and arthritic conditions, as opposed to fresh gum guggul, which was believed to have the opposite effect of increasing body weight.[1]

Other important traditional Ayurvedic uses for guggul have included the treatment of skin disorders (such as psoriasis) and cervical spondylosis (a type of arthritis that affects the spine), stimulation of immune function, and improvement of appetite and digestion. It has been administered topically to abraded skin as an astringent and antiseptic. Guggul is also employed as a mouthwash to treat mouth and dental conditions and as an inhalation for upper respiratory symptoms. Tibetan medicine uses a mixture of guggul and other herbs in the treatment of skin disorders, anemia, and edema (fluid retention).[1] A close relative of myrrh, an important fragrance plant, guggul has also been added to incense and perfumes.

Concerted modern interest in guggul began in India in the mid-1960s. Satyavati's early work on guggul launched a two-decade period of intense investigation by both government scientists and independent Indian investigators into its cholesterol-lowering activity and chemical properties.

INTERNATIONAL STATUS

Guggul is approved by the Indian government.

BOTANY

Guggul *(Commiphora mukul)* and its close relative myrrh *(Commiphora molmol)* are members of the botanical family Burseraceae, a group of plants characterized by the presence of resin ducts in the bark. Guggul is a small, spiny tree that grows in arid, rocky regions of India and Bangladesh. It attains heights of 4 to 6 feet and is characterized by an ash-colored, flaky outer bark, alternate leaves, and sharp spines. It has small, pulpy, roundish fruits, and flowers that appear singly or in clusters. Guggul's medicinal oleo gum resin, also known as Indian Bdellium, is harvested during the cold season from incisions made in the bark of plants aged 5 years or older. The yellow fluid emanating from these cuts hardens into a reddish brown resin within a week or two, after which it is harvested.[1]

BENEFITS

- Helps reduce and maintain cholesterol levels
- Increases the level of HDL ("good") cholesterol
- Protects the heart against atherosclerosis
- Reduces inflammation
- May regulate metabolism through effects on the thyroid

SCIENTIFIC SUPPORT

A number of human trials have demonstrated the effectiveness and safety of guggul in the treatment of high cholesterol. According to studies, the purified extract of guggul, called guggulipid, can improve and maintain the ratio of HDL cholesterol to LDL and very low density lipoprotein (VLDL) cholesterol levels. Most, if not all, of the clinical research on guggul has been performed in India, where the Central Drug Research Institute has extensively researched the herb's effects and mode of action.[2] Guggul has also reduced cholesterol, triglycerides, and total lipid levels when taken in combination with pushkarmool *(Inula racemosa),* a traditional Ayurvedic remedy for angina.[3]

In clinical studies comparing guggulipid with clofibrate, a synthetic cholesterol-lowering drug, guggulipid showed an equal or superior ability to lower serum cholesterol and triglyceride levels.[4,5] Guggulipid also increased levels of HDL cholesterol, an activity that was not demonstrated by clofibrate.[4] In a laboratory experiment, isolated E- and Z-guggulsterones—active compounds in guggulipid—showed an ability to inhibit platelet aggregation (clumping) in a fashion similar to clofibrate, thereby potentially reducing the risk of heart attack and other cardiovascular disease.[6]

Results of at least two laboratory studies suggest that Z-guggulsterone may activate the thyroid gland.[7,8] This stimulation of the thyroid may be at least partially responsible for guggul's lipid- and cholesterol-lowering effects, as well as its unconfirmed anti-obesity activity.

Not all patients with elevated lipid levels respond to guggul therapy. One study showed that people with type IIb and type IV hyperlipoproteinemia (elevated cholesterol and triglycerides) experienced the most benefit.[9] In a study that compared the effects of guggulipid and the drug clofibrate, patients with elevated cholesterol responded better to guggulipid, while those with elevated triglycerides responded better to clofibrate.[4] In these studies, beneficial effects became apparent after an initial treatment period of 2 to 4 weeks, and lasted two to five months beyond completion of treatment.[4,9]

Finally, animal and laboratory experiments have demonstrated that guggulipid possesses some anti-inflammatory activity, offering support for the herb's traditional use for arthritis and other inflammatory conditions.[10,11] In one study in mice, guggul extract was as effective as ibuprofen and phenylbutazone in reducing experimentally induced rheumatoid arthritis. Results indicated that all three of the test substances were effective in reducing joint swelling after 5 months of treatment.[10]

SPECIFIC STUDIES

Elevated Cholesterol and Triglycerides: Clinical Study (1989)

Two studies, one an open trial and the other a double-blind crossover trial, demonstrated guggulipid's ability to significantly reduce serum cholesterol and lipid levels in a manner comparable or superior to that of clofibrate, a synthetic cholesterol-lowering drug. In the open trial, researchers observed a significant lowering of serum cholesterol and triglyceride levels in 70 to 80 percent of 205 patients undergoing 12 weeks of treatment with guggulipid (500 mg three times daily). Mean reductions in serum cholesterol and serum triglycerides were 21.59 percent and 24.61 percent respectively, a statistically significant lowering.

In a subsequent double-blind crossover trial, guggulipid was compared with the synthetic drug clofibrate in 233 people with elevated cholesterol or triglyceride levels or both. Patients with high cholesterol showed a better reaction to guggulipid, and patients with elevated triglyceride levels responded better to clofibrate. Patients with both conditions responded comparably to the two medications: 88 percent responded to guggulipid treatment and 83.3 percent to clofibrate. LDL cholesterol decreased significantly with both treatments, but only patients taking guggulipid demonstrated an increase in beneficial HDL cholesterol. Only one person taking guggul reported gastro-intestinal side effects. The lipid-lowering effects of both guggulipid and clofibrate persisted for approximately 20 weeks after the end of treatment.[4]

Elevated Cholesterol and Triglycerides: Clinical Study (1988)

In this placebo-controlled, randomized trial, 40 people with hyperlipidemia (elevated cholesterol and triglyceride levels) received treatment with either gum guggul or placebo. The 20 patients who took 4.5 grams daily of purified gum guggul showed statistically significant lowering of levels of certain lipids associated with the development of coronary artery disease. All patients were between 40 and 60 years old and had a history of coronary artery disease or myocardial infarction (heart attack). All were also taking antianginal drugs.

In the guggul group, serum cholesterol decreased by 21.75 percent and triglyceride levels by 27.1 percent over the course of the 16-week study. In addition, VLDL and LDL levels decreased significantly, while HDL levels rose significantly, by approximately 26 percent. A statistically significant and persistent effect on these variables was observed within 8 weeks of the beginning of the trial. No adverse effects were reported.[12]

Elevated Cholesterol and Triglycerides: Clinical Study (1986)

A phase I trial assessing the safety of long-term guggul treatment in a group of 21 people with histories of hypertension, ischemic heart disease, gout, or diabetes mellitus concluded that guggul had no adverse effects and was well tolerated by all but one patient. Results of a subsequent small phase II (efficacy) trial showed that cholesterol and/or triglyceride levels were lowered in 15 of 19 people taking guggul. In the phase I trial, guggul was administered at a dosage of 400 mg three times daily for 4 weeks. Twenty of the 21 patients experienced no adverse effects. One patient complained of mild heartburn, which was controlled with oral antacids.

In the phase II trial, 19 patients with suspected or confirmed coronary artery disease and primary hyperlipidemia received placebo for 2 weeks, followed by 500 mg of guggulipid three times daily for 12 weeks, then placebo for 8 weeks. Analysis of blood samples drawn every 4 weeks showed that cholesterol levels were lowered by an average of 17.5 percent and triglycerides by 30.3 percent in the 15 patients who responded to treatment. Researchers observed lipid-lowering effects as early as 4 weeks after treatment started.[9]

HOW IT WORKS

Researchers believe that guggulsterones are the compounds responsible for guggul's cholesterol-lowering activity. A number of studies suggest that guggul lowers cholesterol both by inhibiting cholesterol synthesis in the liver as well as by promoting the breakdown and excretion of cholesterol.[1] In addition, at least one animal study showed that guggulsterones stimulate the thyroid, which may in part account for the lipid- and cholesterol-lowering activity as well as for guggul's traditional use against obesity.[7,8] Further study is needed, however, to investigate the effectiveness of guggul as a weight-control remedy. Gum guggul extracts also inhibit platelet aggregation (abnormal blood clotting), which may further protect cardiovascular health by lowering the risk of stroke and pulmonary embolism.[6]

MAJOR CONSTITUENTS

Guggulsterones, 21- and 27-carbon steroidal compounds; aromatic and nonaromatic acids

SAFETY

Traditional usage and clinical safety studies have demonstrated the safety of standardized guggulipid extract in a dosage of 400 to 500 mg three times a day.

- **Side effects:** A small number of people in some clinical studies reported mild gastrointestinal discomfort, but this side effect was not severe enough to cause them to discontinue the remedy. Ingestion of the crude extract (gum guggul) at clinical doses may produce rashes and gastrointestinal upsets. The standardized extract, guggulipid, has a much better safety record. In very large doses (more than 2 to 4 g), guggulipid may cause kidney irritation and diarrhea.[13]
- **Contraindications:** Guggul should not be used during pregnancy, because studies suggest it may stimulate uterine contractions. Women with excessive uterine bleeding should not take guggul.[13]
- **Drug interactions:** None known.

DOSAGE

The dosages used in clinical studies on cholesterol-lowering effects ranged from 25 mg of guggulsterone three times daily to 400 to 500 mg of guggulipid extract standardized to 5 percent guggulsterones. Today, commercial guggulipid extracts are standardized to

2.5 percent guggulsterones. Clinical trials suggest that for the most effective cholesterol-lowering action, long-term use is needed. In the studies, beneficial effects were seen after 2 to 4 weeks and lasted several months beyond the end of treatment.

- **Standardized extract:** 1,000 mg three times a day of extract standardized to 2.5 percent guggulsterones.

STANDARDIZATION

Guggulipid extract typically contains 2.5 percent guggulsterones.

REFERENCES

1. Satyavati G. Guggulipid: a promising hypolipidaemic agent from gum guggul *(Commiphora wightii).* In: Wagner H, Farnsworth NR, eds. *Economic and Medicinal Plant Research.* Vol. 5. San Diego: Academic Press, 1991.

2. Satyavati G. Gum guggul *(Commiphora mukul)*—The success story of an ancient insight leading to a modern discovery. *Indian Journal of Medical Research* 1988; 87: 327–335.

3. Singh RP, Singh R, Ram P, et al. Use of pushkar-guggul, an indigenous anti-ischemic combination, in the management of ischemic heart disease. *International Journal of Pharmacognosy* 1993; 31(2): 147–160.

4. Nityanand S, Srivastava JS, Asthana OP. Clinical trials with guggulipid: a new hypolipidemic agent. *Journal of the Association of Physicians of India* 1989; 37(5): 323–328.

5. Malhotra SC, Ahuja MMS, Sundaram KR. Long term clinical studies on the hypolipidaemic effect of Commiphora mukul (Guggulu) and Clofibrate. *Indian Journal of Medical Research* 1977; 65(3): 390–395.

6. Mester L, Mester M, Nityanand S. Inhibition of platelet aggregation by "guggulu" steroids. *Planta Medica* 1979; 37: 367–369.

7. Tripathi SN, Gupta M, Sen SP, et al. Effect of a keto-steroid of *Commifora mukul* L. on hypocholesterolemia and hyperlipidemia induced by neomercazole and cholesterol mixture in chicks. *Indian Journal of Experimental Biology* 1975; 13: 15–18.

8. Tripathi YB, Malhotra OP, Tripathi SN. Thyroid stimulating action of Z-guggulsterone obtained from Commiphora mukul. *Planta Medica* 1984; 50: 78–80.

9. Agarwal RC, Singh SP, Saran RK, et al. Clinical trial of guggulipid—a new hypolipidemic agent of plant origin in primary hyperlipidemia. *Indian Journal of Medical Research* 1986; 84: 626–634.

10. Sharma JN, Sharma JN. Comparison of the anti-inflammatory activity of *Commiphora mukul* (an indigenous drug) with those of phenylbutazone and ibuprofen in experimental arthritis induced by mycobacterial adjuvant. *Arzneimittel-Forschung* 1977; 27(2): 1455–1457.

11. Arora RB, Taneja V, Sharma RC, et al. Anti-inflammatory studies on a crystalline steroid isolated from Commiphora mukul. *Indian Journal of Medical Research* 1972; 60: 929–931.

12. Verma SK, Bordia A. Effect of *Commiphora mukul* (gum *guggulu*) in patients of hyper-lipidemia with special reference to HDL-cholesterol. *Indian Journal of Medical Research* 1988; 87: 356–360.

13. McGuffin M, Hobbs C, Upton R, et al., eds. *American Herbal Products Association Botanical Safety Handbook*. New York: CRC Press, 1997.

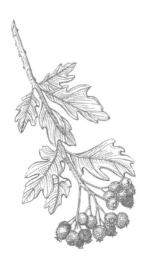

Hawthorn

CRATAEGUS LAEVIGATA
(SYNONYM C. OXYACANTHA)
ROSACEAE

State of Knowledge: Five-Star Rating System

Clinical (human) research	✱✱✱
Laboratory research	✱✱✱
History of use/traditional use	✱✱✱✱
Safety record	✱✱✱✱
International acceptance	✱✱✱✱

PART USED: *Flower, leaf, fruit*

PRIMARY USES

- *Heart health*
- *Mild, chronic congestive heart failure*
- *Cardiac insufficiency*
- *Recovery after heart attack*
- *Aging heart*

Gentle, nontoxic hawthorn fits the classic definition of a health-promoting tonic. One of the premier cardiovascular herbs in the European herbal tradition, hawthorn has a long history of use as a food and as a slow-acting but effective cardiovascular tonic that strengthens the heart muscle, improves blood flow, and enhances the overall efficiency of the circulatory system.

In the last 50 years, clinical experience in Europe has proven that hawthorn can have potent therapeutic effects for heart conditions, including mild congestive heart failure, mild arrhythmia (irregular heart beat), and angina pectoris (chest pain caused by insufficient blood flow to the heart). It is especially appropriate for use in strengthening the function of the heart after a heart attack. Today, hawthorn is widely prescribed for these purposes by physicians in Germany, Switzerland, France, the United Kingdom, and other European nations.

Hawthorn is rich in compounds called *flavonoids,* plant pigments that have been well studied for their powerful antioxidant effects. Flavonoids, which are present in the vast majority of plant tissues, are known for many other healthful effects, including their ability to stabilize and prevent destruction of collagen (the protein that makes up blood vessels), reduce capillary permeability, and help prevent plaque buildup in blood vessels that can lead to atherosclerosis, or hardening and narrowing of the arteries.[1,2]

The benefits of hawthorn are still largely unknown in the United States, where heart disease tops the list of leading causes of death. According to the U.S. National Heart, Lung, and Blood Institute, congestive heart failure is an increasingly common diagnosis in people over age 65 and is expected to become even more common as the population ages. Congestive heart failure occurs as the heart muscle weakens, gradually losing its ability to pump blood to the rest of the body. The condition is twice as common in those with high blood pressure and five times as common in people who have had one or more heart attacks. For those who have already had a heart attack, tonic use of hawthorn may be one of the best steps to take to help head off future heart attacks and prevent the eventual development of congestive heart failure.

Because hawthorn acts slowly, it is not appropriate for cases of acute heart failure, which are treated with strong, fast-acting drugs. But clinical research shows that hawthorn can help improve symptoms and slow the progress of mild, early-stage congestive heart failure that does not yet require drug treatment.

Active heart disease is a serious condition that is not appropriate for self-diagnosis or treatment. If you suspect that you have a heart problem, or are already under treatment for a cardiovascular condition (including high blood pressure), talk to your health-care practitioner before taking hawthorn. In particular, if you have chest pain or pain that spreads from the chest to the arms, neck, or upper abdomen, or if you are having trouble breathing, call your doctor right away.

HISTORY

Widespread European use of hawthorn for the treatment of heart disease began in the late 1800s, when physicians learned of the good results achieved in the treatment of heart disease by an Irish doctor named Green. According to reports from the medical literature of the time, after Dr. Green's death, his daughter revealed that the secret of her father's success was tincture of hawthorn berries. In 1896, this story was reported in *The New York Medical Journal,* and hawthorn quickly became established in American medical practice. Before this time, European physicians seem to have used hawthorn mainly in the treatment of urinary tract problems (including kidney stones), diarrhea and other digestive upsets, and coughs. Hawthorn's astringent properties were well known for centuries.[3]

The traditional Chinese medicine *Shān Zhā* is made from the fruit of the Asian hawthorn species *Crataegus pinnatifida, C. pinnatifida* var. *major,* and *C. cuneata.* Practitioners of traditional Chinese medicine have used hawthorn berries for improving digestion and for treating dyspepsia (indigestion), diarrhea, lack of milk secretion, heart pain, and abdominal distress due to food stagnation.[3,4] In both Europe and China, hawthorn berries have been eaten as a food and were made into wines and jellies. Native Americans used their local hawthorn species for food as well as for the treatment of rheumatism and stomach and bladder problems.

Hawthorn has been called by a variety of different common names throughout history, many of which attest to the plant's role in religious and cultural rituals. In ancient Britain, hawthorn was an important part of springtime May festivals, a use reflected in the common names *mayflower, may bush,* and *mayblossom.* In France, hawthorn sometimes goes by the name *l'epine noble* (the noble thorn), a reference to the belief that the crown of thorns worn by Christ was made of hawthorn branches. Other cultures viewed hawthorn as a symbol of hope, love, and fertility, and often incorporated the plant into wedding ceremonies.

Because of their fast growth habits, hawthorn trees were often used to create living fences to divide property—hence the names quickset and hedgethorn. In fact, the word *haw* is derived from an old word for hedge.

INTERNATIONAL STATUS

In the *German Commission E Monographs,* hawthorn leaf and flower preparations are approved for use in decreasing cardiac output in stage II cardiac insufficiency (congestive heart failure).[5] The berries of the Chinese hawthorns *Crataegus pinnatifida, C. pinnatifida* var. *major,* and *C. cuneata* are listed as official medicines in the *Pharmacopoeia of the People's Republic of China.*[3]

BOTANY

A member of the rose family (Rosaceae), *Crataegus laevigata* is related to many of our best-loved fruit plants, including apples, cherries, plums, and berries such as raspberries, strawberries, and blackberries. The bright red hawthorn fruits themselves, called *haws,* resemble tiny apples or rosehips. Today, extracts made of hawthorn leaf and flower are more widely used than the berries, although some hawthorn preparations contain all three plant parts.

Hawthorn is a small, compact, shrubby tree with white bark, very hard wood, and sharp thorns. As reflected in the common name *mayflower,* the tree puts forth numerous clusters of white or pink blossoms in the spring. The flowers, which are often pollinated by carrion insects, give off a faint smell of decay that these insects find attractive.

Estimates of the number of *Crataegus* species in the world range from about 150 to more than 1,000,[6] depending on how the species are defined by botanists, but the actual number of species is probably closer to 280.[3] Most hawthorns are found in northern temperate zones in Europe, eastern Asia, and eastern North America. Although North American hawthorns have been used in traditional remedies, their medicinal properties have not yet been formally studied.

In scientific and popular literature, *Crataegus laevigata* is often mistakenly called by the outdated name *Crataegus oxyacantha.* Another hawthorn species commonly employed in European medicine is *C. monogyna.*

BENEFITS

- Strengthens the pumping ability of the heart muscle
- Enhances the flow of blood to and from the heart, improving blood supply to the heart
- Dilates and relaxes blood vessels, decreasing the resistance of vessels to blood flow
- Lowers blood pressure
- Protects against free radical damage and lipid peroxidation

SCIENTIFIC SUPPORT

In Germany, where most of the research on hawthorn has been performed, numerous studies of people with chronic congestive heart failure have demonstrated that hawthorn increases exercise tolerance and helps improve typical symptoms such as shortness of breath and fatigue. The effects of hawthorn appear to be dose and time dependent, meaning that better results are achieved with higher doses administered for longer periods of time.[7]

The majority of human studies have investigated the effects of hawthorn in people with stage II and III heart failure, as defined by the classification system of the New York Heart Association (NYHA). In stage II heart failure, patients typically experience symptoms such as shortness of breath, increased heart rate, and a feeling of tightness in the chest upon strenuous physical activity. Symptoms worsen in stage III, occurring even during normal physical activity.

In most of the studies, doctors assessed the effects of hawthorn using a special stationary bicycle that allowed them to measure changes in heart rate, blood pressure, and the working capacity of the heart during exercise. Results of one of these studies showed that hawthorn was as effective as the drug captopril in improving exercise tolerance and reducing heart rate in patients with stage II heart failure (see Specific Studies).[8] Captopril is a type of heart drug commonly known as an ACE inhibitor (short for angiotensin-converting enzyme inhibitor), which is often prescribed to treat high blood pressure and congestive heart failure. Captopril reduces peripheral arterial resistance, thereby lowering blood pressure and increasing blood flow, but also has the potential to cause serious side effects. Hawthorn, on the other hand, has been remarkably well tolerated by patients in clinical trials.

In clinical practice, hawthorn is often used in combination with other botanical remedies for the treatment of heart conditions, including passionflower (*Passiflora incarnata*). European and Asian physicians also employ hawthorn in the treatment of angina pectoris, although only a limited number of studies have investigated this application. Angina pectoris is chest pain caused by restriction of blood flow to the heart. This can occur as a result of atherosclerosis, in which plaque deposits cause narrowing of the blood vessels.

In one controlled German study, there were significant reductions in myocardial ischemia (oxygen deprivation of the heart that causes angina) and improvements in exercise tolerance in patients who took a daily dose of 180 mg of standardized hawthorn extract for 3 weeks (see Specific Studies).[9] In addition, in a double-blind, placebo-controlled Chinese study in 46 patients with angina, 84.8 percent of those taking the Chinese hawthorn

Crataegus pinnatifida at a daily dose of 300 mg reported a decrease in the number of angina attacks per week. Electrocardiogram (ECG) readings demonstrated improvement in 46.4 percent of patients. Of 19 people in the study who depended on nitroglycerin tablets to relieve angina pain, 44.8 percent were able to discontinue nitroglycerin completely while taking hawthorn.[10]

The clinical evidence is well supported by laboratory and animal experiments. Among other effects, these studies have shown that hawthorn and hawthorn constituents relax and dilate coronary arteries, increase the flow of blood in coronary arteries, increase the contractility of the heart, protect against arrythmias, and lower blood pressure.[11-15] In other animal studies, hawthorn and various constituents protected the heart from damage due to oxygen deprivation (ischemia).[15-18] Hawthorn extract has also shown mild sedative effects[6,12] and antioxidant effects in laboratory studies.[12]

SPECIFIC STUDIES

Congestive Heart Failure: Clinical Study (1994)

Hawthorn extract was as effective as the drug captopril in improving exercise tolerance and reducing heart rate in this double-blind study in 132 people with stage II heart failure. The investigators tested patients' tolerance to exercise using an ergometer bicycle, also recording changes in blood pressure, heart rate, and pressure/rate product (a measurement of the heart's capacity to pump blood) during exercise and at rest. In addition, they evaluated changes in a number of clinical symptoms, including breathlessness, fatigability, and edema (swelling due to fluid accumulation). Captopril and hawthorn were equally effective in decreasing heart rate and in improving exercise tolerance and pressure/rate output. The severity of symptoms dropped by about 50 percent in both groups. Unlike captopril, however, hawthorn had no effect on blood pressure in this study.

The dosage of hawthorn extract in this study was 300 mg three times a day, a total daily dose of 900 mg. According to the investigators, this was a much higher dosage than that used in previous studies, many of which employed hawthorn doses of only 200 mg a day. The daily dose of captopril was 12.5 mg. The investigators suggest that because of hawthorn's excellent safety profile, future studies could test doses of up to 2 grams a day in patients with more severe (stage III) heart failure.[8]

Congestive Heart Failure: Clinical Study (1996)

In this randomized, placebo-controlled, double-blind study, 8 weeks of treatment with hawthorn was clearly superior to placebo in improving cardiac performance and symptoms in patients with NYHA stage II cardiac insufficiency. The 136 study participants received either placebo or standardized hawthorn extract at a dosage of one 80-mg capsule twice a day (a total daily dose of 160 mg). The researchers measured therapeutic effectiveness primarily by calculating the difference in pressure/rate product between the hawthorn and placebo groups. They also assessed improvements in typical symptoms and quality of life as reported by patients.

According to changes in pressure/rate product, cardiac performance clearly improved in patients taking hawthorn, but became progressively worse in the placebo group. In addition, significantly greater symptom improvement was seen in the hawthorn group, with 59 percent of people taking hawthorn reporting benefit compared with 44 percent of those taking placebo. Although there was a trend toward improved quality of life among the hawthorn group, this could not be confirmed statistically. There were six adverse effects in the placebo group and three in the hawthorn group, which the investigators did not believe were related to treatment with the herb. The hawthorn extract used in the study was standardized to 15 mg oligomeric procyanidins per 80-mg capsule.[19]

Congestive Heart Failure: Another Clinical Study (1994)

Researchers reported significant improvements in clinical symptoms, blood pressure, heart rate, and working capacity of the heart in people with chronic congestive heart failure after 8 weeks of treatment with standardized hawthorn extract. Participants in the double-blind, placebo-controlled trial were 78 men and women with chronic congestive heart failure (NYHA stage II) who were randomized to receive 8 weeks of treatment with either placebo or hawthorn extract at a daily dose of 600 mg (200 mg three times a day). The investigators measured changes in patients' working capacity with ergometer bicycles and also assessed improvements in typical symptoms, including shortness of breath upon exertion, exhaustion, and general decrease in vitality. Results revealed a statistically significant difference between the hawthorn and placebo groups with regard to improvements in working capacity, systolic blood pressure, and heart rate during exercise. Hawthorn extract had no effect on diastolic blood pressure.[7]

Angina Pectoris: Clinical Study (1983)

In this double-blind, placebo-controlled study, 3 weeks of treatment with standardized hawthorn extract resulted in a significant reduction in the incidence of myocardial ischemia (oxygen deprivation of the heart muscle that causes the chest pain known as angina pectoris). Sixty men and women with stable angina pectoris related to NYHA stage I and II heart disease participated in this trial. Subjects in the hawthorn group took 60 mg of hawthorn extract three times a day, a total daily dose of 180 mg. There was a 25 percent improvement in exercise tolerance in the hawthorn group, whereas no change in exercise tolerance was seen in the placebo group. Among 44 patients who had shown disease-related negative changes in endurance load electrocardiogram (ECG) readings before treatment, the after-treatment ECG readings demonstrated a marked reduction in ischemic changes in 78 percent of subjects taking hawthorn, compared with 29 percent of those taking placebo. No side effects were reported.[9]

HOW IT WORKS

Hawthorn is considered an *inotropic* agent, meaning that it enhances the ability of the heart muscle to contract. Hawthorn's flavonoid and procyanidin constituents are believed to be its most cardioactive compounds; these compounds appear to be concentrated in the flowers and leaves.

Because of their relaxant effect on the smooth muscle tissue of blood vessels, hawthorn flavonoids dilate blood vessels, thereby reducing peripheral arterial resistance and helping to lower blood pressure. In addition, procyanidins in hawthorn inhibit the effects of an enzyme called angiotensin-converting enzyme (ACE). In the body, ACE is responsible for converting angiotensin I into angiotensin II, a powerful blood vessel constrictor.[1]

By improving blood flow and oxygen supply to the heart muscle, hawthorn enhances the heart's production and utilization of energy, helping to increase its contractile force. A contributing factor may be the ability of hawthorn flavonoids to inhibit the enzyme phosphodiesterase, an action associated with improving myocardial perfusion (blood flow into the heart). This effect, which helps protect the heart from ischemic damage, has been demonstrated in animal studies.[13,16,17,20]

MAJOR CONSTITUENTS

Flavonoids (including vitexin 4'-O-rhamnoside, vitexin, quercetin, hyperoside, rutin); oligomeric procyanidins; cardiotonic amines

SAFETY

Hawthorn is generally considered a safe food herb with no known toxicity.

- **Side effects:** None known.[5,21]
- **Contraindications:** None known.[5,21]
- **Drug interactions:** Hawthorn may enhance the effects of digitalis, necessitating a lowered dose of digitalis.[21] Blood pressure should be monitored in those taking beta-blockers.

DOSAGE

Hawthorn is a slow-acting herb and should be used for at least 4 to 8 weeks for full benefit. Doses tested in clinical studies ranged from 160 mg to 900 mg a day of standardized extract.

Note: If you are currently taking any medication for a heart condition, including high blood pressure, it is essential to talk to your doctor before using hawthorn. Hawthorn can enhance the effects of certain heart medications, and your doctor may need to adjust your dosage.

- **Standardized extract:** 120 to 240 mg three times a day[2]
- **Tincture (1:5):** 5 ml (approximately 1 teaspoon) three times a day[1,2]
- **Tea:** 1 to 2 teaspoon of berries steeped for 15 minutes in 1 cup of water[1,2]

STANDARDIZATION

Hawthorn extracts are often standardized to contain 2.2 percent flavonoids or 18.75 percent oligomeric procyanidins.

REFERENCES

1. Murray M. *The Healing Power of Herbs.* Rocklin, CA: Prima Publishing, 1995.

2. Hoffmann D. Hawthorn—the heart helper. *Alternative and Complementary Therapies* April/May 1995; 191–192.

3. Hobbs C, Foster S. Hawthorn: a literature review. *HerbalGram* 1990; 2: 19–33.

4. Bensky D, Gamble A. *Chinese Herbal Materia Medica*. Seattle: Eastland Press, 1986.

5. Blumenthal M, Busse W, Goldberg A, et al., eds. *The Complete German Commission E Monographs*. Austin, TX: The American Botanical Council; Boston: Integrative Medicine Communications, 1998.

6. Sticher O, Meier B. Hawthorn *(Crataegus)*: biological activity and new strategies for quality control. In: Lawson LD, Bauer R, eds. *Phytomedicines of Europe*. Washington, DC: American Chemical Society, 1998.

7. Schmidt U, Kuhn U, Ploch M, et al. Efficacy of the hawthorn *(Crataegus)* preparation LI 132 in 78 patients with chronic congestive heart failure defined as NYHA functional class II. *Phytomedicine* 1994; 1: 17–24.

8. Tauchert M, Ploch M, Hübner W-D. Effectiveness of hawthorn extract LI 132 compared with captopril [in German]. *Münch Medizinische Wochenschrift* 1994; 136(suppl 1): 27–33.

9. Hanak T, Brückel M-H. Treatment of moderately stable forms of angina pectoris with Crataegutt® novo [in German]. *Therapiewoche* 1983; 33: 4331–4333.

10. Weiliang W, Wenqu Z, Fuzai L, et al. Therapeutic effect of Crataegus pinnatifida on 46 cases of angina pectoris—a double blind study. *Journal of Traditional Chinese Medicine* 1984; 4(4): 293–294.

11. Chen ZY, Zhang ZS, Kwan KY, et al. Endothelium-dependent relaxation induced by hawthorn extract in rat mesenteric artery. *Life Sciences* 1998; 63(22): 1983–1991.

12. Bahorun T, Trotin F, Pommery J, et al. Antioxidant activities of *Crataegus monogyna* extracts. *Planta Medica* 1994; 60: 323–328.

13. Schuessler M, Fricke U, Hölzl J, et al. Effects of flavonoids from *Crataegus* species in Langendorff perfused isolated guinea pig hearts. *Planta Medica* 1992; 58(suppl 1): A646–A647.

14. Abdul-Ghani A-S, Amin R, Suleiman MS. Hypotensive effect of *Crataegus oxyacantha*. *International Journal of Crude Drug Research* 1987; 25(4): 216–220.

15. Loew D. Phytotherapy in heart failure. *Phytomedicine* 1997; 4(3): 267–271.

16. Schüssler M, Hölzl J, Rump AFE, et al. Functional and antiischaemic effects of monoacetyl-vitexinrhamnoside in different *in vitro* models. *General Pharmacology* 1995; 26(7): 1565–1570.

17. Rump AFE, Schüssler M, Acar D, et al. Functional and antiischemic effects of luteolin-7-glucoside in isolated rabbit hearts. *General Pharmacology* 1994; 25(6): 1137–1142.

18. Nasa Y, Hashizume H, Ehsanul Hoque AN, et al. Protective effect of *Crataegus* extract on the cardiac mechanical dysfunction in isolated perfused working rat heart. *Arzneimittel-forschung* 1993; 43(2): 945–949.

19. Weikl A, Assmus KD, Neukum-Schmidt A, et al. Crataegus special extract WS 1442. Objective proof of effectiveness for patients with heart failure (NYHA II) [in German]. *Fortschritte Medizin* 1996; 114(24): 291–296.

20. Schüssler M, Hölzl J, Fricke U. Myocardial effects of flavonoids from Cratategus species. *Arzneimittel-forschung* 1995; 45(8): 842–845.

21. McGuffin M, Hobbs C, Upton R, et al., eds. *American Herbal Products Association Botanical Safety Handbook*. Boca Raton, FL: CRC Press, 1997.

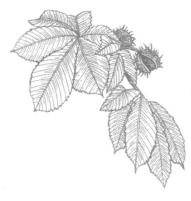

Horse Chestnut

AESCULUS HIPPOCASTANUM

HIPPOCASTANACEAE

State of Knowledge: Five-Star Rating System

Clinical (human) research	✷ ✷ ✷
Laboratory research	✷ ✷ ✷
History of use/traditional use	✷ ✷ ✷
Safety record	✷ ✷
International acceptance	✷ ✷ ✷ ✷

PART USED: *Seed*

PRIMARY USES

- *Chronic venous insufficiency*
- *Capillary fragility*
- *Varicose veins*
- *Hemorrhoids (traditional)*

Varicose veins and other vascular problems are more than just unpleasant symptoms of middle age. They may be a sign that the circulatory system needs some attention through a combination of herbs, good nutrition, and exercise. Much more common in women than men, varicosities (distorted veins) result when the valves of the venous system weaken, making it more difficult for "used" blood to overcome gravity in the legs and return to the heart. More serious problems occur when veins become chronically swollen and inflamed—a condition known as *chronic venous insufficiency* (CVI). People with CVI generally complain of an aching or tired feeling in the legs, which may be accompanied by pain, itching, leg ulcers, changes in skin pigmentation, and other symptoms. Researchers estimate that as many as 20 to 25 percent of women and 10 to 15 percent of men suffer from this condition.

An important measure of the success of any treatment is compliance, the willingness of individuals to adhere to the treatment recommended by the doctor. Standard treatment for CVI generally involves mechanical compression (bandages or support stockings worn around the legs), pharmaceutical drugs, and in some cases surgery. Compression therapy is inconvenient and uncomfortable, leading to a relatively low 47 percent compliance rate.[1] On the other hand, clinical research suggests that horse chestnut is an effective alternative for many cases of CVI with few side effects and a much higher rate of compliance.

HISTORY

Since the late sixteenth century, Europeans have used horse chestnut seeds for varicose veins, fragile capillaries, tendency to bruise easily, thrombophlebitis (venous inflammation with abnormal clotting), and venous congestion. Horse chestnut was one of the first known anticoagulants and was employed as a safer alternative to the drug quinine for painful night leg cramps. Other parts of the plant, including the bark and leaves, were used as an expectorant and astringent for mucus congestion, bronchitis, and whooping cough. Horse chestnut's ability to prevent edema (fluid retention) has led to its application in a wide variety of conditions, including swelling with bruises, fractures, back problems, stroke, and brain trauma. The plant's pain-relieving and anti-inflammatory properties were also used to treat backaches, neuralgia (nerve pain), and rheumatism.

Despite their long history as a food and medicine, unprocessed horse chestnut seeds aren't as user-friendly as many other herbs. Native Americans made horse chestnut bread after first roasting, peeling, mashing, and leaching the seeds in lime for several days to remove toxic constituents. The seeds were also fed to livestock after a similar process of soaking, boiling, rinsing, and drying. Some early cultures buried the seeds in swampy, cold ground over the winter to neutralize the harmful chemicals before use in the spring. Without such special treatment, the crushed, raw seeds made an effective fish poison. Today, it's easy to buy horse chestnut in capsule or tablet form to ensure that the harmful components have been processed out while the active ingredients remain. Horse chestnut is unrelated to the sweet chestnut (*Castanea sativa*), which can be eaten without precautions.

Horse chestnut extract is still widely used for treating varicose veins, capillary fragility, CVI, and hemorrhoids. Naturopathic doctors and herbalists often prescribe the extract along with other cardiovascular tonics, including hawthorn, ginkgo, vitamin C, and grape seed extract, all of which help to strengthen the collagen of the veins.

In Germany, the horse chestnut constituent aescin is a registered drug. Physicians recommend it for many problems associated with local edema, including carpal tunnel syndrome and back injuries. In hospitals, aescin is often given by injection to treat severe head trauma and to reduce swelling after surgery.

INTERNATIONAL STATUS

Horse chestnut seed extract is approved by Germany's Commission E for symptoms of chronic venous insufficiency such as pain, sensation of heaviness in the legs, nighttime leg cramps, itching, and swelling of the legs. In Germany, the isolated constituent aescin is a registered drug.

BOTANY

Native to western Asia, the horse chestnut tree is now a common and beautiful sight in gardens, parks, and city streets throughout Europe and the United States. In summer, the stately trees are covered with fragrant clusters of pink and white flowers. Horse chestnuts are gathered in September as the prickly, ripe fruits turn leathery and fall from the trees. The medicinal seeds are found inside the thick-skinned fruit. The horse chestnut tree has 25 other relatives in temperate parts of North America, including the California buckeye *(A. californica)* and the Ohio buckeye *(A. glabra),* none of which is used medicinally. Poland is a major pro-

ducer of horse chestnut extracts for modern medicine.

BENEFITS

- Strengthens vein walls, increases elasticity, and decreases permeability
- Decreases edema (swelling caused by accumulation of fluid in the veins)
- Reduces venous inflammation
- Stimulates circulation

SCIENTIFIC SUPPORT

Clinical research, much of it conducted in Germany, shows that horse chestnut is beneficial in the treatment of capillary fragility and circulatory problems such as chronic venous insufficiency. A 1998 review article of 13 clinical studies in *Archives of Dermatology* reported that horse chestnut was superior to placebo and just as effective as another complementary therapy (the flavonoid preparation *O*-[beta-hydroxyethyl]-rutosides) in improving the symptoms of CVI. All 13 of these studies were either placebo controlled or compared the effects of horse chestnut against standard therapies. The pooled results showed that horse chestnut reduced edema, pain, fatigue, tenseness and, in some cases, pruritus (itching) in the legs. One study even suggested that horse chestnut was as effective as mechanical compression with bandages and stockings, although the study was not double-blinded (see Specific Studies).[2] Some of the studies also measured leg volumes after "edema provocation," a test which helps researchers estimate horse chestnut's value during "aggravated conditions" such as exercise or long periods of sitting or standing. Horse chestnut also performed well under these conditions.[3] In several of the trials, results were seen within 2 weeks and were maintained for at least 6 weeks after treatment.[2] Research suggests that the mean edema volume can be reduced by up to 25 percent over a 12-week period. Additional edema reductions may be possible when treatment is extended.[1] Preliminary clinical investigations suggest that horse chestnut may be a valuable topical treatment for the pain and tenderness associated with impact injuries.[4,5] In addition, a clinical study of 142 accident victims with severe craniocerebral trauma found that intravenous injections of the constituent aescin over a period of several days were more beneficial than steroid therapy alone in reducing intracranial pressure and lowering mortality rates. Follow-up examinations 2 to 3.5 years after the accident showed that individuals in the aescin group had a higher rehabilitation rate, compared to those who only received steroids.[6]

Scientists are currently investigating horse chestnut's potential for reducing alcohol absorption and lowering blood sugar and for its antiviral effects. So far, these experiments are preliminary and have only been conducted in animals.

SPECIFIC STUDIES

Chronic Venous Insufficiency: Clinical Study (1996)

Horse chestnut was just as effective as standard compression therapy in relieving edema associated with CVI, in a partially blinded, randomized, placebo-controlled study of 240 people. Fifty-five percent of the participants had suffered from CVI for 5 or more years, and 29 percent had already had venous surgery. The men and women were given either horse chestnut extract (containing 50 mg of aescin twice daily), placebo, or compression therapy for 12 weeks. Those in the compression therapy group also took a diuretic (25 mg hydrochlorothiazide and 50 mg triamterene daily) for seven days, to ensure the best possible stocking fit. The results showed that horse chestnut was equivalent to compression therapy in relieving edema, as measured by a statistically significant reduction in fluid volumes in the lower legs at 4, 8, and 12 weeks. Subjects in the placebo group experienced an increase in edema. No serious side effects were reported in either the horse chestnut or compression therapy group.[1]

Chronic Venous Insufficiency: Another Clinical Study (1996)

In this study, horse chestnut seed extract relieved the symptoms of grade II CVI nearly as well as oxerutins, with only a slight tendency toward superior results in the oxerutin group. The randomized, double-blind, placebo-controlled study included 137 postmenopausal women, more than 90 percent of whom suffered from CVI in both legs. During the first 4 weeks of the study, the women took either horse chestnut extract (two 300-mg capsules daily of extract standardized to 50 mg aescin each), oxerutins (1,000 mg daily), or placebo. During the second 12-week treatment period, only the dosage for the oxerutin group was reduced, from 1,000 mg to 500 mg daily. During the third stage of the trial, all treatments were discontinued in order to allow researchers to evaluate possible carry-over effects. The water displacement method was used to measure changes in fluid volume in the legs, and the Visual Analog Scale (VAS) was employed to evaluate improvement of subjective symptoms such as sensations of tingling or heaviness in the legs.

At the end of the study, both the horse chestnut and oxerutin groups demonstrated a statistically significant decrease in mean leg volumes. The women also reported an alleviation of subjective symptoms. Improvement in the oxerutin group was slightly greater, but carry-over benefits were observed in both groups. Patients reported a higher number of side effects such as stomach upset, headache, and dizziness in the oxerutin group (9 versus 2 reports in the horse chestnut group). Researchers concluded that both treatments are effective in treating CVI and that results were comparable to those of previous studies with compression therapy.[7]

Chronic Venous Insufficiency: Clinical Study (1992)

Horse chestnut seed extract was more effective than placebo in relieving edema and other symptoms caused by stage II CVI in a randomized, double-blind study of 39 men and women. During the 6-week study, subjects took either two capsules of horse chestnut seed extract (each 369 to 412 mg capsule standardized to 75 mg aescin) or placebo daily. The main outcome measured was leg volume, but researchers also tracked subjective symptoms before therapy and after each week of treatment. Leg volumes were also measured after "edema provocation," to estimate the effectiveness of the treatments during conditions such as exercise or long periods of sitting or standing. At the end of treatment, researchers observed that leg volumes had decreased by a statistically significant degree in the group taking horse chestnut, as compared with placebo. The differences were just as marked during edema provocation. The people taking horse chestnut also reported a dramatic improvement in subjective symptoms, including feelings of heaviness, tension, fatigue, and paresthesia (burning and pricking sensations) in the legs. The only symptom that was not eased in either group was itching.

There were no serious side effects in the horse chestnut group. The researchers concluded that horse chestnut is a useful adjunct to compression therapy.[3]

HOW IT WORKS

Horse chestnut contains the active constituent aescin, a complex mixture of saponin compounds. Aescin is considered to be 600 times stronger than rutin, a flavonoid that helps strengthen weak capillaries and veins.[8] Like many herbs, horse chestnut is also rich in flavonoid compounds.

Clinical research shows that aescin can help prevent capillary fragility and permeability by decreasing the activity of three enzymes (beta-N-acetylglucosaminidase, beta-glucuronidase, and arylsulphatase) that break down proteoglycans, the molecules that give tone and structural support to the capillary walls. Researchers report that blood levels of these three damaging enzymes are between 60 and 120 percent higher in people with varicose veins, compared with healthy individuals.[9]

According to *in vitro* research, aescin also inhibits the damaging effects of the enzymes elastase and hyaluronidase, which are often abnormally high in areas affected by chronic venous insufficiency.[2] In addition, aescin improves circulation and prevents edema by enhancing fluid drainage from tissues into the capillaries.[8]

MAJOR CONSTITUENTS

Aescin (also spelled *escin*), a triterpene saponin; flavonoids; tannins; and coumarin glycosides (aesculin and aesculetin)

SAFETY

Based on the results of clinical trials, this herb can be considered reasonably safe for most adults at recommended therapeutic doses. However, if you have horse chestnut trees in your yard, make sure that children do not eat the seeds, twigs, leaves or any other parts of the plant, because they can be poisonous if ingested in large enough quantities.

- **Side effects:** Side effects are infrequent but may include pruritus (itching), nausea, headache, dizziness, calf spasm, and stomach upset.[10]
- **Contraindications:** Because of its blood-thinning action, horse chestnut should not be used immediately before or after surgery or by anyone with a bleeding disorder such as hemophilia. The gel or ointment should not be applied to broken skin.
- **Drug interactions:** Although no drug interactions have been reported, horse chestnut is not recommended for use in combination with aspirin or other blood-thinning medications.

DOSAGE

Because of the potential seriousness of vascular problems, it is important to get an accurate diagnosis from a health practitioner before using horse chestnut. Horse chestnut can be taken in capsule or tablet form. Do not eat or make a tea out of raw, unprocessed horse chestnut seeds. The dosages listed here are for initial use and can often be reduced following improvement.

- **Standardized extract:** The dosage used in clinical studies was 300 mg twice a day. This is also the dosage recommended by the Commission E.
- **Capsules/tablets:**
  300 mg twice a day.

STANDARDIZATION

Horse chestnut is typically standardized to contain 16 to 20 percent triterpene saponins (calculated as aescin), or 50 mg aescin per tablet or capsule. Topical gels generally contain 2 percent aescin.

REFERENCES

1. Diehm C, Trampisch HJ, Lange S, et al. Comparison of leg compression stocking and oral horse chestnut seed extract therapy in patients with chronic venous insufficiency. *The Lancet* 1996; 347: 292–294.
2. Pittler MH, Ernst E. Horse chestnut seed extract for chronic venous insufficiency. *Archives of Dermatology* 1998; 134: 1356–1360.
3. Diehm C, Vollbrecht D, Amendt K, et al. Medical edema protection: clinical benefit in patients with chronic deep vein incompetence. *Vasa* 1992; 21(2): 188–192.
4. Hess H, Groher W, Lenhart P, et al. Efficacy and safety of an aescin plus diethylamine-salicylate combination gel in patients with sports impact injuries. *Deutsche Zeitschrift für Sportmedizin* 1996; 47(7/8): 423–430.
5. Calabrese C, Preston P. Report of the results of a double-blind, randomized, single-dose trial of a topical 2% escin gel versus placebo in the acute treatment of experimentally-induced hematoma in volunteers. *Planta Medica* 1993; 59: 394–397.
6. Put T. Advances in the conservative treatment of acute traumatic cerebral edema [in German]. *Münch Medizinische Wochenschrift* 1979; 121(31): 1019–1022.
7. Rehn D, Unkauf M, Klein P, et al. Comparative clinical efficacy and tolerability of oxerutins and horse chestnut extract in patients with chronic venous insufficiency. *Arzneimittel-Forschung* 1996; 46(1): 483–487.
8. Weiss RF. *Herbal Medicine*. Portland, OR: Medicina Biologica, 1988.
9. Kreysel HW, Nissen HP, Enghofer E. A possible role of lysosomal enzymes in the pathogenesis of varicosis and the reduction in their serum activity by Venostasin®. *Vasa* 1983; 12(4): 377–382.
10. Blumenthal M, Busse W, Goldberg A, et al., eds. *The Complete German Commission E Monographs*. Austin, TX: American Botanical Council; Boston: Integrative Medical Communications, 1998.

Kava

PIPER METHYSTICUM
PIPERACEAE

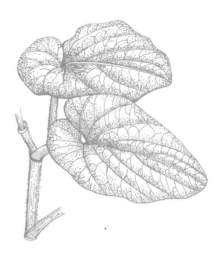

State of Knowledge: Five-Star Rating System

Clinical (human) research	✱ ✱ ✱
Laboratory research	✱ ✱ ✱
History of use / traditional use	✱ ✱ ✱ ✱
Safety record	✱ ✱ ✱
International acceptance	✱ ✱ ✱

PART USED: *Root*
PRIMARY USES

- *Anxiety*
- *Stress and restlessness*
- *Muscle tension (experimental)*
- *Mild pain (experimental)*

The "happiest and friendliest people in the world" live in the South Pacific, according to anthropologists. Many of these people also happen to be regular kava users. In the Pacific islands, kava is taken to relax the mind and muscles, stimulate good conversation, and heighten the senses during ceremonies and social gatherings. The plant's calming, slightly euphoric properties have only recently been discovered in the Western world. In fact, until the early 1900s, Westerners employed kava mainly for urinary tract infections. Today, kava extract is becoming increasingly popular in the United States and Europe for relieving anxiety and stress. One of the root's most useful qualities is its ability to calm the mind without affecting productivity or concentration levels, making it as helpful in the workplace as in the home. Because of the root's mild muscle relaxant and pain-relieving properties, some health practitioners also recommend kava for a variety of other health complaints, such as back pain, chronic tension headaches, and fibromyalgia.

273

HISTORY

The name *kava* comes from the Greek word for "intoxicating." In the South Pacific, kava's relaxing properties have played an integral role at weddings, tribal meetings, and other events for centuries. During welcoming ceremonies, many famous guests have sipped the thick, traditional kava brew, including Lady Bird Johnson and Pope John Paul II. Kava has also been used for bronchitis, rheumatism, urinary tract problems, and as an aphrodisiac. Small pieces of root are chewed for sore throats and toothaches. For hundreds of years, kava was prepared by young people with strong teeth who crushed the woody, fibrous root by chewing it before soaking the pulp in cold water or coconut milk. Today the roots are just as likely to be pounded or grated.

The first kava products appeared in Europe during the 1860s. By 1920, German pharmaceutical-grade extracts were being administered for gonorrhea, chronic cystitis and other urinary tract infections, menstrual problems, and migraine headaches. Kava was also used in combination with pumpkinseed extract for irritable bladder syndrome. As antibiotics and other pharmaceuticals appeared on the market, kava use in Europe and the United States declined. After the Second World War, however, Westerners discovered kava's calming properties. Incidentally, South Pacific cultures have also used kava for resolving arguments peacefully—another possible application for the Western world.

INTERNATIONAL STATUS

Kava is approved by Germany's Commission E for conditions of anxiety, stress, and restlessness.

BOTANY

Kava has been cultivated for so many centuries that its exact botanical birthplace has been forgotten. A member of the pepper (Piperaceae) family, *Piper methysticum* may have originated in New Guinea or Indonesia, spreading to other Pacific islands through trade and exploration. Captain Cook and his botanists discovered the plant during their first expedition to the South Pacific in 1768. Kava is a sprawling, perennial shrub that may reach heights of 20 feet, although it is commonly harvested at 7 or 8 feet. The plant has large, heart-shaped leaves and flowers that resemble small ears of corn. Kava grows best at 300 to 1,000 feet above sea level, in moist, sunny highlands or wet forests.

Today, 118 different kava cultivars are carefully selected and grown for their unique effects. Though all of these cultivars arose from the wild ancestor *Piper wichmanii,* they differ chemically. Kava is grown commercially on many tropical Pacific islands, including Fiji, Samoa, Tonga, and Vanuatu, the center of distribution. In Hawaii, struggling family farmers are striving to cultivate kava in a sustainable fashion, aided by a rural economic assistance program.

BENEFITS

- Calms the nervous system by binding to GABA sites in the brain and by exerting generalized effects on the brain's limbic system
- Relaxes skeletal and smooth muscle tissue in many parts of the body (experimental)
- May help relieve mild pain (experimental)
- May help people recovering from stroke because of its ability to protect the brain from damage caused by oxygen deprivation (experimental)
- May be a useful adjunct treatment in epilepsy due to its anti-convulsant properties (experimental)

SCIENTIFIC SUPPORT

In at least seven high-quality clinical studies, kava has been helpful in the treatment of anxiety, nervousness, and stress in the general population and in menopausal women. Several trials have found kava to be just as effective as the benzodiazepine antianxiety drug oxazepam—without affecting concentration, alertness, or causing some of the more serious side effects associated with standard sedatives.

Although clinical research is lacking, kava has also demonstrated important muscle-relaxing and pain-relieving properties in animal and pharmacological studies.[1,2] This supports the traditional use of kava as an analgesic by medicine men in the South Pacific. Preliminary research also suggests that kava has anti-convulsant activity, but there is still a need for clinical studies that test kava against placebo and prescription anti-convulsants.[3] The plant's ability to protect the brain against ischemia (lack of oxygen) may be related to its anti-convulsant effects.[4] At least four clinical investigations have shown that kava has no negative effects on accuracy, reaction time, or memory during letter-matching tests and memory recognition tests. Two of these studies found that the sedative drug oxazepam impaired subjects' performance, whereas kava did not. One comparative study also measured specific cognitive and motor processes through electrical scalp recordings. Researchers found that oxazepam had a negative effect on the parts of the brains that are responsible for attention and processing capacity, whereas kava did not.[5,6]

SPECIFIC STUDIES

Daily Stress and Anxiety: Clinical Study (1998)

In a randomized, double-blind, placebo-controlled study of 60 people, standardized kava extract was significantly more effective than placebo in reducing everyday stress and anxiety. During the 4-week trial, participants took either 2 capsules of a standardized kava extract (60 mg kavalactones per capsule) or placebo twice daily. Participants were assessed five times during the study using the Daily Stress Inventory (DSI) and State Trait Anxiety Inventory (STAI) tests. The DSI covers five areas of daily stress including interpersonal problems, personal competency, cognitive stressors, environmental hassles, and varied stressors of urban life. Only the kava group experienced significant improvement in all five areas. Anxiety levels continued to decrease as the study proceeded, suggesting a possible cumulative effect. No side effects were reported.[7]

Neurotic Disorders:
Clinical Study (1990)

Kava relieved anxiety just as effectively as the benzodiazepine antianxiety drug oxazepam in 38 outpatients with neurotic or psychosomatic disorders causing physical symptoms such as nausea and vomiting. During the randomized, double-blind, placebo-controlled study, the kava group took one 200-mg capsule of kava extract three times daily, plus 1 placebo capsule twice daily. The placebo group took 1 capsule of oxazepam twice daily, in addition to 1 placebo capsule three times daily. All subjects began the trial with scores of 40 or greater on the Anxiety Status Inventory (ASI).

During the 28-day treatment period, both groups experienced an equivalent reduction in ASI scores, although there was a greater reduction in fear in the kava group and greater relief of psychosomatic nausea and vomiting in the drug group. Both treatment groups reported significant improvement on the Self-Evaluation Anxiety Scale (SAS), although kava users were less likely to experience faintness and oxazepam users had fewer sleep disturbances. Both treatments led to a significant drop in blood pressure. A physician rated the efficacy of the medications as "very good" in 55 percent of the kava group and 71 percent of the oxazepam group. Tolerability was "very good" in 75 percent of the kava subjects and 82 percent of the oxazepam group. There were no side effects in either group.[8]

General Anxiety:
Clinical Study (1996)

Kava significantly reduced symptoms of anxiety and increased feelings of well-being in a randomized placebo-controlled study of 58 people with general anxiety syndromes. For 4 weeks, the participants took three daily doses of kava extract (100 mg each) or placebo. Results were measured after 1, 2, and 4 weeks of treatment using the Hamilton Anxiety Scale (HAMA) and the Adjectives Check List. The kava group experienced improvement in symptoms such as nervousness and tension after just 1 week of treatment, compared with placebo. Improvement continued with no side effects for the duration of the study.[9]

Anxiety and Depression in Menopause: Clinical Study (1991)

Kava significantly improved psychological symptoms such as anxiety and depression, in a randomized, double-blind, placebo-controlled study of 40 menopausal and post-menopausal women. The kava group took 100 mg of kava extract three times daily, and the placebo group took an identical-looking pill three times daily for 8 weeks. All subjects began the study with scores of 18 or greater on the Hamilton Anxiety Scale. During the first week of treatment, HAMA scores dropped to 9 in the kava group, with a further drop to 5 after 4 weeks, compared with only slight changes in the placebo group. In the kava group, 17 out of 20 women improved on the Depression Status Inventory test (DSI) within 4 weeks, compared with just 7 in the placebo group.

Kava users also reported greater subjective improvements after 3 weeks, according to the Kupperman Index of menopause symptoms and personal diaries, in contrast with only slight improvement in the placebo group. Six women in the placebo group reported side effects, compared with only four in the kava group. Seven patients in the placebo group withdrew from the study due to a lack of effectiveness, compared with just two in the kava group.[10]

HOW IT WORKS

Although kava is often compared with sedative drugs, its actions are much more complex. Researchers haven't determined exactly how kava reduces anxiety, but a 1994 study helped shed some light on the issue. In this animal study, researchers discovered that kava extract binds to gamma-aminobutyric acid (GABA) receptors in the brain, which are responsible for promoting relaxation. However, they also concluded that kava acts more indirectly at GABA sites than barbiturate drugs, which may help explain why long-term use does not cause dependence.[11,12] It is interesting to note that whole extracts of kava interact more strongly with GABA receptors than isolated kavalactones.[13] This suggests that kavalactones are not the only important constituents involved in the plant's calming effects. In another important animal study, scientists tested the effects of kava on EEG patterns. They found that the plant exerts most of its effects on the limbic system, and particularly the amygdala, a part of the brain that influences the emotions and other activities.[14] A more recent study reported that kava helps prevent the uptake of noradrenaline, a hormone that initiates the stress response. This new evidence may also help explain kava's relaxing effects.[15]

The results of *in vitro* studies suggest that kava relaxes muscle tissue in a nonspecific manner. It appears to have a direct effect on muscle contractility, as opposed to inhibiting neuromuscular transmission.[15,16] Kava's analgesic effects appear to be distinct from its sedative and muscle-relaxing activity. Researchers have also determined that kava does not relieve pain by the same pathway as that used by opiate drugs. This is reassuring because it lends additional support to kava's long-term safety.[2] An earlier study tested the analgesic activity of two kava constituents, dihydrokavain (DHK) and dihydromethysticin (DHM). Researchers found that DHK was weaker in pain-relieving ability than morphine but stronger than aspirin. When DHK was given with aspirin, the combination had greater effects than either medicine alone. These results are useful but limited because the study was conducted in animals rather than people.[17]

In vitro studies show that kava also has important anti-convulsive activity. Like antiepileptic drugs, kava appears to reduce nerve conduction by blocking sodium channels in the brain. This may make kava a useful adjunct therapy for epilepsy, though it probably isn't potent enough for use by itself. Researchers have not determined whether kava's effects on sodium channels also play a role in the plant's antianxiety activity.[3] In addition, kava helps protect the brain from ischemic damage (lack of oxygen due to impaired blood flow), giving the plant a possible role in recovery from stroke. In an animal study, kava extract was just as effective as the anticonvulsive drug memantine in decreasing the size of brain lesions during ischemia, possibly through a direct action on neurons. The kava constituents methysticin and dihydromethysticin were the most important in this process. This suggests a relationship between kava's anticonvulsive and neuroprotective activity, although researchers still are not clear on the exact mechanism of action.[4]

MAJOR CONSTITUENTS

Kavalactones, including kavain, dihydrokavain (DHK), methysticin, and dihydromethysticin (DHM)

SAFETY

Traditional use and clinical studies have confirmed kava's safety when the herb is used in moderate amounts. Some people feel that kava should not be taken for longer than 3 months without medical advice.[18]

- **Side effects:** There were occasional reports of stomach upset in clinical studies using kava extracts. In large doses, the extract may cause dilation of the pupils and dizziness.[18] Additional side effects may be related to the use of crude preparations of kava root (not kava extracts) over an extended period of time. Excessive use of crude preparations may lead to a temporary discoloration of the skin, hair, and nails, a side effect that disappears when kava is discontinued.[18]

- **Contraindications:** Kava should not be used by pregnant or nursing women or by those with endogenous depression (depression of biological origin). Do not use kava while driving or operating heavy machinery.[18,19] At least one case of "driving under the influence" of kava has been prosecuted in Utah.
- **Drug interactions:** Kava should not be used with other substances that act on the central nervous system, such as alcohol, barbiturates, and medications for psychological disorders.[18]

DOSAGE

Kava can be taken several times during the day for stress and anxiety. As a sleep aid, the daily quantity can be taken in a single dose 30 to 60 minutes before bed.

Note: Teas extract the water-soluble constituents of kava but not other important compounds such as kavalactones—unless you follow the traditional preparation method of chewing the roots before extracting them into water!

- **Standardized extract:** 70 mg of kavalactones, two to three times a day. (By comparison, a traditional kava drink contains about 250 mg of kavalactones.)
- **Capsules/tablets:** 400- to 500-mg capsules or tablets up to six times a day.[20]

- **Tinctures (1:2 ratio):** 15 to 30 drops in water up to three times a day.[20]

STANDARDIZATION

Kava extracts are typically standardized to contain 30 to 70 percent kavalactones.

REFERENCES

1. Singh YN. Effects of kava on neuromuscular transmission and muscle contractility. *Journal of Ethnopharmacology* 1983; 7: 267–276.
2. Jamieson DD, Duffield PH. The antinociceptive actions of kava components in mice. *Clinical and Experimental Pharmacology and Physiology* 1990; 17: 495–508.
3. Gleitz J, Beile A, Peters T. Kava inhibits veratridine-activated voltage-dependent Na+-channels in synaptosomes prepared from rat cerebral cortex. *Neuropharmacology* 1995; 34(9): 1133–1138.
4. Backhauss C, Krieglstein J. Extract of kava (*Piper methysticum*) and its methysticin constituents protect brain tissue against ischemic damage in rodents. *European Journal of Pharmacology* 1992; 215: 265–269.
5. Munte TF, Heinze HJ, Matzke M, et al. Effects of oxazepam and an extract of kava roots (*Piper methysticum*) on event-related potentials in a word recognition test. *Pharmacoelectroencephalography* 1993; 27: 46–53.
6. Heinze HJ, Münthe TF, Steitz J, et al. Pharmacopsychological effects of oxazepam and

kava extract in a visual search paradigm assessed with event-related potentials. *Pharmacopsychiatry* 1994; 27: 224–130.

7. Singh NN, Ellis CR, Singh YN, et al. A double-blind, placebo controlled study of the effects of kava (Kavatrol) on daily stress and anxiety in adults. *Alternative Therapies in Health and Medicine* 1998; 4(2): 97–98.

8. Lindenberg VD, Pitule-Schoedel H. DL-Kavain in comparison with oxazepam in anxiety states: double blind clinical study [in German]. *Fortschritte der Therapie* 1990; 108(2): 31–34.

9. Lehmann E, Kinzler E, Friedemann J, et al. Efficacy of a special kava extract *(Piper methysticum)* in patients with states of anxiety, tension, and excitedness of non-mental origin—a double blind placebo-controlled study of four weeks treatment. *Phytomedicine* 1996; 3(2): 113–119.

10. Warneke VG. Neurovegetative dystonia in the female climacteric: studies on the clinical efficacy and tolerance of kava extract WS 1490 [in German]. *Fortschritte der Therapie* 1991; 109(4): 119–122.

11. Jussofie A, Schmiz A, Hiemke C. Kavapyrone enriched extract from *Piper methysticum* as modulator of the GABA binding site in different regions of rat brain. *Psychopharmacology* 1994; 116: 469–474.

12. Duffield PH, Jamieson D. Development of tolerance to kava in mice. *Clinical and Experimental Pharmacology and Physiology* 1991; 18: 571–578.

13. Davies LP, Drew CA, Duffield P, et al. Kava pyrones and resin: studies on GABA-A, GABA-B, and benzodiazepine binding sites in rodent brain. *Pharmacology and Toxicology* 1992; 71: 120–126.

14. Holm E, Staedt U, Heep J, et al. Studies on the profile of neurophysiological effects of D,L-Kavain: cerebral sites of action and sleep-wakefulness-rhythm in animals [in German]. *Arzneimittel-Forschung* 1991; 41(2): 673–683.

15. Seitz U, Schule A, Gleitz J. [3H]-Monoamine uptake inhibition properties of kava pyrones. *Planta Medica* 1997; 63: 548–549.

16. Seitz U, Ameri A, Pelzer H. Relaxation of evoked contractile activity of isolated guinea pig ileum by kavain. *Planta Medica* 1997; 63: 303–306.

17. Bruggenmann F, Meyer HJ. Studies on the analgesic efficacy of the kava constituents dihydrokavain (DHK) and dihydromethysticin (DHM) [in German]. *Arzneimittel-Forschung* 1963; 13: 407–409.

18. Blumenthal M, Busse W, Goldberg A, eds. *The Complete German Commission E Monographs.* Austin, TX: American Botanical Council; Boston: Integrative Medical Communications, 1998.

19. McGuffin M, Hobbs C, Upton R, Goldberg A, eds. *American Herbal Products Association Botanical Safety Handbook.* Boca Raton and New York: CRC Press LLC, 1997.

20. Foster S. *101 Medicinal Herbs.* Loveland, CO: Interweave Press, 1998.

Lavender

LAVANDULA ANGUSTIFOLIA
LAMIACEAE

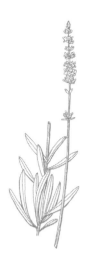

State of Knowledge: Five-Star Rating System

Clinical (human) research	✶
Laboratory research	✶✶
History of use / traditional use	✶✶✶✶
Safety record	✶✶
International acceptance	✶✶✶✶

PART USED: *Flower*

PRIMARY USES

- *Sedative effects (traditional)*
- *Insomnia (traditional)*
- *Digestive system support*
- *Headache (traditional)*
- *Mood enhancement (traditional)*

Few plants have as pleasing an aroma and as many traditional uses as lavender. Lavender flowers have a strong traditional reputation for mood enhancement, and many claim that the sweet scent of the purple flowers evokes uplifting and inspiring thoughts. The herb has a long history of use for clearing the mind, keeping mild depression at bay, and easing anxiety. A sweet-smelling sachet of dried lavender blossoms tucked under a pillow is a favorite traditional remedy for insomnia.

Although thousands may swear by lavender, there is little scientific verification of its effects. However, recent laboratory studies on the essential oil distilled from the flowers have generated excitement. Preliminary results suggest that perillyl alcohol, a compound found in lavender essential oil, may prove to be a powerful anticancer agent against soft tissue tumors. In addition, a small number of clinical trials in people with anxiety and sleep disorders suggest that some of the most important traditional uses of lavender may one day be validated by modern scientific methods. One 1997 study that used short-term electroencephalogram (EEG) testing to compare the effect of herbs and Valium concluded that lavender and the herb valerian had strikingly similar effects on brain waves (see Specific Studies).[1]

HISTORY

The word *lavender* stems from the Latin word *lavare,* meaning "to wash." Fittingly, lavender has traditionally been employed for cleansing and purification of homes and bodies. The ancient people of Greece and Rome used the plant for bathing and to sanctify their temples.

During the Middle Ages, Europeans spread lavender on the floor to scent rooms and protect against insect infestations. Although there have been many improvements in personal hygiene since then, as well as significant reductions in bed-bug infestations, lavender can still be used to perfume a room. Simply sprinkle some flowers on a rug, vacuum them up, and enjoy the refreshing aroma.

Medicinal applications of lavender in the European herbal tradition included nervousness, muscle spasms, and headaches, and a lavender compound prescribed for these purposes was listed in the *British Herbal Pharmacopoeia* for more than 200 years.[2] Traditional herbalists consider lavender a carminative herb, useful in relieving flatulence, colic, and digestive upsets. Lavender essential oil has been commonly applied externally to help heal burns and wounds, to soothe sore joints, and to relieve headache pain when rubbed on the temples.

Lavender's reputation for supporting digestive function is reflected in its many food uses. The small, bitter-tasting flowers have traditionally been added to salads, honey, wine, cheese, butter, and poultry dishes. In England, lavender flower scones are greedily devoured, and French lavender flower sorbet is enjoyed as a refreshing treat on hot summer nights.

Lavender was a favorite herb of the Victorian era in England. Women carried lavender sachets to inhale when they felt faint or were faced with unpleasant odors, and used the distilled water from the flowers in toilet waters and cosmetic lotions. The blossoms remain a favorite ingredient of fine soaps.

INTERNATIONAL STATUS

Lavender flower is listed as an approved herb in the *German Commission E Monographs,* indicated for mood disturbances such as restlessness or insomnia; functional abdominal complaints, including nervous stomach irritations and intestinal discomfort; and for use as a bath additive in the treatment of functional circulatory disorders.[3]

BOTANY

A native plant of the Mediterranean region, lavender is small and shrublike, with mildly scented, oval-shaped leaves that range in color from grayish green to blue-green. Lavender plants in bloom are a beautiful sight to behold. Each slender stalk is encircled by deliciously scented, velvety purple flowers. The sweet perfume is irresistible to the plant's favorite pollinator, the bee. Lavender is a member of the mint family (Lamiaceae), a large family of plants known for their aromatic qualities.

Many different species and varieties of lavender are grown in herb gardens throughout the world. Easy to grow, lavender likes warm weather, a sunny location, and moderate watering. In cold climates, however, it may not survive the winter. The classic lavender aroma varies among species and varieties as well as with different growing conditions and times of harvest. *Lavandula angustifolia* (formerly known as *L. vera* or *L. officinalis*) is the species that is most commonly available commercially and that yields the highest-quality essential oil. Other common lavender species include *L. stoechas* (Spanish lavender) and *L. latifolia* (spike lavender). The essential oil of these plants is very different from that of *L. angustifolia*.

The essential oil of *Lavandula angustifolia* is distilled from the fresh flowers and stalks at harvest time. When harvesting lavender, it is important to gather the flowers on a sunny day because the sun helps to concentrate the essential oils in the flowers. Cut the lavender where the leaves meet the stalk, tie the stalks into small bundles, and hang upside down to dry in a dark place with good air circulation.

BENEFITS

- Sedative and antianxiety effects (flowers and essential oil)
- Potential antitumor activity (perillyl alcohol from essential oil)

SCIENTIFIC SUPPORT

The flowering parts of lavender have long been used as a traditional folk healing remedy, but there has been little scientific research to validate these traditional applications. Laboratory and clinical tests using isolated constituents of the essential oil show great promise for many conditions, and it is possible that the strongest medicinal benefits of lavender lie within its highly concentrated essential oils.

In one clinical study, gentle massage with lavender essential oil reduced anxiety for people in a hospital intensive care unit.[4] A double-blind preliminary investigation on insomnia used lavender essential oil to induce sleep and provide temporary relief from some of the side effects of sedative medications.[1] In another study, lavender essential oil diffused into the air helped to restore restful sleep for participants who had previously been taking prescription sleeping medications for insomnia.[5]

Perhaps more exciting, compounds isolated from lavender essential oil have shown promise in studies designed to investigate their antitumor potential. The essential oil of lavender is made up of a complex combination of constituents, including monoterpenes and alcohols. Monoterpenes are important flavor and aroma compounds in the essential oils of many plants, fruits, and vegetables. In laboratory experiments, a monoterpene in lavender called *limonene* inhibited a number of soft tissue cancers. Clinical research on limonene derived from orange peel is currently underway in the United Kingdom.[6]

Perillyl alcohol, another monoterpene, occurs naturally in lavender and a number of other plants, including mints, citrus, and cranberries. It appears to be less toxic and more effective in smaller doses than limonene.[7] Based on preliminary findings, perillyl alcohol from lavender essential oil is believed to inhibit carcinomas of the soft tissue, including the pancreas, liver, breast, and prostate.[8–10] In laboratory investigations using human cancer cells, perillyl alcohol was effective in inhibiting the growth of pancreatic cancer cells.[8,11] In animal studies, perillyl alcohol caused regression of mammary gland tumors[9,12] and inhibited the growth of colon and liver tumors.[13,14] Although the results of the laboratory tests have been promising, more research is needed to determine effective and safe dosages for humans. Currently, perillyl alcohol is being studied clinically in the United States for its antitumor effectiveness.[15]

SPECIFIC STUDIES

Cancer: Clinical Study (1998)

In preliminary clinical studies designed to assess the effectiveness of perillyl alcohol as an anticancer agent, 18 patients with advanced tumors took oral doses of perillyl alcohol three times a day. The patients had a variety of different cancers, including prostate, ovarian, sarcoma, and breast cancer. Doses ranged from 800 mg to 2,400 mg given three times a day. Researchers studied plasma and urine samples to determine the solubility of perillyl alcohol at the different doses. Although the doses were generally well tolerated, some patients experienced side effects, mostly gastrointestinal in nature but also including mild fatigue. These side effects appeared to be dependent on the amount of perillyl alcohol taken. According to the investigators, disease stabilization for up to 6 months was seen in some of the patients. However, no objective tumor responses were noted. Further research is needed to determine safe and effective dosages and duration of treatment.[15]

Sleep Disorders: Pharmacology Study (1997)

This double-blind study used electroencephalogram testing to compare the effects of valerian *(Valeriana officinalis)*, lavender *(Lavandula angustifolia)*, kava *(Piper methysticum)*, and passionflower *(Passiflora incarnata)* with those of the drug diazepam (Valium) and placebo in 23 women suffering from sleep disorders. Using caffeine as a stimulant, researchers were able to track the effects of each substance on brain waves during the short, 180-minute test. Results showed that each of the herbs had markedly different effects, except for valerian and lavender, which appeared to act similarly in the brain. The study was conducted using 1,200 mg of lavender extract. Researchers are planning more experiments to further define the therapeutic uses of each plant.[1]

Insomnia: Clinical Study (1995)

This small study assessed the sedative effects of ambient lavender essential oil (diffused into the air) on people with insomnia. The researchers were interested in determining whether lavender oil could be considered a replacement therapy for insomnia drugs, which are generally used long term and often have side effects. Even though the study involved only four people, the encouraging results suggest that future studies in this area are warranted. Three of the participants were tapering off prescription medications (temazepam, promazine hydrochoride, or chlormethiazole), whereas the fourth person had taken no insomnia medications prior to the experiment. For the first 2 weeks of the study, measurements of sleep patterns were made; during the next 2 weeks, the subjects were monitored as they withdrew from their sedative medications. For the final 2 weeks, the participants were exposed to ambient essential oil of lavender.

Results showed that the subjects experienced increased insomnia after withdrawal from their medications, but that with lavender treatment, sleep time returned to what it had been when they were taking the sedative medications. Participants were also less restless during sleep with lavender treatment. The investigators concluded, "The study suggests that ambient lavender oil might be used as a temporary relief from continued medication for insomnia."[5]

Anxiety: Clinical Study (1995)

A British study showed that massage with lavender essential oil was effective in improving mood and reducing anxiety in 93 people admitted to an intensive care unit. The participants were experiencing acute physical crisis as well as a distorted sense of smell due to the use of oral and nasal tubes. The randomized controlled trial was designed to compare the effects of aromatherapy massage using lavender oil, massage without lavender oil, and periods of rest. Participants in the massage groups were gently massaged a maximum of three times with either plain grape seed oil or a 1 percent dilution of lavender essential oil (5 to 6 drops of essential oil per ounce of grape seed oil). Subjects in the other group were allowed to rest undisturbed for 30 minutes. Patients were assessed using a 4-point scale for measuring levels of anxiety, mood, and ability to cope with their present situation.

Although the researchers found no statistically significant differences among the three groups in physiological stress indicators, the participants who received massage with lavender reported greater improvements in mood and anxiety levels compared with subjects in the rest group. Patients reported that they felt less anxious and more positive immediately after the essential oil therapy, although the effects were not maintained long term. On the other hand, rest was as effective as grape seed oil massage in reducing anxiety and improving mood, and as effective as the lavender massage treatment with regard to improvements in ability to cope. The nurses who organized this study noted that the 1 percent dilution of lavender employed in the study is very low and that future research within intensive care units should use a higher dilution of 2 percent (10 to 12 drops of essential oil per ounce of carrier oil).[4]

HOW IT WORKS

Because the amount of research so far has been limited, little is known about how lavender works. We do know that lavender essential oil can be absorbed into the body through the skin[16] and by direct inhalation. Researchers believe that when inhaled, the fragrant volatile molecules of an essential oil directly affect the olfactory nerve in the brain. Laboratory studies that demonstrated a sedative effect in mice showed that inhalation of essential oils, including lavender, directly affected the central nervous system.[17] These findings lend credence to the traditional folk use of lavender as a sedative and relaxing plant.

Monterpenes have been shown to inhibit the development of cancer at both initiation and progression stages. A number of mechanisms have been proposed to explain the antitumor effects of perillyl alcohol and limonene. In animal tests, limonene and perillyl alcohol were found to inhibit the growth of tumors of the liver by promoting apoptosis (programmed cell death) of tumor cells.[14] In addition, based on a study of rats with experimentally induced breast cancer, researchers theorized that perillyl alcohol caused tumor regression partly by fostering redifferentiation of tumor cells, meaning that it helped convert the cancer cells back into normal cells.[18]

MAJOR CONSTITUENTS

Volatile oil (linalyl acetate, linalol, borneol, geraniol, camphor, limonene, perillyl alcohol), tannins, flavonoids, coumarin

SAFETY

Lavender flowers are considered safe when used appropriately.[19] Lavender essential oil is also generally considered gentle and safe. However, essential oils are highly concentrated, and even a well-tolerated oil such as lavender could be toxic if used inappropriately. Do not take lavender essential oil internally unless under the supervision of a qualified health-care practitioner.

- **Side effects:** There have been no reported side effects from use of lavender flowers.[3] Some people have reported minor skin irritation from use of undiluted essential oil.[20]
- **Contraindications:** None known.[3]
- **Drug interactions:** None known.[3]

DOSAGE

Lavender flowers may be used for tea, tincture, or in the bath. For external use of lavender essential oil, be sure to dilute the essential oil in a carrier oil (such as almond or grape seed oil) before applying. For a 1 to 2 percent dilution, add 5 to 12 drops of essential oil to 1 ounce of carrier oil. For a lavender essential oil bath, add 3 to 15 drops of the essential oil per bath.

- **Tincture:** Up to 2 ml three times a day

- **Tea:** 1 to 2 teaspoons of flowers per cup of water[3]
- **Bath:** Brew a pot of tea using 1 to 2 cups of flowers per bath. Strain before adding to bath.[3]

STANDARDIZATION

Lavender is not available in standardized form.

REFERENCES

1. Schulz V, Hübner W-D, Ploch M. Clinical trials with phyto-psychopharmacological agents. *Phytomedicine* 1997; 4(4): 379–387.
2. Keville K. *The Illustrated Herb Encyclopedia.* New York: Mallard Press, 1991.
3. Blumenthal M, Busse W, Goldberg A, eds. *The Complete German Commission E Monographs.* Austin TX: American Botanical Council; Boston: Integrative Medicine Communications, 1998.
4. Dunn C, Sleep J, Collett D. Sensing an improvement: an experimental study to evaluate the use of aromatherapy, massage and periods of rest in an intensive care unit. *Journal of Advanced Nursing* 1995; 21: 34–40.
5. Hardy M, Kirk-Smith MD, Stretch DD. Replacement of drug treatment for insomnia by ambient odour. *The Lancet* 1995; 346(8976): 701.
6. Vigushin DM, Poon GK, Boddy A, et al. Phase I and pharmacokinetic study of D-limonene in patients with advanced cancer.

Cancer Chemotherapy and Pharmacology 1998; 42(2): 111–117.

7. Kelloff GJ, Boone CW, Crowell JA, et al. New agents for cancer chemoprevention. *Journal of Cellular Biochemistry* 1996; 26S: 1–28.

8. Bronfen JH, Stark MJ, Crowell PL. Inhibition of human pancreatic carcinoma cell proliferation by perillyl alcohol. *Proceedings of the American Association for Cancer Research* 1994; 35: 431. Abstract.

9. Gould MN. Prevention and therapy of mammary cancer by monoterpenes. *Journal of Cellular Biochemistry* 1995; 22(suppl): 139–144.

10. Jeffers L, Church D, Gould M, et al. The effect of perillyl alcohol on the proliferation of human prostatic cell lines. *Proceedings of the American Association for Cancer Research* 1995; 36: 303. Abstract.

11. Stark MJ, Burke YD, McKinzie JH, et al. Chemotherapy of pancreatic cancer with the monoterpene perillyl alcohol. *Cancer Letters* 1995; 96: 15–21.

12. Haag JD, Gould MN. Mammary carcinoma regression induced by perillyl alcohol, a hydroxylated analog of limonene. *Cancer Chemotherapy and Pharmacology* 1994; 34: 477–483.

13. Reddy BS, Wang C-X, Samaha H, et al. Chemoprevention of colon carcinogenesis by dietary perillyl alcohol. *Cancer Research* 1997; 57: 420–425.

14. Mills JJ, Chari RS, Boyer IJ, et al. Induction of apoptosis in liver tumors by the monoterpene perillyl alcohol. *Cancer Research* 1995; 55: 979–983.

15. Ripple GH, Gould MN, Stewart JA, et al. Phase I clinical trial of perillyl alcohol administered daily. *Clinical Cancer Research* 1998; 4(5): 1159–1164.

16. Jäger W, Buchbauer G, Jirovetz L, et al. Percutaneous absorption of lavender oil from a massage oil. *Journal of the Society of Cosmetic Chemists* 1992; 43: 49–54.

17. Buchbauer G, Jirovetz L, Jäger W, et al. Aromatherapy: evidence for sedative effects of the essential oil of lavender after inhalation. *Zeitschrift für Naturforschung* 1991; 46c: 1067–1072.

18. Shi W, Gould MN. Induction of differentiation in neuro-2A cells by the monoterpene perillyl alcohol. *Cancer Letters* 1995; 95: 1–6.

19. McGuffin M, Hobbs C, Upton R, et al., eds. *American Herbal Products Association Botanical Safety Handbook.* Boca Raton and New York: CRC Press, 1997.

20. Tisserand R, Balacs T. *Essential Oil Safety—A Guide for Health Care Professionals.* London: Churchill Livingstone, 1995.

Licorice

GLYCYRRHIZA GLABRA
FABACEAE

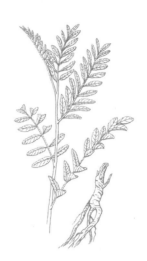

PART USED: *Root, rhizome*

PRIMARY USES

Deglycyrrhizinated licorice (DGL)
- *Peptic and duodenal ulcers*
- *Canker sores*

Whole root
- *Adrenal weakness (traditional)*
- *Coughs (traditional)*

Glycyrrhetinic acid (topical)
- *Psoriasis*
- *Eczema*

Named from the Greek words for "sweet root," licorice has always been loved as much for its taste as for its medicinal value. The roots have been used for coughs and respiratory problems since ancient times, but their antiulcer properties were discovered only recently. In 1946, a Dutch pharmacist noticed that licorice cough syrups were more effective in ulcer patients than their regular ulcer medications, spurring publication of the first scientific studies of the herb in the *Journal of the American Medical Association* and *The Lancet*. Unfortunately, licorice in its whole-plant form also caused water retention in about 20 percent of these patients because of a natural compound in the root called *glycyrrhizin*. By the 1970s, researchers had developed a safe, effective form of licorice for treating ulcers—*deglycyrrhizinated licorice*

(DGL), an extract from which 97 percent of the glycyrrhizin has been removed.

Today, scientific evidence shows that DGL is more effective for treating ulcers than Tagamet (cimetidine), one of the most widely prescribed drugs in the world. Although effective in the short term in relieving ulcer symptoms, Tagamet has many long-term disadvantages. Because it disrupts digestion and alters the structure and function of the cells in the intestinal tract, the drug may increase the chances of ulcer relapse. Unpleasant side effects and reliance on the medication are particularly common in older people. Like most drugs, Tagamet also burdens the liver and kidneys, interacts dangerously with a wide range of drugs, and interferes with the liver's ability to metabolize other drugs. Unlike Tagamet, DGL actually helps protect and heal the lining of the digestive tract for safer, more permanent results.

HISTORY

Licorice is 50 times sweeter than sucrose and was especially prized before the advent of refined sugar. In ancient Egypt, King Tutankhamun and other rulers were buried with licorice roots so they could take their sweets along with them to the next world. Alexander the Great and his troops chewed the roots to quench thirst. Today, Americans still favor licorice primarily for its flavor. Ninety percent of the licorice crop imported to the United States is used as an additive in tobacco products because of licorice's sweet, soothing action. Certain pharmaceutical drugs, including throat lozenges, contain licorice for the same reasons. Although licorice candies from Europe often contain extracts of licorice root, many American brands are actually flavored with anise oil.

For more than 3,000 years, licorice has been one of China's most useful medicinal herbs because of its ability to mask the flavor of unpleasant-tasting herbs while increasing their absorption. According to the principles of Chinese medicine, licorice replenishes "chi" (vital energy), clears heat, removes toxins, moistens the lungs, controls coughs, relieves spasms and pain, and strengthens digestion. The root also has a long history of use in Ayurveda, the traditional healing system of India.

For centuries, Native Americans used indigenous licorice species such as *G. lepidota* for diarrhea, stomach upset, and fever in children, passing their knowledge on to the early settlers. Around the turn of the twentieth century, the Eclectic physicians (a group of prominent American doctors who practiced at that time) prescribed licorice for female complaints and for respiratory problems such as asthma, dry cough, sore throat, and laryngitis.

INTERNATIONAL STATUS

Licorice is approved by Germany's Commission E for treating upper respiratory tract problems and gastric and duodenal ulcers. It is also an approved plant in the United Kingdom, Belgium, and France.

BOTANY

A graceful member of the pea family (Fabaceae), licorice grows 3 to 7 feet tall and has oval-shaped leaflets covered with sticky hairs. During the summer, the blue-violet flowers bloom in clusters, which later become flat pods containing one to six seeds. Licorice has a deep, yellowish-brown taproot that sends out numerous thin, horizontal rhizomes. Native to the Mediterranean and parts of Asia, licorice is now grown commercially in temperate areas of Turkey, Greece, and Asia. The most common species include *Glycyrrhiza glabra* and the Chinese variety *G. uralensis*. Although the plant is easy to grow, the roots cannot be harvested until the fall of the third or fourth year. Licorice favors rich soil and sunny, warm locations.

BENEFITS

- DGL helps treat duodenal and stomach (gastric) ulcers by increasing the healing rate, relieving pain, preventing relapse, and reducing the need for surgery
- Whole licorice root has a soothing, expectorant, and anti-inflammatory effect on sore throats, coughs, and other respiratory problems
- Whole licorice helps treat adrenal weakness because of its similarity to cortisol
- Topical glycyrrhetinic acid may help relieve eczema, psoriasis, contact dermatitis (such as poison oak), and allergic dermatitis, because of its anti-inflammatory action
- A mouthwash containing DGL may be helpful in treating canker sores

SCIENTIFIC SUPPORT

Clinical research shows that DGL helps in the treatment of peptic and duodenal ulcers by relieving pain, aiding the healing process, reducing the number of relapses, and often preventing the need for surgery—even in severe cases. Numerous studies have proven the safety of DGL, even at fairly high doses, during short-term treatment and maintenance therapy lasting up to 2 years. Although two studies suggested that DGL was no more effective than placebo, they have been widely criticized for being too short to adequately test for results. Most ulcers require at least 6 to 8 weeks to heal, and these trials were just 4 weeks long.[1,2]

In addition, researchers demonstrated that licorice reduces gastrointestinal bleeding and damage to the stomach lining caused by aspirin use.[3] This is important since at least 20 percent of gastric ulcers may be linked to use of aspirin, nonsteroidal anti-inflammatory drugs (NSAIDs), and other substances that harm the integrity of the stomach lining.[4]

Researchers have also found DGL highly effective for treating painful mouth ulcers known as canker sores. In one study, 75 percent of the subjects using DGL solution as a mouthwash (200 mg of powdered DGL dissolved in 200 ml warm water) experienced a 50 to 75 percent improvement within 1 day. Complete healing took just 3 days.[5] The plant's anti-inflammatory properties have also led to its application as an external treatment for eczema, psoriasis, and allergic dermatitis. One study showed that topical glycyrrhetinic acid was more effective than hydrocortisone in relieving symptoms of these conditions.[6]

Preliminary studies suggest that glycyrrhizin may significantly improve immune function in HIV-positive individuals when taken at doses of 150 to 225 mg daily over a period of several years. In these trials, the patients in the control groups who did not take licorice had declining immune function, measured as a decrease in levels of helper T-cells, total T-cells, and antibodies. In addition, several patients in the control groups developed AIDS.[7,8]

Japanese research shows that glycyrrhizin may also be effective in improving liver function in up to 40 percent of patients with acute and chronic hepatitis B and C.[9,10] Alpha-interferon, the standard drug for hep-atitis, is effective in 45 to 50 percent of cases, but is associated with unpleasant side effects such as fever, joint pain, nausea, and flu-like symptoms. Although these studies used intravenous injections of glycyrrhizin, some naturopathic doctors believe that oral formulations are absorbed just as effectively.[11] The main challenge in using glycyrrhizin for HIV and hepatitis is preventing side effects such as elevated blood pressure.

SPECIFIC STUDIES

Peptic Ulcer: Clinical Study (1982)

Researchers found deglycyrrhizinated licorice just as effective as cimetidine (Tagamet) in a single-blind study of 100 people with peptic ulcers. Patients in the licorice group were given 760 mg of DGL three times daily, whereas those in the drug group took 200 mg of cimetidine three times daily and an additional 400 mg dose at night. In both groups, 63 percent of ulcers healed within 6 weeks, and 91 percent within 12 weeks. Both groups experienced similar levels of daytime pain relief during the first 2 weeks, although at first the cimetidine group reported more relief.

During a 1-year maintenance period, the subjects reduced their dosages to either 760 mg DGL twice daily or 400 mg cimetidine at night, leading to just four ulcer recurrences in each treatment group within 6 months. Those patients who were taking anti-inflammatory drugs such as aspirin or prednisone before the study tended to have larger ulcers and higher rates of acute gastrointestinal bleeding than those who had not taken such medications. Two patients in the cimetidine group showed signs of liver stress, measured as a transient rise in serum transaminase levels.[12]

Duodenal Ulcer: Clinical Study (1985)

Licorice (DGL) was just as effective as an antacid (aluminum-magnesium hydroxide), the drug Tagamet (cimetidine), and the European drug Gefarnate (geranylferensylacetate) in a randomized study of 874 patients with duodenal ulcers. Researchers found no difference in the relapse rate, the need for surgery, or side effects after 12 weeks, although the antacid treatment initially showed better results. Dosages used in the study were 380 mg of DGL three times daily; 3 grams of aluminum-magnesium hydroxide daily; 200 mg Tagamet three times daily, with an additional 400 mg at night; or 50 mg Gefarnate three times daily.[13]

Chronic Duodenal Ulcer: Clinical Study (1973)

Researchers found licorice (DGL) highly effective in aiding healing in a study of 40 patients with severe, chronic duodenal ulcers. All of the subjects had suffered symptoms for 4 to 12 years, had experienced more than six relapses in the past year, and had been referred for surgery due to debilitating pain and frequent vomiting. Antacids and anticholinergic drugs had become ineffective over time, even at high doses. One group of 20 subjects was given 8 tablets (3 g) of DGL daily for 8 weeks, while the other group took 12 tablets (4.5 g) of DGL daily for 16 weeks. Out of 40 participants, 35 reported a greater sense of well-being within 5 days of treatment. All of the patients showed dramatic improvement, but those taking the higher dose of DGL tended to heal more quickly and had fewer relapses. During the year of follow-up, no one required surgery. There were no side effects, even with patients taking the higher dose of DGL.[14]

HOW IT WORKS

Anti-Ulcer Effects

Deglycyrrhizinated licorice helps heal ulcers by increasing the levels of prostaglandins in the stomach that promote the secretion of protective mucus and new cell growth.[15,16] Aspirin and other NSAIDs suppress the secretion of these protective prostaglandins, increasing the risk of gastrointestinal ulceration, hemorrhage, and perforation. DGL also supports the healing process by increasing blood flow to the intestinal lining and by reducing muscle spasms.[17,18]

Adrenal-Strengthening Effects

Whole licorice root contains a constituent called glycyrrhizin that is structurally similar to cortisol, a hormone produced by the adrenal cortex that helps the body deal with long-term stress. For this reason, many naturopathic doctors and herbalists prescribe whole licorice root for general burn-out and adrenal weakness. Licorice may also be useful in the treatment of Addison's disease, a serious condition characterized by very low production of adrenal cortex hormones, although there has been no research in this area.[11]

According to laboratory studies, glycyrrhizin asserts its adrenal effects by blocking the enzyme 5-beta-reductase, which would normally convert cortisol into cortisone. Cortisol has adrenal effects but cortisone does not.[19]

Glycyrrhizin also mimics a second adrenal cortex hormone, the mineralocorticoid known as aldosterone. As the name suggests, mineralocorticoids help regulate mineral balance in the body, especially potassium and sodium levels. This explains why chronic use of licorice can lead to hypertension, potassium loss, and water retention in certain people.[20] Although licorice can help people recover from intense periods of adrenal stress, it is not an herb to overuse.

Other Hormonal Effects

Like soy and red clover, licorice contains isoflavones (phytoestrogens) that may help balance levels of estrogen and progesterone in the body.[21] Today, naturopathic doctors and herbalists often prescribe licorice for premenstrual syndrome (PMS) and menopause in combination with other herbs.[11]

MAJOR CONSTITUENTS

Glycyrrhizin (also known as glycyrrhizic acid or glycyrrhizinic acid), glycyrrhetinic acid, flavonoids, phytosterols, coumarins

SAFETY

Whole licorice root can be safely used in small amounts for short periods of time. Deglycyrrhizinated licorice has not been associated with side effects in ulcer patients, even when used long term.

- **Side effects:** Chronic use of isolated glycyrrhizin or whole licorice root may cause hypertension, sodium and water retention, hypokalemia (potassium loss), edema (swelling), headache, dizziness, and impaired kidney function.[22] Side effects disappear when licorice treatment is discontinued.

   Note: According to many naturopathic doctors, people who consume a high-potassium, low-sodium diet generally do not develop these side effects.[11] Most reports of side effects have occurred in people who consumed large quantities of real licorice candy or highly concentrated licorice extracts, not whole licorice root.

- **Contraindications:** Do not use glycyrrhizin or whole licorice root if you have hypertension, diabetes, hypertonia (extreme tension of the muscles or arteries), severe kidney insufficiency, hypokalemia (low potassium levels), cirrhosis of the liver, or cholestatic liver disorders (low bile production). Do not use during pregnancy.[22,23]
- **Drug interactions:** Avoid taking glycyrrhizin or whole licorice root with thiazide diuretics, stimulant laxatives, or other drugs that contribute to potassium loss. Individuals taking licorice may be more sensitive to digitalis glycosides and cortisol.[22,23]

DOSAGE

For the treatment of ulcers, DGL tablets should be taken between meals or 20 minutes before eating. DGL needs to mix with the saliva and is not effective in capsule form. Long-term maintenance therapy may be necessary. Consult a health-care practitioner for an accurate diagnosis before trying DGL.

Do not take more than 100 mg glycyrrhizin or 3 g of whole licorice root daily for longer than 4 to 6 weeks. Licorice root can be added to herbal teas in small amounts with no adverse effects. When using licorice root

for PMS, start taking it on day 14 of the cycle and continue until menstruation begins.

- **DGL:** Six to eight 250-mg chewable tablets a day
- **Capsules:** 400 to 500 mg up to six times a day[24]
- **Tincture:** 20 to 30 drops up to three times a day[24]
- **Powdered root:** 1 g up to three times a day

STANDARDIZATION

Licorice is not currently available in standardized form.

REFERENCES

1. Feldman H, Gilat T. A trial of deglycyrrhizinated liquorice in the treatment of duodenal ulcer. *Gut* 1971; 12: 449–451.
2. Bardhan KD, Cumberland DC, Dixon RA, et al. Clinical trial of deglycyrrhizinised liquorice in gastric ulcer. *Gut* 1978; 19: 779–782.
3. Rees WDW, Rhodes J, Wright JE, et al. Effect of deglycyrrhizinated liquorice on gastric mucosal damage by aspirin. *Scandinavian Journal of Gastroenterology* 1979; 14: 605–607.
4. Morgan AG, Pacsoo C, McAdam WAF. Maintenance therapy: a two year comparison between Caved-S and cimetidine treatment in the prevention of symptomatic

gastric ulcer recurrence. *Gut* 1985; 26: 599–602.

5. Das SK, Das V, Gulati AK, et al. Deglycyrrhizinated liquorice in apthous ulcers. *Journal of the Association of Physicians of India* 1989; 37(10); 647–648.

6. Evans FQ. The rational use of glycyrrhetinic acid in dermatology. *The British Journal of Clinical Practice* 1958; 12(4): 269–274.

7. Ikegami N, Yoshioka K, Akatani K. Clinical evaluation of glycyrrhizin on HIV-infected asymptomatic hemophiliac patients in Japan. Paper presented at the Fifth International Conference on AIDS: The Scientific and Social Challenge; June 4–9, 1989; Montreal, Canada. Abstract W.B.P 298. Cited in *AIDS Treatment News,* May 18, 1990.

8. Ikegami N, Akatani K, Imai M, et al. Prophylactic effect of long-term oral administration of glycyrrhizin on AIDS development of asymptomatic patients. Paper presented at the IX International Conference on AIDS and the IV STD World Congress; June 6–11, 1993; Berlin, Germany.

9. Eisenburg VJ. Treatment of chronic hepatitis B. Effect of glycyrrhizinic acid on the course of illness [in German]. *Fortschritte der Medizin* 1992; 110: 395–398.

10. Acharya SK, Dasarathy S, Tandon A, et al. A preliminary open trial on interferon stimulator (SNMC) derived from *Glycyrrhiza glabra* in the treatment of subacute hepatic failure. *Indian Journal of Medical Research* 1993; 98: 69–74.

11. Murray M, Pizzorno J. *Encyclopedia of Natural Medicine.* Rocklin, CA: Prima Publishing, 1998.

12. Morgan AG, McAdam WAF, Pacsoo C, et al. Comparison between cimetidine and Caved-S in the treatment of gastric ulceration, and subsequent maintenance therapy. *Gut* 1982; 23: 545–551.

13. Kassir ZA. Endoscopic controlled trial of four drug regimens in the treatment of chronic duodenal ulceration. *Irish Medical Journal* 1985; 78(6): 153–156.

14. Tewari SN, Wilson AK. Clinical trials: deglycyrrhizinated liquorice in duodenal ulcer. *The Practitioner* 1973; 210: 820–823.

15. Van Marle J, Aarsen PN, Lind A, et al. Deglycyrrhizinised liquorice (DGL) and the renewal of rat stomach epithelium. *European Journal of Pharmacology* 1981; 72: 219–225.

16. Robbers JE, Tyler VE. *Tyler's Herbs of Choice.* New York and London: The Haworth Press, 1999.

17. Johnson B, McIssac R. Effect of some anti-ulcer agents on mucosal blood flow. *British Journal of Pharmacology* 1981; 1: 308.

18. Tewari SN, Trembalowicz FC. Some experience with deglycyrrhizinated liquorice in the treatment of gastric and duodenal ulcers with special reference to its spasmolytic effect. *Gut* 1968; 9: 48–51.

19. MacKenzie MA, Hoefnagels WHL, Jansen RWMM, et al. The influence of glycyrrhetinic acid on plasma cortisol and cortisone in healthy young volunteers. *Journal of Clinical Endocrinology and Metabolism* 1990; 70(6): 1637–1643.

20. Stormer FC, Reistad R, Alexander J. Glycyrrhizic acid in liquorice: evaluation of health hazard. *Food and Chemical Toxicology* 1993; 31(4): 303–312.

21. Kumagai A, Nishino K, Shimomura A, et al. Effect of glycyrrhizin on estrogen action. *Endocrinologia Japonica* 1967; 14(1): 34–38.

22. Blumenthal M, Busse W, Goldberg A, eds. *The Complete German Commission E Monographs.* Austin, TX: American Botanical Council; Boston: Integrative Medical Communications, 1998.

23. McGuffin M, Hobbs C, Upton R, et al., eds. *American Herbal Products Association Botanical Safety Handbook.* Boca Raton, FL: CRC Press, 1997.

24. Foster S. *101 Medicinal Herbs.* Loveland, CO: Interweave Press, 1988.

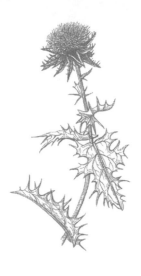

Milk Thistle

SILYBUM MARIANUM
ASTERACEAE

State of Knowledge: Five-Star Rating System

Clinical (human) research	✳ ✳ ✳
Laboratory research	✳ ✳ ✳ ✳
History of use/traditional use	✳ ✳ ✳ ✳
Safety record	✳ ✳ ✳ ✳
International acceptance	✳ ✳ ✳

PART USED: *Seed*

PRIMARY USES

- *Liver health*
- *Protection against harmful chemicals, drugs, and pollution*
- *Digestive aid*
- *Acute and chronic hepatitis*
- *Alcoholic and other liver damage*
- *Gallbladder symptoms*

Prickly thistles may not be as "approachable" as softer plants, but appearances can be deceiving. Not only does this group of plants contain no poisonous members, but many thistles have the ability to protect our livers against harmful substances, including poisons present in our daily environment. The thistle that stands out most in this regard is milk thistle. This remarkable plant has earned a worldwide reputation as an antioxidant and liver protectant that can even help repair and regenerate injured liver cells.

As the word *liver* suggests, maintaining the health of this essential organ is key to the overall quality of life. The liver, the body's second largest organ, processes nutrients, drugs, toxins, and any other substance entering the body through the intestines, lungs, or skin. Savvy Europeans have long recognized this, taking milk thistle extract as a daily form of health insurance against pollution, over-the-counter drugs such as acetaminophen, and even the self-inflicted damage of overindulgence in rich foods and alcohol. In Germany, milk thistle extracts accounted for over $180 million in herb product sales during 1998.

Health practitioners also prescribe milk thistle to treat a variety of problems you might not normally connect with liver health, including poor digestion, female hormonal problems, constipation, mood disorders, hemorrhoids, varicose veins, atherosclerosis (hardening and narrowing of the arteries), and skin conditions such as psoriasis and acne. Today, regular use of milk thistle extract can be considered a modern necessity—every bit as important as a healthful diet, exercise, rest, and the most common vitamin supplements.

HISTORY

Milk thistle has been used to support liver health for more than 2,000 years. As early as A.D. 23, Pliny the Elder recommended a mixture of milk thistle juice and honey for improving digestion by stimulating the flow of bile. During the sixteenth century, the British herbalist Gerard called milk thistle "the best remedy that grows against all melancholy diseases." Melancholy (what we might call depression today) gets its name from the Greek words for "black bile" and was historically treated with liver herbs as

well as mood-enhancing plants. During the seventeenth century, British herbalist Nicholas Culpeper prescribed milk thistle seeds for jaundice (yellow discoloration of tissues due to excessive amounts of bile), gallstones, and obstructions of the liver and spleen.

Milk thistle became popular in American medicine around the turn of the twentieth century, when the Eclectic physicians (a prominent group of American doctors who practiced at that time) adopted it as a treatment for varicose veins, menstrual problems, and liver and kidney ailments. The plant gradually fell out of favor later in the century—except in Germany, where herbs have always enjoyed widespread acceptance. During the 1970s and 1980s, German scientists began testing the plant to validate its many centuries of application as a liver herb. Today, milk thistle is a popular treatment in Germany for many liver problems, including hepatitis and cirrhosis. Intravenous silymarin (a complex of important milk thistle constituents) is also a life-saving emergency room treatment used throughout Europe in cases of poisoning.

Like its cousin the globe artichoke (*Cynara scolymus*), milk thistle has a long history as a delicious and nutritious food. When boiled, young milk thistle flowerheads look and taste much like a savory artichoke. All parts of the plant are edible, including the roots and young stalks and leaves. To incorporate the benefits of milk thistle seeds into your daily diet, herbalist Christopher Hobbs suggests making a seasoning salt by soaking milk thistle seeds overnight, draining the water, grinding the seeds into a powder using a coffee grinder, lightly toasting them in the oven, and then mixing them with salt or other spices.[1] Milk thistle seeds are high in protein and the essential fatty acid linoleic acid, a healthy fat that can help reduce chronic inflammation, balance the female menstrual cycle, and improve heart health.

INTERNATIONAL STATUS

Milk thistle seeds are approved in the *German Commission E Monographs* as a supportive treatment for inflammatory liver conditions such as cirrhosis, hepatitis, and fatty infiltration caused by alcohol and other toxins.[2]

BOTANY

Herbalist Michael Moore describes milk thistle as "a bulldog with a spiked collar" because of the plant's prickly appearance. The plant grows to heights of 5 to 10 feet and is dangerous looking—right down to the sharp spines on its reddish purple flowers. Milk thistle's common name comes from the white markings on the leaves, its milky white sap, and its traditional use by nursing mothers to increase lactation. The humble plant is closely related to other common thistles, including blessed thistle *(Cnicus benedictus),* which has similar medicinal properties but is not as well researched.

Milk thistle is native to Europe, southern Russia, Asia, and North Africa. When the English colonists brought it to North America, the plant quickly became a common weed in many parts of the United States. Today, large fields of milk thistle are cultivated in Texas and Argentina, with an eye toward developing cultivation methods that yield the highest amounts of silymarin. If you decide to grow milk thistle in your own garden, watch out! The plant lives up to its reputation as a weed, spreading easily on its many parachutelike seeds. Milk thistle is an annual or biennial and favors sunny locations and well-drained soils, though it generally tolerates harsher conditions. The seeds can be harvested in July or August after the flowers have blossomed.

BENEFITS

- Protects the liver from damage by guarding liver cell membranes
- Acts as a powerful antioxidant in the liver, stomach, and intestines
- Helps repair and regenerate liver cells by stimulating protein synthesis
- Aids digestion and elimination by stimulating the flow of bile (needed to break down fats)

SCIENTIFIC SUPPORT

One of the best-studied herbs, milk thistle has been the subject of more than 300 clinical and laboratory trials. In cases of acute hepatitis, milk thistle extract helps people recover more quickly and prevents the condition from becoming chronic. Improvement is often apparent within 5 days, and even greater benefits are seen after 3 weeks. Milk thistle is also useful for treating chronic hepatitis when taken over a period of 3 to 12 months. Studies show that it can help reverse liver cell damage, normalize elevated levels of liver enzymes, and improve symptoms such as abdominal discomfort, decreased appetite, and fatigue. Standard therapy for hepatitis usually involves the drug alpha-interferon, which has many unpleasant side effects, including flu-like symptoms, fatigue, and irritability. Research has also demonstrated that milk thistle can slow the advancement of cirrhosis (chronic liver damage) and increase life span in people with cirrhosis, particularly alcoholics.

Preliminary research shows that milk thistle may help prevent gallstones by reducing cholesterol levels in the bile. In one study, a daily dose of 420 mg of silymarin taken for 1 month led to a reduction of bile cholesterol in people with a history of gallstones and gallbladder surgery.[3]

Exciting breakthrough research suggests possible antioxidant benefits in another area: nonmelanoma skin cancer. A number of preliminary laboratory investigations indicated that silymarin could reduce the rate of tumor formation and tumor size at all three stages of development—initiation, promotion, and complete carcinogenesis. Silymarin's effects were most dramatic in the later stages of skin cancer. Clinical studies are necessary to determine how these results apply to humans.[4]

Another area of current research is milk thistle's possible anti-allergenic effects. *In vitro* research indicates that silymarin and silybin may help prevent allergic reactions by inhibiting the release of histamine from mast cells in animals and from blood basophils in humans.[5]

SPECIFIC STUDIES

Liver Protection: Clinical Study (1994)

Silymarin provided protection against the toxic effects of long-term treatment with psychotropic drugs (used in mental illness) in a randomized, double-blind, placebo-controlled clinical study of 60 people. Before the study began, all of the participants had been taking the psychotropic drugs phenothiazine or butyrophenone, or both, for at least 5 years. Subjects were divided into four groups for the 3-month trial: group I took psychotropic drugs and a high dose of silymarin (800 mg per day), group II took psychotropics with placebo, group III took silymarin only (800 mg per day), and group IV took placebo. Silymarin provided liver protection to group I by reducing blood levels of malon-dialdehyde (MDA), an indicator of liver damage that increases during long-term treatment with psychotropics. Not surprisingly, the decrease in MDA levels was even greater in the group taking silymarin alone (group III). Patients in group II continued to experience rising levels of MDA, whereas those who took placebo had declining MDA levels until the psychotropics were reinstated. There were no adverse effects associated with milk thistle treatment.[6]

Active Cirrhosis:
Clinical Study (1992)

Silymarin was just as effective as the bile acid ursodeoxycholic acid (UDCA) in improving symptoms of active cirrhosis in a randomized, controlled, crossover study involving 21 people. During the 6-month trial, subjects took either 420 mg of silymarin or 600 mg of UDCA daily. In the UDCA group, liver function improved significantly, measured as a 30 percent drop in serum aspartate amino transferase (AST) levels and a 22 percent drop in alanine amino transferase (ALT) levels. Serum levels of gamma-glutamyltranspeptidase (γ-GT) also demonstrated a beneficial decline. Those in the silymarin group had a 15 percent drop

in AST and a 23 percent decline in ALT levels, with no change in γ-GT levels.

During the second half of the study, 20 of the 21 original participants took either combined treatment (UDCA and silymarin) or no treatment. Combination therapy caused a beneficial decrease in liver enzymes over a 12-month period. On the other hand, those who received no treatment experienced a rise in mean levels of serum transminases and γ-GT, similar to pretreatment values. No side effects were reported for UDCA or silymarin.

Lastly, researchers tested UDCA in relation to hepatitis C virus (HCV). They found that UDCA was not as effective in lowering ALT and AST levels in people who were positive for anti-HCV antibodies, compared to those who were negative for these antibodies. The researchers concluded that both UDCA and silymarin are safe and effective in treating active cirrhosis of the liver. However, UDCA treatment should be restricted to people who test negative for anti-HCV antibodies.[7]

Cirrhosis:
Clinical Study (1989)

Long-term treatment with silymarin significantly increased survival rates in a randomized, double-blind, placebo-controlled study of 105 people with cirrhosis. Subjects took either 420 mg of silymarin daily or placebo during the study, which lasted for approximately 41 months. Over a 4-year period, the mortality rate in the placebo group was twice that of the silymarin group. Silymarin showed the greatest benefit in those with alcohol-related cirrhosis. There appeared to be no difference in the results of liver function tests (transminases, bilirubin, SGGPT, and other liver enzymes) between the two groups. No side effects were reported.[8]

HOW IT WORKS

Milk thistle prevents toxins from entering the liver by guarding the organ's numerous doorways—the membranes of liver cells. By slowing the rate at which the liver absorbs harmful substances, the toxins are excreted through the kidneys before they can cause liver damage.[9] The most dramatic example of this is milk thistle's ability to block poisons from the deathcap mushroom *(Amanita phalloides),* one of the most notorious liver toxins known to humans. In a group of 49 patients with *Amanita* poisoning, physicians rated the results "amazing" and "spectacular," after patients were given injections (20 mg/kg daily) of silybin, a major constituent in milk thistle. All of the patients survived, even though they were treated 24 to 36 hours after poisoning, when liver and kidney damage had already occurred. The death rate in emergency rooms from *Amanita* poisoning is usually 30 to 40 percent.[10] Milk thistle acts in a similar fashion to detoxify other synthetic chemicals that find their way into our bodies, from acetaminophen and alcohol to heavy metals and radiation.[9]

Much of milk thistle's protective effect is due to the flavonoid complex silymarin, which acts as a powerful antioxidant, combining with and thus neutralizing harmful free radicals that result from normal metabolic processes and from the breakdown of toxic substances. At least 10 times as potent as vitamin E, silymarin also helps increase levels of two additional antioxidants, glutathione and superoxide dismutase (SOD).[11] A laboratory study showed that silymarin may increase glutathione content in the liver and intestines by up to 50 percent.[12] Silymarin also increases the activity of SOD in erythrocytes (red blood cells) and lymphocytes (white bood cells) formed in the lymphatic tissue in patients with liver disease.[13] Because silymarin is a potent antioxidant in the stomach and intestines, it may also have a role to play in treating inflammatory conditions such as colitis and ulcers.[14]

When damage has already been done, milk thistle aids the liver in repairing injured cells and generating new ones. It does this by stimulating protein synthesis through the enzyme RNA polymerase I. Protein is a basic building block of cell walls, cell structures, and enzymes that are vital to all body processes. Recent evidence (molecular modeling) suggests that the constituent silybin may be responsible for stimulating protein synthesis, because it imitates a steroid hormone. Silybin increases protein synthesis by up to 25 to 30 percent, compared with controls.[9] Milk thistle's regenerative ability is essential for treating serious conditions such as chronic hepatitis, cirrhosis, and toxic fatty deposits in the liver.

Recent evidence suggests that silymarin may be just as important for kidney health. Silymarin concentrates in kidney cells, where it aids in repair and regeneration by increasing protein and nucleic acid synthesis. One study showed that it increased cell replication by 25 to 30 percent.[9]

Of the many compounds that make up the silymarin complex, silybin and silychristin are the two most potent ones, according to current pharmacological studies.[9] Unfortunately, these compounds are relatively poorly absorbed by the gastrointestinal tract. Some studies suggest an absorption rate of just 20 to 50 percent, which explains why it is so important to take standardized milk thistle extracts to ensure high concentrations of the active ingredients.[15] Some manufacturers claim that combining milk thistle with phosphatidylcholine increases absorption.

MAJOR CONSTITUENTS

Silymarin (a flavonoid complex that includes silybin, silychristin and silydianin)

SAFETY

Milk thistle has been safely used as a food herb and medicine for centuries.

- **Side effects:** No side effects have been reported during clinical trials. Milk thistle may initially have a mild laxative effect in certain people because of its stimulating effects on bile secretion.[2]
- **Contraindications:** Milk thistle is considered safe for use during pregnancy and has a long history of use by nursing women.[16] People with diabetes who are taking milk thistle should carefully monitor their blood glucose and may require reduction in standard antihyperglycemic agents.[17]
- **Drug interactions:** None known.[2]

DOSAGE

Standardized milk thistle products are strongly recommended to ensure therapeutic levels of silymarin. There is no research on milk thistle as a tincture or tea. In any case, milk thistle does not make an effective tea because the main constituents do not dissolve easily into water. For maintaining overall health, begin with the full dosage of milk thistle for 6 to 8 weeks, followed by a reduction to 280 mg daily. Those with liver problems should continue the full dosage for at least 4 to 8 weeks. Long-term therapy may be required in serious or chronic cases.

- **Standardized capsules/tablets:** 420 mg silymarin, divided into two to three doses a day
- **Tincture (unstandardized):** 10 to 25 drops up to three times a day

STANDARDIZATION

Milk thistle is typically standardized to contain 70 to 80 percent silymarin.

REFERENCES

1. Hobbs C. *Milk Thistle: The Liver Herb.* Capitola, CA: Botanica Press, 1992.
2. Blumenthal M, Busse W, Goldberg A, eds. *The Complete German Commission E Monographs.* Austin, TX: American Botanical Council; Boston: Integrative Medical Communications, 1998.
3. Nassuato G, Iemmolo RM, Strazzabosco M, et al. Effect of silibinin on biliary lipid composition: experimental and clinical study. *Journal of Hepatology* 1991; 12(3): 290–295.
4. Katiyar SK, Korman NJ, Mukhtar H, et al. Protective effects of silymarin against photocarcinogenesis in a mouse skin model. *Journal of the National Cancer Institute* 1997; 89(8): 556–566.
5. Miadonna A, Tedeschi A, Leggieri E, et al. Effects of silybin on histamine release from human basophil leucocytes. *British Journal of Clinical Pharmacology* 1987; 24: 747–752.
6. Palasciano G, Portincasa P, Palmieri V, et al. The effect of silymarin on plasma levels of malon-dialdehyde in patients receiving long-term treatment with psychotropic drugs. *Current Therapeutic Research* 1994; 55(5): 537–545.
7. Lirussi F, Okolicsanyi L. Cytoprotection in the nineties: experience with ursodeoxycholic acid and silymarin in chronic liver disease. *Acta Physiologica Hungarica* 1992; 80(1–4): 363–367.
8. Ferenci P, Dragosics B, Dittrich H, et al. Randomized controlled trial of silymarin treatment in patients with cirrhosis of the liver. *Journal of Hepatology* 1989; 9: 105–113.
9. Sonnenbichler J, Sonnenbichler I, Scalera F. Influence of the flavonolignan silibinin of milk thistle on hepatocytes and kidney cells. In: Lawson L, Bauer R, eds. *Phytomedicines of Europe: Chemistry and Biological Activity.* Washington, DC: American Chemical Society, 1998.
10. Farkas L, Gabor M, Kallay, F, eds. Flavonoids from natural red resins. *Proceedings of the International Bioflavonoid Symposium, September 6–9, 1981.* Amsterdam, Oxford, and New York: Elsevier Scientific, 1982.
11. Hikino H, Kiso Y, Wagner H, et al. Antihepatotoxic actions of flavonolignans from

Silybum marianum fruits. *Planta Medica* 1984; 50: 248–250.

12. Valenzuela A, Aspillaga M, Vial S, et al. Selectivity of silymarin on the increase of the glutathione content in different tissues of the rat. *Planta Medica* 1989; 55: 420–422.

13. Muzes G, Deak GY, Lang I, et al. Effect of the bioflavonoid silymarin on the in vitro activity and expression of superoxide dismutase (SOD) enzyme. *Acta Physiologica Hungarica* 1991; 78(1): 3–9.

14. Brown D. Phytotherapy review and commentary: silymarin educational monograph. *Townsend Letter for Doctors* November 1994; 1282–1285.

15. Robbers JE, Tyler VE. *Tyler's Herbs of Choice: The Therapeutic Use of Phytomedicinals.* New York and London: The Haworth Press, 1999.

16. McGuffin M, Hobbs C, Upton R, et al., eds. *American Herbal Products Association Botanical Safety Handbook.* Boca Raton, FL: CRC Press, 1997.

17. Velussi M, Cernigoi AM, Viezzoli L, et al. Silymarin reduces hyperinsulinemia, malondialdehyde levels, and daily insulin need in cirrhotic diabetic patients. *Current Therapeutic Research* 1993; 53 (5): 533–545.

Nettle

URTICA DIOICA
URTICACEAE

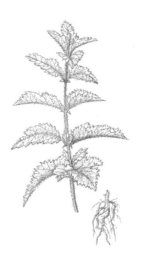

State of Knowledge: Five-Star Rating System

Clinical (human) research	✶✶
Laboratory research	✶✶
History of use/traditional use	✶✶✶✶
Safety record	✶✶✶✶
International acceptance	✶✶✶

PART USED: *Root, Leaf*

PRIMARY USES

Nettle root

- *Benign prostatic hyperplasia (BPH)*
- *Prostatitis*

Nettle leaf

- *Arthritis*
- *Diuretic effects*
- *Nutritive tonic*
- *Allergies (traditional)*

Anyone who has ever taken a careless stroll through a nettle patch understands the origin of the plant's botanical name, *Urtica,* which means "to sting" in Latin. Nettle's infamous sting causes a painful, itchy skin irritation that may last for hours. Yet in the European herbal tradition, this "noxious weed" has a long history of use as a nutritive tonic and for the treatment of numerous ailments, including arthritis, asthma, allergies, urinary tract conditions, and skin problems. Even the nettle sting itself has been employed as a folk remedy for arthritis pain, in a traditional practice that requires the arthritis sufferer to intentionally allow nettle plants to sting affected joints. Believers report that nettle stings can relieve arthritis pain for weeks at a time, and the practice has even received some recognition from modern physicians,[1] but no clinical studies have confirmed its effectiveness. However, preliminary clinical studies do support the traditional role of nettle leaf taken internally for the treatment of arthritis.

In Europe today, nettle root is a remedy of choice for treating the early symptoms of benign prostatic hyperplasia (BPH), commonly known as prostate enlargement. BPH, which causes symptoms such as increased frequency of urination and obstructed urine flow, is a common condition that affects about half of men between the ages of 40 and 60. Substantial clinical evidence has confirmed the ability of nettle root to relieve symptoms of BPH, particularly in the early stages of the condition. For treating BPH, nettle root is often taken in combination formulas with other herbs such as saw palmetto *(Serenoa repens),* pygeum *(Prunus africana,* also known as African prune), and pumpkinseed *(Cucurbita pepo).*

Nettle leaf has a history of use for the treatment of allergic rhinitis—commonly known as hay fever—but this application has not been extensively studied. Nettle leaf also has a strong reputation as an effective diuretic.[2,3] German herbalists recommend it for treating kidney infections and inflammations of the lower urinary tract.[4]

Traditionally, nettle has been used as a "spring tonic" plant to help increase energy and metabolism and prepare the body for the busy spring season after a winter of inactivity. Nettle's diuretic action also stimulates urination, possibly helping to move toxins out of the body—another benefit of the spring tonic.[5] Young nettle shoots do not have the stinging capabilities of mature plants and are a well-loved early spring food in many different cultures. Gather the young leaves when the shoots are about 6 inches high and prepare them like spinach. They may be simmered in water, sauteed with butter or oil, or added to salads and soups. Nettle is an excellent source of many vitamins and minerals and may in fact be one of the most nutrient-rich herbs available.[6]

HISTORY

Nettle has been applied medicinally and eaten as a food since ancient times and has a rich history of traditional use throughout Europe. Its extensive medicinal applications have been documented since the first century, when Pliny the Elder noted the ability of nettle leaf to stop bleeding. In the first and second centuries, the physicians Dioscorides and Galen, respectively, recommended nettle as a diuretic, to stop nosebleeds, and for infected wounds.[7] For centuries, nettle has been administered in Europe to treat arthritis, skin conditions, and kidney disease. Because of the plant's high iron content, Europeans have also used nettle to treat anemia.[4]

In folk medicine, nettle roots and leaves have been employed to relieve coughing and asthma, to both initiate menstruation and stem excessive menstrual flow, to stop bleeding, and to heal infected sores. The seed has also been used as a diuretic in the treatment of urinary, bladder, and kidney disorders. In turn-of-the-century America, nettle was used to treat diarrhea, hemorrhoids, eczema, and colon disease.[6] Native American women took the herb during pregnancy to strengthen the fetus and make childbirth easier. Nettle also has been used traditionally to restore hair or increase hair growth, though there has been no modern scientific research substantiating this application. The use of nettle root for treating BPH is relatively new and was probably popularized by German research in the 1950s.[6]

In a written account from the 1600s, the British physician Nicholas Culpeper mentions the folk practice of applying fresh nettles to relieve the pain of gout, sciatica, or arthritis. This practice, traditionally known as *urtication,* apparently continues today. In 1994, a British physician writing to the *British Journal of General Practice* related stories of two patients who claimed they obtained relief from arthritis pain of the hip and fingers by applying nettle leaves.[1] This traditional arthritis treatment has not yet been scientifically investigated.

Nettle fiber, said to be similar to that of flax or hemp, was historically employed in weaving.[8] During the Bronze Age in the region that is now northern Europe, people wove burial shrouds out of nettle fiber. Later, nettle was used by Europeans to make sailcloth, fishing lines, and even clothing. More recently, nettle cloth served as a substitute for cotton in Germany during the First World War.

INTERNATIONAL STATUS

In the *German Commission E Monographs,* nettle root is approved for the treatment of difficult urination due to benign prostatic hyperplasia (stages I and II). Nettle leaf is listed as an approved herb for supportive therapy for rheumatic ailments, as irrigation therapy for inflammatory diseases of the lower urinary tract, and for the prevention and treatment of kidney stones. The leaf is approved in the United Kingdom and France for internal and external use in the treatment of rheumatic conditions.

BOTANY

There are approximately 50 *Urtica* species in the botanical family Urticaceae, the best known being *Urtica dioica,* or stinging nettle. The plant is native to Europe, and there are six North American varieties of an American subspecies called *U. dioica* subsp. *gracilis.*[4] North American nettles differ from their close European relatives in that they are *monoecious,* meaning that male and female flowers occur on the same plant. European strains are *dioecious,* meaning that individual plants have either male or female flowers.[4] In fact, the species name *dioica* is derived from the word *dioecious.* Another commonly used nettle is *Urtica urens,* also known as small nettle or dog nettle.

Stinging nettle (also called great nettle) stands 2 to 3 feet tall, with an erect stalk, dark, drooping, green leaves, and small, inconspicuous white flowers during summer. Nettles often grow in groups in shady soils or disturbed ground. Fine, hollow, silica-tipped hairs cover the entire plant. When touched, the syringelike hairs break off and deliver chemicals that cause the classic skin irritation. These hairs are inactivated during processing (including drying or cooking); thus, people taking the herb internally do not get stung. Young nettle shoots are edible and contain carotene (a precursor to vitamin A) and vitamin C in the same quantities as spinach.[9] The entire plant is also rich in chlorophyll, carotenoids, and minerals, including iron, potassium, and magnesium.

BENEFITS

- **Root:** Improves urine flow, reduces urinary frequency and nocturia (nighttime urination), and decreases volume of residual urine in early stage BPH
- **Leaf:** May relieve arthritis pain by altering the inflammatory response

SCIENTIFIC SUPPORT

Considerable clinical and laboratory research supports the use of nettle root, either alone or with other herbs, to treat symptoms of the early stages of prostate enlargement (be-

nign prostatic hyperplasia, or BPH), including difficult and frequent urination and nighttime urination (nocturia). In one clinical study, frequency of nighttime urination was significantly reduced in patients with mild prostatic enlargement who took 5 ml of a nettle root water extract three times a day, although no changes were observed in prostate size.[10] In an open study involving more than 4,000 men with BPH, patients in all stages of the disease experienced a significant decrease in the frequency of nighttime urination after 8 weeks of treatment with nettle root extract at a daily dose of 1,200 mg.[11] Other favorable results from nettle root treatment include improvements in urinary flow and reductions in the amount of residual urine left in the bladder after urination.[12] In addition, in one small study, significant symptomatic improvement was seen in patients treated with beta-sitosterol, a mixture of phytosterols found in nettle root.[13]

A number of other investigations have demonstrated the effectiveness of nettle root used in combination with other herbs for the treatment of BPH.[14–16] One recent double-blind study using a combination of saw palmetto and nettle root showed that the herbal preparation was at least as effective as finasteride, a synthetic drug commonly used in treating BPH, with fewer side effects (see Specific Studies).[14] Both nettle root and saw palmetto have had an excellent safety record in clinical trials, causing a very low incidence of side effects.

There is also preliminary evidence that supports nettle leaf as a treatment for arthritis. Encouraging results from two clinical studies suggest that stewed nettle leaf may enhance the effectiveness of nonsteroidal anti-inflammatory drugs (NSAIDs) commonly used to ease the pain and inflammation of arthritis. In these studies, combination treatment with nettle leaf and a low dose of NSAIDs afforded pain relief comparable with that from a full dose of the drug alone (see Specific Studies).[17,18] Nettle's anti-inflammatory activity has been demonstrated in at least one laboratory study,[19] but further research is needed to determine exactly how it works.

Nettle's reputation for preventing and treating hay fever has not been fully investigated. However, in one clinical study, people taking freeze-dried nettle leaf reported moderate relief from allergy symptoms. Fifty-two percent of those taking the daily dose of 300 mg nettle said they would use it again, whereas only 15 percent preferred the placebo.[20] Though not extensively researched, it is possible that histamine, a constituent of nettle, may be responsible for the plant's observed anti-allergenic effects.[21]

SPECIFIC STUDIES

Benign Prostatic Hyperplasia: Clinical Study (1997)

Results from this randomized, double-blind study showed that a combination of saw palmetto and nettle root extracts performed as effectively as the synthetic drug finasteride in improving symptoms of BPH. The herbal formula contained 120 mg nettle root extract and 160 mg saw palmetto extract. Participants took either 2 capsules of the herbal preparation or 1 capsule (5 mg) of finasteride daily for 48 weeks. The investigators monitored changes in maximum urine flow rate and volume and recorded patient reports of improvements in quality of life and symptom severity. The herbal preparation and finasteride were equally effective in improving urinary flow rate and other symptom scores. However, the saw palmetto and nettle root combination seemed to be better tolerated than finasteride, causing fewer side effects. The researchers concluded that the herbal preparation should be the therapy of first choice in patients with early-stage BPH.[14]

Benign Prostatic Hyperplasia: Clinical Study (1986)

Fifty-five percent of participants in this open trial reported reductions in urinary frequency and nighttime urination after 10 weeks of treatment with nettle root extract. Increased frequency of nighttime urination (nocturia) is one of the most common symptoms of BPH, and all patients in this study had experienced the need to urinate at least twice during the night at the beginning of the study. The 83 patients were divided into three groups based on the number of episodes of nocturia they experienced at the start of the study. In the two groups of subjects reporting the highest number of nighttime urination episodes, approximately 54 percent reported improvement in this symptom by the end of the 10-week study, with 77 percent of all patients rating the effects of the herbal treatment as "good" or "very good." The dosage of nettle root extract tested in the study was two 300-mg tablets twice daily. Seven people reported mild side effects.[22]

Osteoarthritis: Clinical Study (1997)

This open randomized clinical study showed that a combination of nettle leaf and a low dose of a conventional anti-inflammatory drug was as effective at relieving arthritis pain as a full dose of the drug alone. Forty patients suffering from acute arthritis attacks participated in the 2-week study. Subjects took either 200 mg of diclofenac (a nonsteroidal anti-inflammatory drug) or 50 mg diclofenac plus 50 g of stewed *Urtica dioica* leaves. Clinical symptom scores improved by about 70 percent in both treatment groups, and a dramatic decrease in levels of C-reactive protein (a chemical associated with acute arthritis) was noted in both groups.

The typical daily dose of diclofenac is 150 to 200 mg, and previous studies have shown that 75 mg per day of diclofenac is inadequate to control arthritis pain in most patients.

Therefore, the researchers concluded it was unlikely that the 50-mg drug dose administered with the stewed nettle was responsible for the profound pain-relieving effects seen in patients taking the herb/drug combination. Future studies should investigate the possibility that acute arthritis attacks will respond to treatment with stewed nettle leaf alone. The stewed nettle used in the study was prepared by heating up a prefrozen nettle leaf puree. Three people in each of the treatment groups reported mild gastrointestinal upset.[17]

HOW IT WORKS

Relief of BPH Symptoms

Several theories have been proposed to explain how nettle root works to relieve symptoms of prostate enlargement. In animals, nettle root extracts inhibited the enzymes 5-alpha-reductase and aromatase, although it is not known which nettle compounds produced this effect.[23] In the body, 5-alpha-reductase acts on testosterone to produce dihydrotestosterone, a chemical that appears to play a role in prostate enlargement. (The drug finasteride specifically inhibits 5-alpha-reductase.) Estrogen may also stimulate prostatic enlargement. In men, estrogen likely is produced by conversion of androstenedione to estrone and estradiol by aromatase. However, some researchers question whether aromatase is present in prostate tissue, so it is uncertain whether nettle's inhibition of the enzyme is responsible for the beneficial effects.[23]

The compounds responsible for nettle root's effects on the prostate have not been fully identified. A group of plant sterols known as beta-sitosterols effectively reduced symptoms in patients with BPH and have been proposed as the "active ingredients" of nettle root, but a number of different compounds have demonstrated antiprostatic activity in laboratory studies. A lignan compound in nettle root appears to reduce the binding ability of sex hormone binding globulin (SHBG), a protein that stores and transports sex hormones and may play a role in the development of BPH.[24,25] Nettle root may also affect the prostate by blocking prostaglandin and leukotriene synthesis, pathways involved in the inflammatory response.[26] Preliminary laboratory experiments suggest that polysaccharides and lectins in nettle root have anti-inflammatory effects.[26,27] In addition, some researchers believe that growth factors may influence prostatic enlargement. A laboratory study showed that a lectin in nettle root may prevent a cell growth factor from binding to its receptor, which in theory might diminish prostate cell proliferation.[28]

Anti-Arthritis Effects

Laboratory tests suggest that the effects of nettle leaf against the pain and inflammation of arthritis may be due to at least three factors. First, possibly because of its caffeic malic acid content, nettle has demonstrated an ability to inhibit reactions affecting chemicals called cyclooxygenase and 5-lipoxygenase, which are involved in the body's inflammatory response.[19] Furthermore, nettle leaf may inhibit cytokine release and stimulate the release of interleukin-6 (IL-6), two other chemical pathways that are involved with initiating and perpetuating inflammation.[29] Cytokines are known to play a key role in the inflammatory destruction of bone and cartilage and other processes that occur with degenerative arthritis. IL-6 works against one such cytokine by decreasing prostaglandin E2, a hormone-like substance involved in the inflammatory response, so stimulating the release of IL-6 may be another method by which nettle decreases inflammation and pain.

What Puts the Sting in Stinging Nettle?

Anyone who has had a close encounter with live nettles can attest to the unpleasant sting they deliver. Tiny, syringelike hairs break off when touched, delivering a mixture of chemicals that inflame the skin and cause pain, numbness, and itching that can last anywhere from a few minutes to longer than a day, depending on the sensitivity of the individual.[6] Several compounds in nettle are responsible for the prickly, stinging sensation caused by contact with the hairs on the plant's leaves and stems.[4] Histamine, acetylcholine and 5-hydroxytryptamine are the main components, along with small amounts of formic acid—the same chemical that red ants use in inflicting their painful bites. The traditional antidote for nettle rash is rumored to be the juice of the nettle itself or of other plants, including yellow dock *(Rumex crispus)* or jewel weed *(Impatiens capensis),* although there is no solid evidence that this remedy works.

MAJOR CONSTITUENTS

Lignans, beta-sitosterol (a group of plant sterols), other plant sterols, polysaccharides, caffeic malic acid, lectins (including agglutinin), histamine, acetylcholine, 5-hydroxytryptamine, formic acid, vitamins and minerals

SAFETY

Nettle leaf has a long history of traditional use as a food and is generally considered safe when taken appropriately.[30] In clinical studies, nettle root was associated with a very low incidence of side effects.

- **Side effects:** Occasional mild gastrointestinal upset has been reported with nettle root.[31] There have been rare reports of allergic reaction to nettle leaf.[3]

- **Contraindications:** Nettle leaf should not be used as a diuretic by people with edema (fluid retention) due to heart or kidney problems.[31]
- **Drug interactions:** None known.[31]

DOSAGE

Before using nettle root, it is important to see a doctor to get a diagnosis of BPH and rule out more serious conditions, such as prostate cancer.

Nettle root

- **Extract:** Up to 1,200 mg a day, taken in divided doses.
- **Tincture:** 2 to 5 ml ($^1/_2$ to 1 teaspoon) three times a day.[6]
- **Tea:** Simmer 1 teaspoon dried root in a cup of water. Drink 2 to 3 cups a day.

Nettle leaf

- **Tincture:** 2 to 5 ml ($^1/_2$ to 1 teaspoon) three times a day.[6]
- **Tea:** 2 to 3 teaspoons of dried herb per pint of boiling water. Drink 2 to 3 cups a day.

STANDARDIZATION

Currently, nettle root and leaf products are not available in standardized form.

References

1. Randall CF. Stinging nettles for osteoarthritis pain of the hip [letter]. *British Journal of General Practice* November 1994; 533–534.

2. Bisset N, ed. *Herbal Drugs and Phytopharmaceuticals.* Boca Raton, FL: CRC Press, 1994.

3. Bradley PR, ed. *British Herbal Compendium.* Vol. 1. Dorset, England: British Herbal Medicine Association, 1992.

4. Foster S. Inconspicuous until touched: stinging nettle. *The Business of Herbs* September–October 1996; 14–15.

5. Theiss B, Theiss P. *The Family Herbal.* Rochester, VT: Healing Arts Press, 1989.

6. Yarnell E. Stinging nettle: a modern view of an ancient healing plant. *Alternative and Complementary Therapies* June 1998; 180–186.

7. Bombardelli E, Morazzoni P. *Urtica dioica* L. *Fitoterapia* 1997; 68(5): 387–402.

8. Grieve M. *A Modern Herbal.* New York: Dover Publications, 1931.

9. Foster S, Tyler V. *Tyler's Honest Herbal,* 4th ed. New York and London: The Haworth Herbal Press, 1999.

10. Belaiche P, Lievoux O. Clinical studies on the palliative treatment of prostatic adenoma with extract of *Urtica* root. *Phytotherapy Research* 1991; 5: 267–269.

11. Stahl HP. The treatment of prostatic nycturia with standardized extract of Radix Urticae (ERU) [in German]. *Zeitschrift Allgemeiner Medizin* 1984; 60: 128–132.

12. Dathe G, Schmid H. Phytotherapy for benign prostatic hyperplasia (BPH): double-blind study with extract Radicus Urticae (ERU) [in German]. *Urologe B* 1987; 27: 223–226.

13. Berges RR, Windeler J, Trampisch HJ, et al. Randomised, placebo-controlled, double-blind clinical trial of β-sitosterol in patients with benign prostatic hyperplasia. *The Lancet* 1995; 345: 1529–1532.

14. Sökeland J, Albrecht J. A combination of Sabal and Urtica extract vs. finasteride in BPH. Comparison of therapeutic effectiveness in a 1-year, double-blind study [in German]. *Urologe A* 1997; 36(4): 327–333.

15. Schneider H, Honold E, Masuhr T. Treatment of benign prostatic hyperplasia: results of a treatment study with the phytogenic combination of Sabal extract WS 1473 and Urtica extract WS 1031 in urologic specialty practices [in German]. *Fortschritte der Medizin* 1995; 113(3): 37–40.

16. Krzeski T, Kazon M, Borkowski A, et al. Combined extracts of *Urtica dioica* and *Pygeum africanum* in the treatment of benign prostatic hyperplasia: double-blind comparison of two doses. *Clinical Therapeutics* 1993; 15(6): 1011–1020.

17. Chrubasik S, Enderlein W, Bauer R, et al. Evidence for antirheumatic effectiveness of Herba *Urtica dioicae* in acute arthritis: a pilot study. *Phytomedicine* 1997; 4(2): 105–108.

18. Ramm S, Hansen C. Stinging nettle extract for arthrosis and rheumatoid arthritis [in German]. *Therapiewoche* 1996; 28: 1575–1578.

19. Obertreis B, Giller K, Teucher T, et al. Anti-inflammatory effect of *Urtica dioica* folia extract in comparison to caffeic malic

acid [in German]. *Arzneimittel-Forschung* 1996; 46(1): 52–56.

20. Mittman P. Randomized, double-blind study of freeze-dried *Urtica dioica* in the treatment of allergic rhinitis. *Planta Medica* 1990; 56: 44–46.

21. Brinker FJ. *Eclectic Dispensary of Botanical Therapeutics.* Sandy, OR: Eclectic Medical Publications, 1995.

22. Vandierendounck EJ, Burkhardt P. The extract of *Radicus Urticae* for fibromyadenoma of the prostate with nightly pollakiuria. Study for testing the effect of ZY 15095 (Simic®) [in German]. *Therapiewoche Schweiz* 1986; 10: 892–895.

23. Hartmann RW, Mark M, Soldati F. Inhibition of 5-reductase and aromatase by PHL-00801 (Prostatonin®), a combination of PY 102 *(Pygeum africanum)* and UR 102 *(Urtica dioica)* extracts. *Phytomedicine* 1996; 3(2): 121–128.

24. Schöttner M, Gansser D, Spiteller G. Lignans from the roots of *Urtica dioica* and their metabolites bind to human sex hormone binding globulin (SHBG). *Planta Medica* 1997; 63: 529–532.

25. Hryb DJ, Khan MS, Romas NA, et al. The effect of extracts of the roots of the stinging nettle *(Urtica dioica)* on the interaction of SHBG with its receptor on human prostatic membranes. *Planta Medica* 1995; 61: 31–32.

26. *ESCOP Monographs on the Medicinal Uses of Plant Drugs.* Vol. 2. The Netherlands: European Scientific Cooperative on Phytotherapy, 1996.

27. Wagner H, Willer F, Samtleben R, et al. Search for the antiprostatic principle of stinging nettle *(Urtica dioica)* roots. *Phytomedicine* 1994; 1: 213–224.

28. Wagner H, Geiger WN, Boos G, et al. Studies on the binding of Urtica dioica agglutinin (UDA) and other lectins in an in vitro epidermal growth factor receptor test. *Phytomedicine* 1995; 4: 287–290.

29. Obertreis B, Ruttkowski T, Teucher T, et al. Ex-vivo in-vitro inhibition of lipopolysaccharide stimulated tumor necrosis factor-alpha and interleukin-1 beta secretion in human whole blood by extractum urticae dioicae foliorum [in German]. *Arzneimittel-Forschung* 1996; 46(4): 389–394.

30. McGuffin M, Hobbs C, Upton R, et al., eds. *American Herbal Products Association Botanical Safety Handbook.* Boca Raton, FL: CRC Press, 1997.

31. Blumenthal M, Busse W, Goldberg A, et al., eds. *The Complete German Commission E Monographs.* Austin, TX: The American Botanical Council; Boston: Integrative Medical Communications, 1998.

Red Clover

TRIFOLIUM PRATENSE
FABACEAE

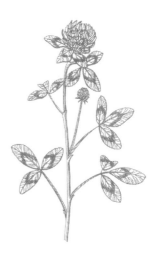

State of Knowledge: Five-Star Rating System

Clinical (human) research	✶
Laboratory research	✶✶
History of use / traditional use	✶✶✶✶
Safety record	✶✶✶
International acceptance	✶✶

PART USED: *Flower, leaf*

PRIMARY USES

- *Menopause*
- *Heart health*
- *Skin disorders such as psoriasis and eczema (traditional)*
- *Cancer (traditional / experimental)*
- *Nutritive tonic (traditional)*

Why do Asian and Mediterranean women generally breeze through menopause, whereas Western women suffer from hot flashes, depression, insomnia, and other unpleasant symptoms? Researchers are discovering that the differences may be dietary. For centuries, women in Asian and Mediterranean cultures have benefited from the effects of plant phytoestrogens (also called *isoflavones*) consumed in the form of soybeans, chickpeas, split peas, lentils, and other legumes. Today, studies show that these important plant compounds may help bridge the hormonal gap as natural estrogen levels decline with menopause.

Population studies show that people in Asian cultures take in at least 40 mg of isoflavones daily, compared with just 2 to 5 mg consumed by Americans. Cross-cultural data also suggest that men who eat isoflavone-rich foods have lower rates of prostate cancer and benign prostatic hyperplasia (BPH), an enlargement of the prostate that can lead to urinary problems as men get older.[1] Standardized red clover extracts are currently being marketed for improvement of both menopausal symptoms and prostate health. Like soy, red clover may also help lower cholesterol levels, increase bone mass during menopause, and protect against various cancers because of its isoflavone content and other constituents.

Although there are many studies on isoflavones, research on red clover itself is still in the early stages. Recent evidence does show that red clover helps improve heart health in menopausal women.[2] This is important because as estrogen levels decline, women's cardiovascular risk factors approach those of men, who have a higher risk of heart attack earlier in life. Promising research on red clover's ability to relieve menopausal hot flashes is expected to be published soon.

HISTORY

Aside from the lucky "four-leaf" variety, clover species have several other historical associations with good fortune. The familiar Irish shamrock and the suit of clubs on playing cards both come from this plant. Because of its three-part leaves, clover was also an early Christian symbol of the Trinity. The plant's importance to ancient cultures stems from its value as a forage crop for cattle, horses, sheep, and other animals. The blossoms are also an important source of nectar for bees and wildflower honey for people.

Red clover itself has a long history of application as a "blood-cleansing" herb that thins the blood, aids digestion, and stimulates detoxification through the liver and gallbladder. The plant has been used as a purifying "spring tonic"—a remedy to increase energy and metabolism for spring following a winter of inactivity—and as a treatment for skin problems such as psoriasis and eczema, often in combination with herbs such as yellow dock (*Rumex crispus*) and dandelion root (*Taraxacum officinalis*). People from more than 30 countries around the world have used red clover both internally and externally for treating cancer. The leaves and flowers were also taken as an expectorant and antispasmodic for colds, bronchitis, asthma, whooping cough, and tuberculosis. Even today, compresses made from red clover blossom tea are applied externally to treat athlete's foot, sores, burns, and ulcers. When eaten in salads, soup stocks, or prepared as tea, red clover acts as a general tonic due to its rich vitamin and mineral content.

Red clover, the state flower of Vermont, has a colorful history of use in the United States as well. Native Americans traditionally ate the leaves and the beautiful, sweet flowers either raw or cooked. They used red clover as a blood purifier, a salve for burns, an eyewash, and as a treatment for a variety of gynecological problems. Around the turn of the twentieth century, a line of remedies called Trifolium Compounds became popular with the Eclectic physicians (a prominent group of American doctors who practiced around that time) for respiratory problems, cancer, and syphilis, and as a mild sedative. Red clover was also the backbone of Harry Hoxsey's controversial alternative cancer therapy, which is still used in some Mexican cancer clinics. The plant was listed in the *The United States Pharmacopoeia* as a treatment for skin diseases until 1946. However, by the early twentieth century, the American Medical Association had begun its attack on many herbal remedies, including Trifolium Compounds.

INTERNATIONAL STATUS

In the United Kingdom, red clover is approved for use in skin problems such as psoriasis, eczema, and rashes; coughs and bronchitis; and as an antispasmodic. It is also approved in Australia and Sweden.

BOTANY

Although the Latin name *Trifolium* means "three leaves," if you're lucky you may find an occasional four-leaf clover. Like other members of the pea family (Fabaceae), red clover leaves are compound and usually composed of three leaflets. Of more than 80 species of clover indigenous to the United States, the two most common include red clover *(Trifolium pratense)* and white clover *(Trifolium repens)*. Many other clover species are native to Europe and the temperate parts of Asia and Africa. During the summer, red clover is easily recognized by its characteristic pinkish-red flowers, which are gathered when in full bloom from May to September. In other seasons, the whitish V-shaped marking on each leaflet is the plant's most distinctive characteristic. When not in bloom, red clover is often mistaken for alfalfa, which also grows from 18 to 36 inches tall and has similar-looking foliage.

Red clover and other members of the pea family help improve the health of soil by fixing nitrogen, breaking up compacted earth, and bringing trace minerals to the surface for absorption by other plants. For these reasons, farmers have traditionally plowed it under as a soil-enriching green manure. Red clover is an easy plant to grow in any sunny location with moist, well-drained soil. Today, large-scale commercial cultivation is centered in Australia. (Helpful hint: you'll have more luck finding a four-leaf clover if you hunt in beds of big-head clover, which flaunt up to nine leaflets in the western United States.)

BENEFITS

- Helps relieve hot flashes and night sweats during menopause

- Improves cardiovascular health during menopause by protecting the elasticity of the large arteries
- May help lower cholesterol levels due to its isoflavone content (experimental)
- May help treat skin disorders such as psoriasis because of its "blood-purifying" action (traditional)
- May help prevent and treat cancers due to its "blood-purifying" action, phytoestrogen content, and other constituents (traditional/experimental)
- May be useful as a relaxing expectorant for respiratory problems (traditional)

SCIENTIFIC SUPPORT

Although clinical research on red clover is still in its early stages, a 1999 study suggests that the extract may help protect cardiovascular health during menopause. At this time of life, a decline in estrogen levels often leads to a rise in blood pressure and cholesterol levels, prompting some women to begin hormone-replacement therapy (HRT). Now research suggests that herbs such as red clover may help protect heart health just as effectively. The results of this study showed that red clover extract improved arterial compliance, a measure of elasticity in the large arteries, just as successfully as soy or HRT did in earlier studies.[2]

Two forthcoming double-blind placebo-controlled studies show that red clover may also decrease the incidence and severity of hot flashes during menopause. In both of these 12-week trials, there was a strong correlation between increasing urinary levels of isoflavones and relief from hot flashes. The participants also experienced a beneficial rise in levels of high-density lipoprotein (HDL) cholesterol, which lowers the risk of heart disease.[3,4]

SPECIFIC STUDIES

Cardiovascular Health During Menopause: Clinical Study (1999)

In a randomized, double-blind, placebo-controlled study involving 17 postmenopausal women, researchers found that standardized red clover extract significantly improved arterial compliance (a measure of elasticity of the large arteries). After an initial 3 to 4 week run-in period and a 5-week placebo period for all 17 participants, the women were divided into two treatment groups for an additional 10 weeks. During the first 5 weeks, 14 women took one red clover tablet (40 mg isoflavones) and one placebo tablet daily. The placebo group took two placebo tablets daily. During the final 5 weeks, the dosage for the red clover group was increased to two tablets (80 mg isoflavones) daily. At the beginning of the study, all women were free of obvious cardiovascular disease. Participants were required to discontinue the use of any drugs or supplements that might affect cardiovascular health for at least 6 weeks prior to treatment, and were instructed to avoid eating isoflavone-rich legumes throughout the study. At the end of each period (run-in, placebo, and two active periods), researchers measured arterial compliance using ultrasound, as well as isoflavonoid absorption and serum cholesterol levels.

The results of the study showed a statistically significant increase in arterial compliance in the red clover group, compared with the placebo group (a value of 23.7 versus 16 in the placebo group). Treatment with the higher isoflavone dose did not appear to be more effective than the lower dose. The red clover group also demonstrated a 10 percent downward trend in the ratio of harmful low-density lipoprotein (LDL) cholesterol (which decreased) versus healthful HDL cholesterol levels (which increased), although this trend was not statistically significant. Urinary excretion of isoflavones increased in those taking red clover, compared with the placebo group.

One important drawback in this study was the small sample size of 17 participants, which included a placebo group of just 3 women. Researchers did not subject data from the placebo group to statistical analysis, due to the group's small size. Interestingly, the placebo group originally included 5 women before 2 dropped out, citing a return of "intolerable menopausal symptoms requiring hormone-replacement therapy."

No side effects were reported in the red clover group.[2]

HOW IT WORKS

Much of the research on the isoflavones genistein and daidzein outlined in "Soy," also applies to red clover. Please see "Soy" for a discussion of how red clover and soy may both help lower cholesterol and protect against various types of cancer.

Limited research has been conducted on red clover itself and on some specific red clover constituents—coumarins and the isoflavones formononetin and biochanin. Preliminary clinical research suggests that red clover may improve cardiovascular health by supporting the elasticity of arteries during menopause. Although researchers don't know exactly how red clover does this, they believe that the plant's isoflavone content helps relax the smooth muscle lining the arteries. Diminished elasticity in the arteries is thought to contribute to heart disease by increasing blood pressure and coronary artery insufficiency and impairing the function of the left ventricle of the heart.[2]

Unlike soy, red clover also contains the isoflavones formononetin and biochanin, which some researchers believe may provide additional health benefits. A recent pharmacokinetic study indicated that when 2 tablets of red clover extract (a total of 80 mg isoflavones) were taken daily over a period of 2 weeks, the body rapidly converted most of the formononetin into daidzein and biochanin into genistein. However, small amounts of formononetin and biochanin remained in unchanged form.[4]

Researchers have not determined exactly what health-protective effects formononetin and biochanin may have. Recent laboratory experiments suggest that biochanin, like genistein, may help prevent the growth of human prostate cancer cells and stomach cancer cell lines.[5,6] A whole red clover extract also had a protective effect against the common carcinogen benzopyrene *in vitro,* an effect attributed mostly to the plant's biochanin content.[7] Benzopyrenes are carcinogens commonly found in grilled or barbecued foods.

The evidence on formononetin is limited to two studies in which the compound demonstrated no estrogenlike effects. In these studies, the isoflavone failed to bind to estrogen receptor sites in mice or in human breast cancer cell lines. This signifies that formononetin may not offer estrogen-like benefits during menopause.[8,9]

Red clover also contains coumarins, compounds found in several medicinal plants that have been linked to protective effects against cancer and edema (swelling due to fluid accumulation), as well as antioxidant, blood-thinning, and cholesterol-lowering actions.[10] More studies are needed to determine the health benefits of the specific coumarins found in red clover.

MAJOR CONSTITUENTS

Isoflavones, including daidzein, genistein, formononetin, and biochanin; coumarins

SAFETY

Red clover is included in the Food and Drug Administration's list of herbs that are generally recognized as safe (GRAS) and has traditionally been used over long periods of time.

- **Side effects:** No side effects have been reported in clinical studies. Although red clover has been associated with infertility in grazing sheep, researchers say there is little cause for concern in people. Sheep have a different body chemistry than humans, consume much larger amounts of red clover, and are far more sensitive to phytoestrogens.[11]
- **Contraindications:** Red clover should not be used during pregnancy.[12] Because of its coumarin content, the plant probably should not be used if you have a blood clotting disorder. For the same reason, red clover should not be used immediately before or after surgery, although no adverse effects have been reported.
- **Drug interactions:** Red clover should not be used in combination with blood-thinning drugs. Women who are

taking birth control pills or other hormonal drugs should consult a health practitioner before using red clover.

DOSAGE

The active constituents in red clover are soluble in water and alcohol. Teas and home-made vinegars also provide a wide array of vitamins and minerals that cannot be extracted by alcohol.

- **Standardized tablets:** 1 to 2 tablets a day
- **Capsules:** Up to five 430-mg capsules a day[13]
- **Tincture:** 15 to 30 drops, up to four times a day[13]
- **Tea:** 1 cup three to four times a day
- **Vinegar:** 1 tablespoon two to three times a day

To make a medicinal vinegar, cover fresh red clover blossoms and leaves with organic apple cider vinegar in a glass jar. Make sure the plant material is completely submerged to avoid fermentation. Let the jar sit, covered, in a cool, dark place for several days. Strain, refrigerate, and enjoy on salads, pasta dishes, or right off the spoon.

STANDARDIZATION

Standardized red clover tablets contain 40 mg of total isoflavones, including daidzein (3.5 mg), genistein (4 mg), biochanin (24.5 mg), and formononetin (8 mg).

REFERENCES

1. Holt S. Prostatic health. Part 1: the optimal diet. *Alternative and Complementary Therapies* September/October 1996; 302–305.
2. Nestel PJ, Pomeroy S, Kay S, et al. Isoflavones from red clover improve systemic arterial compliance but not plasma lipids in menopausal women. *The Journal of Clinical Endocrinology and Metabolism* 1999; 84(3): 895–898.
3. Husband AJ, Howes JB, Knight DC, et al. The correlation between phenolic estrogen levels and menopause symptoms in women. In press.
4. Husband AJ, Howes JB, Howes LG, et al. Pharmacokinetic analysis of urine and plasma levels of isoflavones after acute and chronic administration of a purified red clover extract. In press.
5. Peterson G, Barnes S. Genistein and biochanin A inhibit the growth of human prostate cancer cells but not epidermal growth factor receptor tyrosine autophosphorylation. *The Prostate* 1993; 22: 335–345.
6. Yanagihara K, Ito A, Toge T, et al. Antiproliferative effects of isoflavones on human cancer cell lines established from the gastrointestinal tract. *Cancer Research* 1993; 53: 5815–5821.
7. Cassady JM, Zennie TM, Chae YH, et al. Use of a mammalian cell culture

benzo(a)pyrene metabolism assay for the detection of potential anticarcinogens from natural products: inhibition of metabolism by biochanin A, an isoflavone from *Trifolium pratense* L. *Cancer Research* 1988; 48: 6257–6261.

8. Wong E, Flux DS. The oestrogenic activity of red clover isoflavones and some of their degradation products. *Journal of Endocrinology* 1962; 24: 341–348.

9. Martin PM, Horwitz KB, Ryan DS, et al. Phytoestrogen interaction with estrogen receptors in human breast cancer cells. *Endocrinology* 1978; 103(5): 1860–1867.

10. Hoult JRS, Payá M. Pharmacological and biochemical actions of simple coumarins: natural products with therapeutic potential. *General Pharmacology* 1996; 27(4): 713–722.

11. Beckham N. Phyto-oestrogens and compounds that affect oestrogen metabolism—part II. *Australian Journal of Medical Herbalism* 1995; 7(2): 27–33.

12. McGuffin M, Hobbs C, Upton R, et al., eds. *American Herbal Products Associations Botanical Safety Handbook*. Boca Raton and New York: CRC Press LLC, 1997.

13. Foster S. *101 Medicinal Herbs*. Loveland, CO: Interweave Press, 1998.

Saw Palmetto

SERENOA REPENS
ARECACEAE

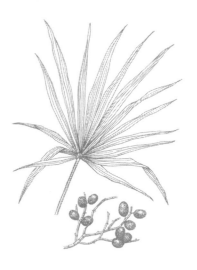

State of Knowledge: Five-Star Rating System

Clinical (human) research	✶✶✶
Laboratory research	✶✶✶
History of use/traditional use	✶✶✶✶
Safety record	✶✶✶✶
International acceptance	✶✶✶✶

PART USED: *Berry*

PRIMARY USES

- *Prostate health maintenance*
- *Benign prostatic hyperplasia (BPH), especially mild or moderate cases*
- *Nonbacterial prostatitis (chronic inflammation of the prostate)*

Traditionally called "the old man's friend," saw palmetto was used as a male tonic long before people understood how it helps support prostate health. The ripe, purplish berries were an important Native American food, valued for their nutritive and health-enhancing benefits. Men have also historically taken saw pal-metto as a natural treatment for urinary symptoms associated with prostate enlargement. A common condition, prostate enlargement affects roughly 50 to 60 percent of men between the ages of 40 and 60, and almost 90 percent of men by age 85. When men begin to experience symptoms such as difficult urination or more frequent urge to urinate, doctors use a more technical term to describe the condition: *benign prostatic hyperplasia* (BPH).

Recent clinical studies show that saw palmetto is a safe, effective alternative to standard drug therapy and surgery in treating the uncomfortable symptoms of BPH, either by itself or in combination with nettle root *(Urtica dioica),* pumpkinseed *(Cucurbita pepo),* or pygeum *(Prunus africana).* Saw palmetto has been found effective in roughly 90 percent of men, usually within 4 to 6 weeks. In contrast, fewer than 50 percent of men have success with the common drug finasteride (Proscar) even after a year of treatment.[1] Side effects with drug therapy and surgery can include incontinence, impotence, and decreased sexual desire and performance—not to mention financial stress due to the high cost of these therapies!

Throughout the world, saw palmetto is quickly becoming the treatment of choice for improving male reproductive health. In Germany, Austria, Italy, France, and many other European countries, the extract is widely prescribed by physicians as a safe, effective, and inexpensive treatment for mild to moderate BPH. American urologists are also increasingly recommending saw palmetto to their patients, based on a favorable 1998 review of eighteen clinical studies published in the *Journal of the American Medical Association.*[2]

HISTORY

Native Americans used saw palmetto berries as a tonic and a treatment for urinary problems long before the arrival of Europeans in North America. The plant's first introduction into American medicine came in an 1879 issue of the *American Journal of Pharmacy.* Within 20 years, saw palmetto was a common treatment for prostate enlarge-

ment. Although primarily an herb for men, the plant has also been used to treat mammary gland disorders in women. During the 1930s, European physicians began prescribing saw palmetto for irritations of the bladder, urethra, and prostate. Saw palmetto's historical reputation as an aphrodisiac only added to its popularity as a male tonic.

The plant has also traditionally been recommended for conditions such as bronchitis, because of its soothing action on mucous membranes in many parts of the body. After the Second World War, American use of saw palmetto declined at the same time that German researchers began taking an avid interest in the herb. Scientific studies followed from Italy, Spain, Belgium, France, and many other European countries. Today, saw palmetto is widely taken by men in Europe and in the United States, where it is the sixth best-selling herb.

INTERNATIONAL STATUS

Saw palmetto is approved in the *German Commission E Monographs* for urinary problems caused by stage I or II BPH.

BOTANY

Saw palmetto is a member of the palm family (Arecaceae), but is much shorter than the palm trees common in Florida and

California. If you've ever spent time in the southern United States, you may have seen dense saw palmetto thickets covering large areas of South Carolina, Louisiana, Georgia, and Florida. You may even have personally encountered the sharp, sawlike leaves that give saw palmetto its name. The relatively small bushes grow from 6 to 9 feet tall, with leaves having 20 or more leaf blades that fan out more than 2 feet. Between August and October, the fruits turn purple black and ripen. In the South, large saw palmetto colonies serve as an important habitat and food source for several animal species. Saw palmetto *(Serenoa repens)* was formerly known by the botanical name *Sabal serrulata*.

Today, wildcrafters pick saw palmetto berries throughout central and southern Florida, southern Georgia, and Alabama. As of 1999, there is no large-scale cultivation of this important medicinal plant. Recent attempts to grow saw palmetto have resulted in bushes that failed to produce berries even after 6 years, according to well-known herbalist Steven Foster. The University of Florida is currently conducting a 3-year agricultural study of saw palmetto's cultivation and harvesting needs. Although the plant does not appear to be in immediate danger of over harvesting, Florida state officials are concerned about the possible effects of over harvesting on indigenous wildlife and ecosystems.[3] In 1998, Florida wildcrafters harvested an estimated 2,000 tons of saw palmetto berries, primarily for export to Europe.[4]

BENEFITS

- Relieves many symptoms of BPH, including difficult urination, urinary frequency (frequent urge to urinate), nocturia (frequent urination during the night), and residual urine (incomplete emptying of the bladder), while strengthening urinary flow
- Improves BPH by counteracting inflammation, muscle spasms, and edema (swelling) of the prostate
- May reduce the need for prostate surgery

SCIENTIFIC SUPPORT

Saw palmetto has been studied in nearly 3,000 men with BPH in more than 18 clinical trials. Sixteen of these studies were double-blinded.[2] Clinical research indicates that saw palmetto is superior to placebo and at least as effective as the drug finasteride (Proscar) in relieving symptoms of BPH. Since treatment of an enlarged prostate is usually an ongoing process, many of the longer-term clinical studies are especially important. Several recent studies demonstrate sustained benefits from saw palmetto use for a period of 14 months to 2.5 years after discontinuation of the therapy.[5] Saw palmetto has been used successfully in combination with nettle root, pumpkinseed, and pygeum in clinical studies lasting up to 1 year.

SPECIFIC STUDIES

Benign Prostatic Hyperplasia: Clinical Study (1996)

A standardized saw palmetto extract (320 mg daily) was just as effective as the drug finasteride (5 mg daily) in reducing symptoms of moderate BPH in a 6-month double-blind randomized study of 1,098 men. In both treatment groups, two-thirds of the participants experienced improvement in frequency, nocturia, urinary hesitancy, volume of residual urine, peak urinary flow, and overall quality of life. Fewer than 2 percent of men in the saw palmetto group experienced mild side effects. The men taking finasteride reported a greater number of negative effects on sexual function, such as impotence, ejaculatory disorders, and decreased libido.[6]

Benign Prostatic Hyperplasia: Another Clinical Study (1996)

In a 3-year multicenter study of 435 men with BPH, the participants experienced a significant reduction in urinary symptoms after taking a standardized saw palmetto extract (320 mg daily). Several symptoms improved, including frequency, nocturia, volume of residual urine, and peak urinary flow. The physicians and patients both rated saw palmetto's effectiveness as "good" or "very good" in 80 percent of cases. There

Tips for Prostate Health

Eating a nutritious diet may be the most powerful step you can take toward good prostate health. Preliminary research suggests that the low rate of prostate problems in many Asian countries is linked to a diet low in saturated fat and refined sugar and high in essential fatty acids, soy foods, and carotene-rich vegetables.[7] See "Soy" and "Flax" for more information.

were minor side effects in just 2 percent of the men.[8]

Benign Prostatic Hyperplasia: Another Clinical Study (1996)

In an uncontrolled 1-year trial involving 42 men with moderate BPH, symptoms improved in 74 percent of those taking 320 mg of standardized saw palmetto extract daily. The participants showed the greatest benefit in three areas: peak urinary flow, frequency, and volume of residual urine. Improvement did not depend on the size of the prostate before or after treatment.[9]

Benign Prostatic Hyperplasia: Clinical Study (1990)

A combination of saw palmetto and pumpkinseed produced statistically significant improvement in BPH symptoms compared with placebo in a randomized, double-blind, placebo-controlled study of 53 men. Subjects took either 160 mg standardized extract composed of equal parts saw palmetto and pumpkinseed (2 tablets three times daily) or placebo. Researchers measured improvement in several objective parameters, including urinary flow rate, voiding time, and residual volume. Participants noted benefits in subjective variables such as difficulty urinating, frequency, and nocturia. No significant side effects were reported.[10]

HOW IT WORKS

Although many theories exist about the causes of prostate enlargement, most researchers now believe that increased levels of dihydrotestosterone (DHT) are the main culprit. As men approach age 50, they begin converting testosterone into DHT, a more potent form of testosterone. DHT is concentrated in the prostate gland, ultimately causing the overproduction of prostate cells, which leads to enlargement.[1]

Finasteride, the most commonly prescribed FDA-approved drug for BPH, helps decrease levels of DHT by inhibiting the enzyme 5-alpha-reductase. Researchers haven't determined exactly how saw palmetto works, but they generally agree that its action is nonhormonal and different from that of finasteride. *In vitro* experiments have shown that saw palmetto does lower DHT levels—

but not at doses that men would normally take. Some researchers believe that saw palmetto may play a more indirect role in decreasing DHT levels, namely, by preventing the hormone from binding to prostate cells.[11]

Many different mechanisms of action have been proposed to explain how saw palmetto alleviates the urinary symptoms of BPH. *In vitro* studies demonstrate that saw palmetto helps reduce inflammation, muscle spasms, and swelling (edema) in the prostate. These actions help decrease the amount of pressure around a man's urethra and bladder, making urination less difficult. The plant's antispasmodic action affects smooth muscle in the prostate and urinary bladder and may be due to an inhibition of calcium influx at the plasma membrane level.[12] Studies show that saw palmetto counteracts inflammation and edema by inhibiting prostaglandins, hormone-like chemicals that cause inflammation.[13] Some researchers believe that saw palmetto works by altering cholesterol metabolism. It is also possible that the plant affects a man's hormone levels by modifying the level of sex-hormone-binding globulin (SHBG).[2]

A recent landmark study showed for the first time that a combination of saw palmetto and nettle root actually helps shrink enlarged prostate tissue. This was the first clinical study to biopsy prostate tissue in men with BPH. The herbal therapy demonstrated the most marked effects on the epithelial tissue of the transition zone (middle layer) of the prostate.[3]

MAJOR CONSTITUENTS

Free fatty acids and sterols (including lauric acid and myristic acid)

SAFETY

Saw palmetto is considered safe for consumption when used appropriately.[14] Most men can successfully use saw palmetto without side effects.

- **Side effects:** There have been some reports of mild stomach upset, which is often resolved by taking the extract with meals.[14,15]
- **Contraindications:** None known.[15] Because many of the symptoms of BPH and prostate cancer are similar, men should consult a physician to get a definitive diagnosis before using saw palmetto. Saw palmetto is not appropriate for symptoms of pain or fever, which may indicate bacterial prostatitis.
- **Drug interactions:** None known.[15]

Note: Saw palmetto does not affect standard blood tests or concentrations of prostate-specific antigen (PSA), so it will not interfere with the blood test for prostate cancer.[16,17] If you are a man over the age of 40, schedule a yearly digital prostate exam to test for prostate enlargement. An annual blood test is also recommended if your family has a history of prostate cancer.

DOSAGE

Saw palmetto can be taken as a capsule, tablet, or tincture. It is much less effective as a tea because the active constituents are not water soluble. Some men experience improvement as quickly as 1 month after beginning therapy with saw palmetto, whereas others require a period of 45 to 90 days. Practitioners generally recommend taking the extract for 4 to 6 months, followed by a checkup to determine whether longer-term use is indicated.

- **Standardized extract:** The dosage used in clinical studies was 160 mg twice a day (total of 320 mg) of standardized extract. Good news for those who forget to take their herbs: A single 320-mg dose of saw palmetto was recently found to be just as effective as a 160-mg dose taken twice a day.[17]
- **Capsules/tablets:** One 585-mg capsule or tablet up to three times a day[18]
- **Tincture (1:2 liquid extract):** 20 to 30 drops up to four times a day[18]

STANDARDIZATION

Saw palmetto is typically standardized to contain 85 to 95 percent fatty acids and sterols.

REFERENCES

1. Murray MT. *Male Sexual Vitality.* Rocklin, CA: Prima Publishing, 1994.
2. Wilt TJ, Ishani A, Stark G, et al. Saw palmetto extracts for treatment of benign prostatic hyperplasia: a systematic review. *Journal of the American Medical Association* 1998; 280(18): 1604–1609.
3. Overmyer M. Saw palmetto shown to shrink prostatic epithelium. *Urology Times* 1999; 27(6): 1,42.
4. Marks LS, Tyler VE. Saw palmetto extract: newest (and oldest) treatment alternative for men with symptomatic benign prostatic hyperplasia. *Urology* 1999; 53: 457–461.
5. Champault G, Bonnard AM, Cauquil J, et al. A double-blind trial of an extract of the plant *Serenoa repens* in benign prostatic hyperplasia. *Actualité Thérapeutique* 1984; 6: 407–410.
6. Carraro JC, Raynaud JP, Koch G, et al. Comparison of phytotherapy (Permixon®) with finasteride in the treatment of benign prostatic hyperplasia: a randomized international study of 1,098 patients. *The Prostate* 1996; 29: 231–240.
7. Wallace E. Natural remedies for the prostate. *Delicious!* September 1995; 60–63.
8. Bach D, Ebeling L. Long-term drug treatment of benign prostatic hyperplasia—results of a prospective 3-year multicenter study using Sabal extract IDS 89. *Phytomedicine* 1996; 3(2): 105–111.
9. Kondas J, Philipp V. *Sabal serrulata* extract (Strogen forte®) in the treatment of symptomatic benign prostatic hyperplasia. *International Urology and Nephrology* 1996; 28: 767–772.
10. Carbin BE, Larsson B, Lindahl O. Treatment of benign prostatic hyperplasia with phytosterols. *British Journal of Urology* 1990; 66: 639–641.
11. Bone K. Saw palmetto—a critical review (parts 1 and 2). *MediHerb Professional Review* 1998; 60 & 61: 1–4.
12. Gutierrez M, Hidalgo A, Cantabrana B. Spasmolytic activity of a lipidic extract from *Sabal serrulata* fruits: further study of the mechanisms underlying this activity. *Planta Medica* 1996; 62: 507–511.
13. Breu W, Hagenlocher M, Redl K, et al. Antiphlogistic activity of an extract from Sabal serrulata fruits prepared by supercritical carbon dioxide: in vitro inhibition of cyclooxygenase and 5-lipoxygenase metabolism [in German]. *Arzneimittel-Forschung* 1992; 42(1): 547–551.
14. McGuffin M, Hobbs C, Upton R, Goldberg A, eds. *American Herbal Products Association Botanical Safety Handbook.* Boca Raton and New York: CRC Press LLC, 1997.
15. Blumenthal M, Busse W, Goldberg A, eds. *The Complete German Commission E Monographs.* Austin, TX: American Botanical Council; Boston: Integrative Medical Communications, 1998.

16. Braeckman J. The extract of *Serenoa repens* in the treatment of benign prostatic hyperplasia: a multicenter open study. *Current Therapeutic Research* 1994; 55(7): 776–785.

17. Braeckman J, Bruhwyler J, Vandekerckhove K, et al. Efficacy and safety of the extract of *Serenoa repens* in the treatment of benign prostatic hyperplasia: therapeutic equivalence between twice and once daily dosage forms. *Phytotherapy Research* 1997; 11: 558–563.

18. Foster S. *101 Medicinal Herbs*. Loveland, Co: Interweave Press, 1998.

Shiitake

Lentinus edodes
Polyporaceae

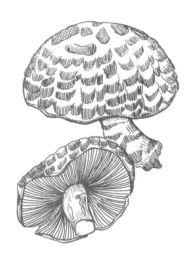

State of Knowledge: Five-Star Rating System

Clinical (human) research	✳
Laboratory research	✳✳✳
History of use/traditional use	✳✳✳✳
Safety record	✳✳✳
International acceptance	✳✳

PART USED: *Fruiting body, mycelium*

PRIMARY USES

- *Immune system support*
- *Cancer (experimental)*
- *Chronic fatigue syndrome (experimental)*
- *HIV (experimental)*
- *High cholesterol (experimental)*
- *Hepatitis and other liver problems (experimental)*

"Fungiphobic." That's how Harvard-trained physician and alternative medicine expert Andrew Weil describes the American public. Until recently, the only mushrooms widely available in U.S. grocery stores were the ubiquitous and rela-tively bland white button mushrooms of the genus *Agaricus*. Across the Pacific, however, Asian cultures have long savored a variety of common and exotic mushrooms, including fragrant and flavorful shiitakes. In traditional Chinese medicine, shiitake and many other fungi have been used to boost immunity for centuries. North American tastes have changed dramatically in the past 10 years, and a much wider variety of mushrooms is appearing in grocery stores. These include portobellos, oyster mushrooms, chanterelles, morels, porcini, maitake, and shiitake.

Often called the "king of mushrooms," shiitake is just one of a number of medicinal mushrooms currently under study at research centers in Germany, the United States, Japan, and China. Shiitake is being used for a wide variety of conditions involving depressed immune function, from frequent colds to cancer. In Japan, physicians prescribe shiitake in two different forms to treat many health conditions, including asthma, hepatitis B, ulcers, high cholesterol, AIDS, kidney inflammation, herpes, and various skin problems. One of these forms of shiitake is called *Lentinus edodes* mycelium (LEM), an extract of the rootlike mass *(mycelium)* that grows underground before the formation of the *fruiting body* that we know as a mushroom. Many shiitake extracts contain both the mycelia and the whole fruiting bodies (stems and caps). In more serious health conditions, physicians give injections of *lentinan,* a polysaccharide from shiitake that is considered one of its main constituents. In Japan, lentinan is one of the eight top-selling drugs for cancer.

Many researchers are now recommending a combination of mushrooms to maximize effects on the immune system. "A complex blend of medicinal fungi can offer a powerful therapeutic punch," says internationally renowned mycologist Paul Stamets, known by some as "Mr. Medicinal Mushroom."[1] Two other mushrooms that hold great therapeutic promise are reishi, or Ling zhi *(Ganoderma lucidum),* and maitake *(Grifola frondosa)*. Because of its reputation as a longevity tonic, reishi (the "mushroom of immortality") is under investigation for its

potential as an anti-aging supplement at the Chinese Academy of Medical Sciences in Beijing. In Japan, the government has officially listed it as an adjunct treatment for cancer. Reishi is also being studied for its effects against arthritis, bronchitis, asthma, acute hepatitis, diabetes, allergies, insomnia, and altitude sickness. In early 1998, American researchers began a phase II pilot study testing the effects of an extract from maitake known as D-fraction in patients with advanced breast and prostate cancers. Maitake is also being administered clinically for uterine fibroids, AIDS, high blood pressure, and weight loss.

HISTORY

Ancient Chinese doctors considered shiitake an essential food and medicine for a long and healthy life. Wu Juei, a Chinese physician from the Ming dynasty (1368 to 1644), claimed that shiitake improved stamina, circulation, and overall good health. For thousands of years, this healing mushroom was also used for arthritis, elevated cholesterol, colds, childhood measles, bronchial inflammation, faintness, dropsy (fluid accumulation in tissues), intestinal worms, smallpox—and even poisoning from toxic mushroom species. Shiitake is prescribed for people of all ages, to protect the young and active from exhaustion and overwork and to rejuvenate older people as they age. With such a long list of impressive applications, it's not surprising that shiitake cultivation also dates back to ancient times.

In the past 10 years, scientists have observed an interesting phenomenon that occurs in shiitake mushrooms after they are harvested. Several studies revealed that when they are placed in direct sunlight for 3 hours a day, their vitamin D content increases by up to five times. The sun's rays also seem to heighten shiitake's sweet flavor and increase the mushroom's amino acid content. This is particularly interesting in light of the mushroom's legendary love for growing in darkness.[2]

INTERNATIONAL STATUS

In Japan, LEM is considered a food supplement, and lentinan is classified as a drug. Both extracts are employed for a variety of conditions characterized by low immune function. Shiitake is not officially approved for use in any European country.

BOTANY

The name *shiitake* comes from the wild mushroom's affinity for growing on fallen Japanese shiia trees. This particular fungus is also fond of other types of broadleaf trees, including chestnut, chinquapin, beech, oak, Japanese alder, sweet gum, maple, walnut, and mulberry. Shiitake mushrooms range in color from light amber to dark brown, with a delicate white overlay. Although they belong to the Polyporaceae family (a name that means "many pores"), shiitakes have gills rather than pores on their undersides. Mycologists now believe that shiitakes and other gilled mushrooms evolved from the more ancient polypores over the millenia. Like most mushrooms, shiitakes have tough cell walls because they contain polysaccharides, the constituents that help strengthen the human immune system.

Shiitakes are native to temperate areas of Japan, China, and other Asian countries, and are not found growing wild in the United States. A related species has been identified in the Costa Rican wilderness. Today, shiitakes are widely cultivated on logs or in sawdust, either indoors or outside. They are Japan's number one agricultural export and are second only to the common table mushroom (*Agaricus bisporus*) in worldwide mushroom production. Shiitake-growing kits are available for fungi fans who desire a plentiful and relatively inexpensive supply in their own homes.

BENEFITS

- May help prevent and treat a variety of conditions associated with lowered immunity by boosting the body's own immune response
- May prolong the survival time of cancer patients by supporting immunity

- May help lower cholesterol levels by increasing the rate at which cholesterol is excreted from the body
- May help normalize liver function in people with hepatitis

SCIENTIFIC SUPPORT

Scientific research on shiitake and other medicinal mushrooms has been conducted primarily in Japan and other Asian countries. Until the 1980s, most of the research was carried out in the laboratory, rather than with human subjects.

Recent clinical studies suggest that lentinan, a polysaccharide from shiitake and one of its main constituents, may be an important adjunct treatment for cancer. In one of the first randomized, controlled, clinical investigations, patients with advanced or recurrent stomach cancer who took lentinan in combination with chemotherapy had longer survival times than those who only had chemotherapy. The results were especially impressive considering the generally poor prognosis and survival time for stomach cancer patients.[3] A more recent trial showed that patients with advanced pancreatic cancer survived longer when lentinan was combined with chemotherapy.[4]

There are still many unanswered questions regarding the use of lentinan in cancer. Much of the research has been done in patients with advanced cancer, but it is possible that lentinan may be even more effective during the beginning stages of tumor development. Scientists still do not know why lentinan is effective against certain types of tumors and not others. According to research, lentinan also strengthens the immune system and prolongs survival times in some individuals but not in others.[4] Efficacy seems to depend, in part, on the dosage and timing of the treatment.[5]

Two preliminary studies of lentinan in people infected with human immunodeficiency virus (HIV) have yielded encouraging results.[6,7] In the first study, lentinan effectively stimulated immunity (as measured by T-cell counts) within 8 weeks in 30 percent of 39 people with HIV.[6] A second randomized placebo-controlled study of 100 HIV-positive people supported these results: Patients who combined lentinan with the drug didanosine experienced a significantly greater increase in immune response than those taking drug therapy alone.[7]

Based on the results of these trials, researchers have recommended testing lentinan in future multi-drug studies in people with HIV. There is a need for alternative AIDS therapies because standard drugs such as zidovudine (commonly known as AZT) and didanosine are very expensive, are associated with serious side effects, and often become less effective over time. Lentinan may be a promising alternative or adjunct treatment because of its overall safety and its potential for raising immunity against both

HIV and opportunistic infections, the cause of death in more than 95 percent of those who die of AIDS-related complications.[8]

Lentinan therapy has also shown promise in the treatment of chronic fatigue syndrome (CFS), a condition marked by long-term fever and fatigue. CFS is still not well understood, but a preliminary study showed that lentinan returned levels of natural killer cells to normal in many of the participants, while improving symptoms such as fatigue.[9]

Shiitake supplements may have some beneficial effects on heart and liver health as well. Several experiments have demonstrated that shiitake (fresh and dried whole mushrooms and an isolated extract of the constituent eritadenine) helps lower cholesterol in animals and humans.[10] Lentinan has also been tested for its effects against hepatitis in at least three clinical trials. In a controlled double-blind study of 72 people with chronic, persistent hepatitis, lentinan improved liver function more effectively than the Chinese herb danshen (Codonopsis pilosula), commonly used in traditional Chinese medicine to treat hepatitis. In two other studies, an extract of Lentinus edodes mycelium (LEM) enhanced liver function in people with chronic hepatitis B.[2]

Until the 1980s, lentinan was administered by injection in most laboratory studies, leading many researchers to believe that it would not be effective when taken orally. More recent evidence shows that oral doses of shiitake are also effective in lowering cholesterol and fighting tumors. This research tested a powdered, dried extract from shiitake fruiting bodies.[5]

SPECIFIC STUDIES

Advanced Pancreatic Cancer: Clinical Study (1997)

A clinical study of 39 patients with advanced pancreatic cancer showed that combining lentinan with chemotherapy significantly prolonged survival in some patients, compared with those who underwent chemotherapy alone. One group of 28 patients received 2 mg of lentinan weekly (injected intravenously) in addition to chemotherapy. The other 11 patients were treated with chemotherapy alone. Researchers performed immunological analyses before and 10 days after administration of lentinan.

Survival time was nearly doubled in 5 people taking lentinan, compared with no change in the chemotherapy group, a result that was statistically significant. The average survival time in people treated with lentinan was 14 months, compared with only 8 months without lentinan. Patients who responded to lentinan demonstrated a 2.5-fold increase in levels of killer T-cells compared with suppressor T-cells (a measure of immune system activity). Positive response was also associated with a decrease in interleukin-6, granulocyte colony-stimulating factor, and prostaglandin E2, factors that are known to lower immune system strength. Researchers concluded that lentinan is a valuable adjunct to chemotherapy in certain patients. The optimal duration of treatment is still unknown.[4]

Stomach Cancer: Clinical Study (1987)

A randomized, controlled study showed that patients with advanced or recurrent stomach cancer had prolonged survival times when they took lentinan in combination with chemotherapy. Patients over 80 years old or with serious complications were not eligible for the study. A total of 77 people were given 2 mg lentinan weekly (injected intravenously), along with the chemotherapeutic agent tegafur (600 mg per day). A second group of 68 people received only tegafur. Investigators analyzed the efficacy of lentinan based on antitumor effects and increased lifespan measured over a 4-year follow-up period.

The response rate for antitumor effects was 16.3 percent in the lentinan group, compared with only 2 percent in the control group, a statistically significant difference. Survival rates at 1, 2, 3, and 4 years among lentinan-treated patients were significantly higher than in the control group. The 2-, 3-, and 4-year survival ratio of the lentinan-treated group was 13.0, 9.5, and 3.8 percent respectively, compared with the typical 0.8 percent stomach cancer survival rate in Japan reported by the investigators. Two patients were free of cancer and alive more than 5 years after the beginning of the study. Side effects associated with lentinan were rare and none were severe enough to warrant discontinuation of treatment. Researchers concluded that lentinan may be beneficial for stomach cancer patients when used in combination with conventional chemotherapies.[3]

HOW IT WORKS

A significant body of research suggests that shiitake can be useful in a variety of conditions associated with lowered immunity. It appears to work by enhancing the body's immune response rather than by directly attacking tumors, viruses, bacteria, and other foreign cells. Its beneficial effects have been attributed mainly to lentinan, a polysaccharide found in the cell walls of shiitake mycelia and in the fruiting bodies. Lentinan appears to strengthen both vital aspects of the immune system: nonspecific immunity, which protects against a wide range of foreign invaders, and specific immunity, which enlists individual antibodies to target specific invaders (antigens).

Anticancer Effects

In a recent clinical study, lentinan prolonged survival times in certain patients with advanced pancreatic cancer by causing a 2.5-fold increase in the ratio of killer T-cells to suppressor T-cells. As part of the specific immune system, killer T-cells are important because they specialize in destroying cancerous and virus-infected cells. Lower levels of suppressor T-cells are desirable in immuno-compromised people, because such cells release chemicals that inactivate the beneficial killer T-cells.[4] Lentinan also activates macrophages (literally, "big eaters"), which engulf foreign particles, making it easier for T-cells to destroy them.[11] In another clinical study of patients with gastric cancer, lentinan significantly increased levels of tumor necrosis factor (a substance that fights tumors) and interleukins 1 and 2, chemicals that stimulate the activity of T-cells and other immune cells.[12]

Anti-HIV Activity

Much of the immune dysfunction associated with AIDS is thought to be due to lowered T-cell and CD4 function. CD4 molecules sit on the membranes of T-cells, helping them bind to and destroy HIV.[8] In a randomized placebo-controlled study of 100 people with HIV, a combination of lentinan and the drug didanosine raised CD4 levels more effectively than drug therapy alone.[7] Standard drugs for the treatment of AIDS raise CD4 levels, but may succeed only temporarily.[8] Lentinan may be more effective at boosting the immune system on a long-term basis. In this trial, lentinan also caused a rise in natural killer (NK) cells, part of the nonspecific immune system. NK cells circulate in the blood and lymph, destroying virus-infected and cancerous cells long before the rest of the immune system is drawn into the battle.[7]

A second clinical trial supported these results. In this study, lentinan raised CD4 levels in 30 percent of people with HIV who had lowered CD4 counts. The mean increase in CD4 cells was from $291/mm3$ to $406/mm3$ after 8 weeks.[6] Studies show that both lentinan and LEM prevent HIV infection of human cells in vitro. Laboratory research also suggests that lentinan potentiates the effects of the AIDS drug zidovudine (AZT) by helping to decrease the rate of viral replication in human blood cell lines.[5]

Antibacterial and Antiviral Activity

Lentinan acts against a variety of viruses and harmful bacteria, mostly due to its effects on the nonspecific immune system. It appears to increase the body's resistance to harmful bacteria by stimulating the activity of complement C3, a chemical that attaches to and ruptures foreign cells. It also stimulates the activity of macrophages, the "big eaters" that help devour invaders. In terms of antiviral activity, lentinan stimulates the production of interferon, a protein that interferes with the ability of viruses to take over uninfected tissue.[5]

Heart Health Benefits

Shiitake's cholesterol-lowering action is due primarily to a compound called eritadenine, which helps increase the rate at which the body excretes blood cholesterol. Dietary fiber present in whole shiitakes may also play a role in this process. Shiitake may also reduce the risk of heart attack by thinning the blood and preventing abnormal clotting (platelet aggregation).[5] Preliminary research suggests that a compound in shiitake known as tyrosinase helps lower blood pressure levels.[2]

MAJOR CONSTITUENTS

Polysaccharides (especially lentinan); eritadenine; tyrosinase

SAFETY

Shiitake is considered safe when used appropriately.[13]

- **Side effects:** Shiitake extract may occasionally cause mild side effects, such as skin rashes or stomach upset. Those who cultivate shiitake mushrooms indoors may develop a respiratory allergy to the spores, a problem that can be partially relieved by wearing a protective mask when tending the fungi.
- **Contraindications:** None known.
- **Drug interactions:** None known.

DOSAGE

Shiitake mushrooms can be found fresh or dried in most grocery stores and are delicious in stir-frys, soups, pilafs, and many other dishes. Shiitake extracts are available in capsule, tablet, and tincture form, often as a combination of the mycelium and whole fruiting body. Some formulas blend shiitake with reishi or maitake mushrooms as well as herbs such as astragalus, Siberian ginseng, and schisandra. According to well-known naturopath Don Brown, vitamin C may help enhance absorption of the complex polysaccharides found in medicinal mushrooms.[14]

For general health maintenance

- **Fresh shiitake mushrooms:** 3 to 4 a day
- **Capsules:** 1 to 5 a day (400 mg each)
- **Tincture:** 1 dropperful two to three times a day

For therapeutic purposes

If you are using shiitake for cancer or other serious health conditions, consult a practitioner to determine the right dosage. According to the scant evidence available from clinical trials, the optimum dosage of LEM may be between 2 and 6 g daily in two or three divided oral doses during the initial stages of AIDS or chronic hepatitis. Once the disease is more stable, the dose may be decreased to around 0.5 to 1 g daily. Lentinan is typically given as an injection either intra-venously or intramuscularly.[2] Currently, lentinan is not available in the United States.

STANDARDIZATION

Standardized shiitake extracts are currently not available. However, LEM extracts may be standardized to 0.3 or 1.5 percent EP-3 (a lignin compound).

REFERENCES

1. Casura LG. "Mr. (Medicinal) Mushroom:" an interview with mycologist Paul Stamets. *Townsend Letter for Doctors and Patients* June 1998: 11–17.
2. Hobbs, C. *Medicinal Mushrooms: An Exploration of Tradition, Healing, and Culture.* Santa Cruz, CA: Botanica Press, 1995.
3. Taguchi T. Clinical efficacy of lentinan on patients with stomach cancer: end point results of a four-year follow-up survey. *Cancer Detection and Prevention* 1987; 1(suppl): 333–345.
4. Matsuoka H, Seo Y, Wakasugi H, et al. Lentinan potentiates immunity and prolongs the survival time of some patients. *Anticancer Research* 1997; 17: 2751–2756.
5. Jong SC, Birmingham JM. Medicinal and Therapeutic Value of the Shiitake Mushroom. *Advances in Applied Microbiology,* Volume 39. New York: Academic Press, 1993.
6. Abrams D, Greco M, Wong R, et al. Results of a phase I/II placebo-controlled dose finding pilot study of lentinan in patients with HIV infection. In: Volume 3 Abstracts, Sixth International Conference on AIDS; June 23–24, 1990; San Francisco, CA.
7. Gordon M, Guralnik M, Kaneko Y, et al. A phase II controlled study of a combination of the immune modulator, lentinan, with didanosine (DDI) in HIV patients with CD4 cells of 200–500/mm3. *Journal of Medicine* 1995; 26: (5,6): 193–207.
8. Berkow R, Fletcher AJ, eds. *The Merck Manual,* 16th ed. Rahway, NJ: Merck Research Laboratories, 1992.
9. Aoki T, Usuda Y, Miyakoshi H, et al. Low natural killer syndrome: clinical and immunological features. *Natural Immunity and Cell Growth Regulation* 1987; 6: 116–128.
10. Jones K. Shiitake: a major medicinal mushroom. *Alternative and Complementary Therapies* February 1998: 53–59.
11. Sakamaki S. Individual diversity of IL-6 generation by human monocytes with lentinan administration. *International Journal of Immunopharmacology* 1993; 15(6): 751–756.
12. Arinaga S, Karimine N, Takamuku K, et al. Enhanced production of interleukin 1 and tumor necrosis factor by peripheral monocytes after lentinan administration in patients with gastric carcinoma. *International Journal of Immunopharmacology* 1992; 14(1): 43–47.
13. McGuffin M, Hobbs C, Upton R, et al., eds. *American Herbal Products Association Botanical Safety Handbook.* Boca Raton, FL: CRC Press, 1997.
14. Brown D. The king lives! Maitake mushroom comes to the United States. *Let's Live* November, 1992; 22–28.

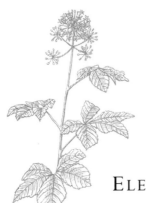

Siberian Ginseng

ELEUTHEROCOCCUS SENTICOSUS
ARALIACEAE

PART USED: *Root, root bark*

PRIMARY USES

- *Energy*
- *Stamina and endurance*
- *Immune system stimulation*

Siberian ginseng is a tonic plant with an ancient reputation for increasing energy levels and enhancing performance and general health. Russian athletes and cosmonauts have used it for decades, and both Chinese and Russian researchers have tested its benefits in numerous clinical and laboratory studies. Ironically, Siberian ginseng is neither Siberian nor ginseng, technically speaking. The plant grows in eastern Russia and northern China, but not in Siberia. And it is not a true ginseng in the genus *Panax,* which contains both Asian ginseng *(Panax ginseng)* and American ginseng *(P. quinquefolius),* although all of these plants are in the Aralia family. Marketers of "real" ginseng tried in vain to banish the common name Siberian ginseng, which has been in use since the 1960s. One botanist suggested "Ussurian thorny pepperbush," which, to nobody's surprise, did not catch on. The name Siberian ginseng stuck, although some refer to the plant as *eleuthero,* and at least one company calls it by its Chinese name, *ciwujia.*

The Chinese have taken the herb for at least 2,000 years to increase longevity and to improve general health, appetite, and memory. A poem by Ye Zhishen from the Qing dynasty includes these lines: "It will keep your virgin face younger/And prolong your life for ever and ever."

There have been more than 1,000 scientific studies on *Eleutherococcus,* most of them Russian investigations dating from the 1960s or earlier. By modern standards, most of these studies cannot be considered compelling, but they do include large populations and cover a variety of different health conditions. Extracts of the root are reported to enhance both physical and mental performance and improve resistance to hot and cold conditions and other environmental stresses. They protect against toxins and boost the immune system, possibly even more than echinacea. The world's leading researcher on the plant was the renowned Russian physician I. I. Brekhman, M.D. He was the first to describe Siberian ginseng as an "adaptogen," a nontoxic substance that has a "nonspecific action" of improving the body's resistance to environmental stress, and a "normalizing" action that can help return body functions to normal, no matter whether above or below normal. By this definition, an herb should be able to lower blood pressure if it is elevated, or raise blood pressure if it is low. The most active and best-studied compounds in Siberian ginseng are called *eleutherosides,* which are similar to the ginsenosides found in *Panax ginseng* in some of their effects.

Siberian ginseng caught the attention of the Russians as an inexpensive and plentiful substitute for ginseng. Today, it is still a popular sports tonic and is favored in Russia by people with occupations that expose them to environmental stresses, such as deep sea divers, mine and mountain rescuers, climbers, explorers, soldiers, pilots, and factory workers.[1]

In spite of the large number of studies already conducted, more definitive research on the performance benefits of Siberian ginseng is still needed. The early experiments produced very impressive results, and some of these studies would be easy and inexpensive to repeat using modern research standards. As an example, in Russian research, telegraph operators had better speed and accuracy when taking Siberian ginseng. This would be an easy experiment to replicate using modern word processing equipment, and one with a potential major impact in the business world.

Eleutherococcus has a strong record of safety research and a long history of use and is backed by intriguing research on a wide range of health-promoting effects. In addition, traditional Chinese and Russian practitioners consider the herb to be appropriate for a wider range of people than *Panax ginseng,* including women and children.

(*Panax ginseng* is traditionally used only by men.)

HISTORY

The first written mention of *ciwujia* (Siberian ginseng) is in the 2,000-year-old *Divine Husbandman's Classic of the Materia Medica,* an ancient Chinese medical text. The Chinese classify the plant as a first-class or superior plant, meaning it is very highly regarded and considered quite safe. Centuries ago it was used in traditional Chinese medicine (TCM) against bronchitis and other respiratory infections and as a general tonic to enhance energy, vitality, and resistance. Russians began studying the plant in the 1950s, and, based on a review completed in 1958, Siberian ginseng was added to the pharmacopoeia of the Soviet Union in 1962.

These early Russian studies focused on performance and resistance, beginning with trials in runners and swimmers. Next, the effects of Siberian ginseng were investigated in people who perform demanding mental work, including telegraph operators and pilots. The effects on human stamina and endurance led to animal experiments that used swimming or rope-climbing tests to compare the effects of different substances that can improve performance. By 1976, an estimated three million Russians were using Siberian ginseng extract.[2]

INTERNATIONAL STATUS

Siberian ginseng is widely used throughout Europe, and is approved by the German Commission E as a "tonic for invigoration and fortification in times of fatigue or debility or declining capacity for work and concentration, also during convalescence." It is in the pharmacopoeias of the Soviet Union and China, and, as with other TCM remedies, those in other Southeastern Asian countries use it as well.

BOTANY

Eleutherococcus senticosus is a hardy, thorny shrub that reaches heights of up to 8 feet. It grows in the brutal climate of the northeastern Chinese province of Manchuria, on the border between China and eastern Russia. The Chinese sometimes refer to it as *Acanthopanax senticosus,* an outdated botanical name. The root of Siberian ginseng is woody and much larger than a *Panax ginseng* root. There are around 30 species in the genus *Eleutherococcus,* mostly prickly trees and shrubs, found in eastern Asia, the Himalayas, and Malaysia. *E. senticosus* usually has several erect spiny stems with light gray or brownish bark, mostly unbranched. Leaves are palmate (palm shaped), similar in appearance to *Panax ginseng* leaves, with five oval leaflets that have serrated margins.

Flowers are in simple round umbels with long stalks. The fruit is a black berry (a drupe). The roots and leaves are used medicinally, and the highest concentrations of eleutherosides occur just before the leaves drop in autumn.

BENEFITS

- Increases resistance to environmental stress
- Enhances physical and mental performance
- Stimulates immune response
- Protects the liver against toxins
- Increases resistance to oxygen deprivation of the heart

SCIENTIFIC SUPPORT

After testing *Eleutherococcus* extract in a "large group of athletes" running a 10-mile race, Dr. Brekhman reported that the runners who took the herb finished the race 5 minutes earlier than the placebo group. His colleague Professor Korobkov conducted trials in 1,500 athletes, confirming that the extract increased endurance and improved reflexes and concentration.[1] Numerous other clinical trials followed, focusing on both physical and mental performance.

Researchers sought to evaluate the effects of Siberian ginseng on people's ability to withstand adverse conditions such as heat and cold, noise, motion sickness, heavy workloads, exercise, and decompression. Several studies involving telegraph operators documented improvements in speed and accuracy. One such experiment also showed that Siberian ginseng enhanced performance in the presence of increased background noise. After taking Siberian ginseng, people from many walks of life experienced benefits: Skiers had better resistance to oxygen deprivation (hypoxemia), and work performance improved in proofreaders, sailors, deep sea divers, office workers, and other healthy individuals.[2]

Russian researchers also tested the effects of Siberian ginseng on people with various illnesses. Dozens of Russian studies performed between 1960 and 1985 were briefly summarized in a review by pharmacognosist Norman Farnsworth, Ph.D., and several of his colleagues from the University of Illinois at Chicago. One such study of 45 patients with atherosclerosis (hardening and narrowing of the arteries) reported that chest pains disappeared, blood pressure dropped, and general well-being increased after treatment with *Eleutherococcus*. Similarly, in 47 patients with kidney disease, kidney function increased, as measured by kidney capacity and excretion of phenol red. Two studies of unreported size showed that Siberian ginseng raised blood pressure in people with hypotension (low blood pressure) and lowered blood pressure in those with hypertension (high blood pressure). In 48 miners with pneumoconiosis, an inflammation of the lungs commonly caused by dust inhalation, the extract reportedly increased lung capacity.[2] Some of Siberian ginseng's adaptogenic benefits may be attributed to its ability to stimulate immune function. According to a placebo-controlled German study, Siberian ginseng caused a "drastic increase" in the number of immune cells in healthy volunteers who took 10 ml Siberian ginseng extract three times a day. In particular, the researchers observed a highly significant increase in the total number of lymphocytes and helper T-cells, as well as increased T-cell activation. Results were measured using flow-cell cytometry, a technique which allows researchers to analyze the characteristics of individual cells in whole blood.[3]

Laboratory experiments in animals demonstrated that Siberian ginseng helped protect the liver against a variety of toxins, such as the pesticides parathion and chlorofos and drugs such as cardiac glycosides, chemotherapy drugs, and others. These tests also documented protective effects against doxorubicin, Thiotepa, 6-mercaptopurine, cyclophosphamide, and sarcolysin, most of which are antitumor drugs. According to the researchers, oral doses of Siberian ginseng extract decreased the toxicity of the drugs and also enhanced their effectiveness. Oral use also protected mice from x-ray damage.[2]

Animal tests bolstered the evidence from human trials in the areas of performance enhancement and stress resistance. Mice could swim longer in cold water, climb ropes for a longer duration before exhaustion, and withstand stress without developing ulcers and with less increase in adrenal weight (a standard measure of stress reaction).[2]

SPECIFIC STUDIES

Exercise Performance: Clinical Study (1986)

In an 8-day study designed to assess the effects of Siberian ginseng on physical working capacity, six healthy adolescent baseball players were tested in a single-blind crossover study comparing the effects of Siberian ginseng extract, placebo, and no treatment. The subjects took 2 ml of Siberian ginseng extract or placebo twice daily. They exercised on an ergometer bicycle that recorded various body function rates, which the investigators used to measure maximum work capacity after treatment. Compared with no treatment, the Siberian ginseng extract was associated with increased maximal oxygen uptake, oxygen pulse, and total work as well as extended time to exhaustion, all to a statistically significant degree. The latter two measurements were also significantly better in the group taking Siberian ginseng than in those taking placebo. A dose of 1 ml of the extract used in the study (as listed in the official Soviet pharmacopoeia) contained 0.53 mg eleutheroside B and 0.12 mg eleutheroside D.[4]

Exercise Performance: Clinical Study (1996)

A double-blind placebo-controlled, 8-week trial in 20 highly trained distance runners found no statistically significant improvements in heart rate, oxygen consumption, or other measures during 10-kilometer races. The athletes took 3.4 ml of Siberian ginseng alcohol extract daily for 6 weeks. These results do not support an ergogenic effect (an ability to increase physical work output) of Siberian ginseng, at least in highly trained athletes.[5]

Health Maintenance: Clinical Study (1977)

Siberian ginseng extract reduced the incidence of illness by 50 percent in 1,000 metallurgical factory employees laboring under harsh climatic and work conditions near the Arctic Circle. Results with Siberian ginseng were compared with those of a control group of workers who did not take the herb but had similar working conditions. Those in the Siberian ginseng group took 4 ml of an alcohol-based extract of *Eleutherococcus* daily every other month for 12 months, except for July and August. Morbidity, or illness,

was 50 percent less in the Siberian ginseng group, and lost workdays were reduced by 40 percent. Ninety-five percent of the workers who took Siberian ginseng reported subjective improvements in overall health.[6]

Mental Performance: Clinical Study (1966)

The radiotelegraph operators who took Siberian ginseng extract in this study substantially improved in typing speed and accuracy. For the placebo-controlled study, 39 radiotelegraph operators took either 2 ml *Eleutherococcus* extract or 2 ml of placebo daily for 1 month. Testing took place before dosing began, after 14 days, and again after 30 days. At the 14-day mark, typing speed in subjects taking Siberian ginseng had increased by 7.7 percent compared with 2.3 percent in the control group. Typing accuracy increased by 23.1 percent, compared with a decrease in the control group of 20.8 percent. By the 30-day mark, the group using Siberian ginseng made only half as many mistakes compared with the initial test, whereas the control group was virtually unchanged in accuracy.[7]

HOW IT WORKS

Little is known about how *Eleutherococcus* works. It appears to increase resistance to stress partly by reducing the adrenal cortex response to stress (the alarm phase reaction). Research on isolated constituents has concentrated mostly on the eleutherosides, which are considered the most active compounds in Siberian ginseng. There are at least 15 eleutheroside compounds, most of them unrelated.

MAJOR CONSTITUENTS

Eleutherosides (including eleutherosides B and D), senticosides, vitamin E, beta-carotene, polysaccharides

SAFETY

Siberian ginseng has been subjected to the most modern types of safety testing. It has virtually no acute toxicity, meaning overdose is virtually impossible (the extrapolated toxic dose for a 60-kilogram or 132-pound human would be over 1,800 grams of powdered dry root—around 4 pounds). No toxic effects have been observed in long-term animal feeding studies. It has also been shown to be harmless to pregnant animals and their offspring.[2] The human history of use is also uneventful, despite long-term and widespread use. The extract has been administered in clinical trials involving over 6,000 people, with no serious adverse reactions reported.

- **Side effects:** Side effects were very uncommon in the Russian studies, and included only rare cases of insomnia, headaches, and elevated blood pressure.[2]
- **Contraindications:** Germany's Commission E recommends against use in those with high blood pressure, possibly based on recommendations from two older Russian studies.[8] However, there is also research indicating that eleutherosides lower blood pressure.[9]
- **Drug interactions:** None known.

DOSAGE

- **Extract:** 2 to 12 ml a day of 33 percent ethanol extract
- **Whole plant:** 2 to 8 g powdered root

STANDARDIZATION

Most research has been done on an unstandardized 33 percent ethanol extract. Some extracts are standardized to total eleutheroside content or to eleutherosides B, D, and E, but research has not yet determined the optimal levels of these constituents.

REFERENCES

1. Fulder, S. The drug that builds Russians. *New Scientist* August 21, 1980; 576–579.

2. Farnsworth NR, Kinghorn AD, Soejarto DD, et al. Siberian ginseng (*Eleutherococcus senticosus*): current status as an adaptogen. In: Wagner H, Hikino H, Farnsworth NR, eds. *Economic and Medicinal Plant Research.* Vol. 1. London: Academic Press, 1985: 155–215.

3. Bohn B, Nebe CT, Birr C. Flow-cytometric studies with Eleutherococcus senticosus extract as an immunomodulatory agent. *Arzneimittel-Forschung* 1987; 37(10): 1193–1196.

4. Asano K, Takahashi T, Miyashita M. Effect of *Eleutherococcus senticosus* extract on human physical working capacity. *Planta Medica* 1986; June (3): 175–177.

5. Dowling EA, Redondo DR, Branch JD, et al. Effect of *Eleutherococcus senticosus* on submaximal and maximal exercise perfor- mance. *Medicine and Science in Sports and Exercise* 1996; 28(4): 482–489.

6. Gagarin IA. Prophylaxis of *Eleutherococcus* on patients in Zanolajpyaj [in Russian]. *Adaptation and Adaptogens* 1977; 2: 128.

7. Baburin EF. The effect of *Eleutherococcus* on the results of work and on auditory sensitivity in radiotelegraphers [in Russian]. *Lek Sredstva Dal'nego Vostoka* 1966; 7: 179–184.

8. Blumenthal M, Busse W, Goldberg A, et al., eds. *The Complete German Commission E Monographs.* Austin, TX: The American Botanical Council; Boston: Integrative Medical Communications, 1998.

9. McGuffin M, Hobbs C, Upton R, et al., eds. *American Herbal Products Association Botanical Safety Handbook.* Boca Raton, FL: CRC Press, 1997.

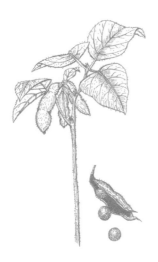

Soy

GLYCINE MAX
FABACEAE

State of Knowledge: Five-Star Rating System

Clinical (human) research	✶✶
Laboratory research	✶✶✶✶
History of use/traditional use	✶✶✶✶
Safety record	✶✶✶
International acceptance	✶✶✶

PART USED: *Seed (bean)*
PRIMARY USES

- *High cholesterol*
- *Menopause (experimental)*
- *Protection against certain cancers (experimental)*
- *Osteoporosis prevention (experimental)*

For at least 5,000 years, the Chinese have called soybeans *ta-tou*, meaning "greater bean." Today this name seems especially appropriate in light of research showing that soy can reduce cholesterol levels. Even the U.S. Food and Drug Administration (FDA) is impressed with soy's potential for improving heart health. In 1999, the government agency approved a new rule that would allow manufacturers to proclaim the cardiovascular benefits of any food containing at least 6.25 grams of soy protein. Although research is still in preliminary stages, there is also scientific evidence that soy may ease menopause symptoms and protect against the development of osteoporosis and certain cancers. Numerous population studies confirm that Asians, who have long known the health secrets of soybeans, have much lower rates of heart disease, menopause-related hot flashes, osteoporosis, and a range of cancers.

What makes soy so special? Of all the legumes, it is highest in isoflavones (also called phytoestrogens) such as genistein and daidzein, compounds with well-researched health benefits. Soybeans also pack in 38 percent protein, which has been shown to help lower cholesterol levels when eaten in place of animal protein. In Asia, the average person consumes 25 to 45 mg of isoflavones daily, primarily derived from soy, compared with just 1 to 3 mg a day in the United States. In Japan, isoflavone intake often reaches 200 mg daily.

Fortunately, many Americans are beginning to see soybeans as more than just bland blocks of tofu. In 1996, sales of all soy foods were expected to top two billion dollars in the United States. Sales of soymilk alone are growing by nearly 40 percent annually.[1] Natural food stores and supermarkets now carry a wide variety of soy products, from chocolate soymilk and barbecued tempeh burgers to Thai peanut tofu and soy sausages. Soy isoflavones are also available in capsule form and in some supplements for bone health. In general, you will find lower amounts of isoflavones in processed soy foods containing soy protein isolate and concentrate, although such foods are usually high in soy protein. These foods include many brands of veggie burgers, meatless dinner entrees, chicken-free nuggets, soy "ice creams," and energy bars.

Tradition still holds a place in the world of soy, however. According to research, fermented soy, present in the ancient foods tempeh and miso, contain a more easily ab-

sorbed form of isoflavone than those found in nonfermented products.[2,3] Interestingly, the isoflavones in opened containers of soymilk and tofu appear to change to this more desirable form as they sit in the refrigerator. At least one company has begun offering a fermented soy supplement in tablet form. Because tempeh and miso are whole foods made from the entire soybean, they also contain high levels of dietary fiber, protein, and a whole range of health-enhancing components—some known and others perhaps still to be discovered.

HISTORY

Before soybeans were a food for people, they were planted on fallow land as a valuable food for the soil. Like other members of the pea family (Fabaceae), soybean plants help turn free nitrogen into a useable form, making them excellent soil builders. The Chinese didn't begin eating soybeans until they discovered fermentation techniques sometime during the Chou dynasty (1134 to 246 B.C.). This natural process causes a chemical change in the soybean that creates more easily digested foods such as tempeh, miso, and tamari soy sauce. From that time on, soy was considered one of the five sacred grains, along with barley, wheat, millet, and rice. Soy was also affectionately known as the "cow of China," because it served as a valuable protein source in a mostly rice-based diet. During the second century B.C., the Chinese added tofu to their repertoire, and from there, soy foods spread to other parts of Asia, including Japan and Indonesia.

In traditional Chinese medicine (TCM), soy is valued for treating fevers, headaches, chest distention, and hyperactivity, and as a tonic for the lungs and stomach. In ancient Chinese medical texts, black soybeans were often favored over the more familiar yellow ones. Asian cultures have also traditionally used soybean straw to manufacture brown paper, an intriguing idea that deserves a closer look as many countries move to preserve the earth's remaining forests.

Europeans discovered soy during the 1700s, but soybeans did not arrive in the United States until the influx of Chinese immigrants began in the early nineteenth century. Large-scale American cultivation started during the Second World War, and today midwestern growers produce 49 percent of the world's supply of soybeans. Unfortunately, more than half of the U.S. soybean crop is exported. The rest is used mainly as livestock feed or in the manufacture of soy oil, margarine, shortening, and industrial products such as paint and leather finishes.

INTERNATIONAL STATUS

Soy lecithin (the phospholipid portion of the soybean) is approved by Germany's Commission E for treating moderate disturbances of fat metabolism, especially cases of high cholesterol that are not responsive solely to dietary or exercise-related measures.

Is Your Veggie Burger Genetically Engineered?

Soy's many health benefits are becoming more well known at the same time that the controversy about genetically engineered (GE) foods is heating up worldwide. Currently soybeans are one of the leading GE crops. To date, no safety studies have been conducted to determine the long-term effects of these foods on human health or the environment. In many European and Asian countries, consumers have vociferously rejected GE foods and have won legislation requiring mandatory labeling. Awareness is growing more slowly in the United States. As of 1999, American farms grew roughly half of the world's supply of soybeans, of which nearly 50 percent are GE.[5] Morover, it is estimated that 60 percent of processed foods in the US now contain genetically modified organisms (GMOs) from soy, corn, and more than 50 other plants.[6] Unfortunately, even certified organic foods may contain GMOs, according to the Organic Trade Association (OTA). Although OTA standards forbid the use of genetically engineered seed stock by organic growers, this standard is not routinely enforced. In addition, GE crops can cross-pollinate with fields of non-GE crops, including those that are being grown organically.

BOTANY

Native to southeastern Asia, soy is an annual, subtropical plant that favors shady, moist climates. It has also been successfully cultivated in temperate regions up to latitudes of 52° North. Soy grows from 1 to 5 feet tall and is covered with short, fine hairs from its stem to its bean pods. The clusters of three to five pods contain two to four yellow-to-brownish colored beans per pod.

Today, farmers cultivate more than 2,500 different varieties of soybeans that vary in size, shape, color, and isoflavone content depending on soil and climate. Soybeans are planted in late spring and harvested from October to November. Much more earth-friendly than beef, soy cultivation yields 25 percent more protein per acre, while also helping to save precious water resources.[4] The plant's botanical name, *Glycine*, comes from the Greek word *glykys*, meaning "sweet."

BENEFITS

- Helps lower total cholesterol and low-density lipoprotein (LDL) cholesterol levels
- Provides a safe and natural source of estrogen-like compounds during menopause (experimental)
- May help protect against certain types of cancer (experimental)
- May help maintain optimal bone mass into old age (experimental)

SCIENTIFIC SUPPORT

Of all the health claims made for soy, its ability to lower cholesterol is backed by the most scientific evidence. Based on more than 40 clinical studies, researchers have concluded that soy protein significantly lowers harmful low-density lipoprotein (LDL) and total cholesterol levels. Studies have demonstrated decreases of up to 20 percent in people with the highest cholesterol levels.[7] Many studies have also shown a slight rise in healthful levels of high-density lipoprotein (HDL) cholesterol, although these changes were not statistically significant. At least 25 grams of soy protein are needed to produce therapeutic effects, and the greatest benefits result when soy is consumed as part of a healthful diet low in saturated fat and cholesterol. Not surprisingly, vegetarians and those with normal cholesterol levels had less impressive declines in cholesterol levels in studies.

Clinical research on soy's ability to reduce hot flashes during menopause is also promising.[8] Soy may provide additional benefits during and after menopause by helping to protect against heart disease, in some cases as effectively as synthetic hormone replacement therapy.[9] Although research on soy and osteoporosis is still in its early stages, one clinical trial showed that 66 postmenopausal women consuming a diet high in soy isoflavones had significant increases in bone mineral content and density in their lumbar spines after 6 months, compared with a control group.[10] This is supported by an animal study which showed that soy helps prevent bone loss associated with estrogen deficiency.[11] Other areas of current research include a potential role for soy in treating diabetes, kidney disease, and autoimmune diseases. Although the evidence for soy's cancer-protective effects comes mostly from population studies and laboratory trials, the results have generated excitement. Currently, researchers are also exploring the possibility of combining genistein with anticancer drugs in order to reduce their dosage and toxicity.[12,13]

of isolated soy protein powder daily (containing 76 mg of isoflavonoids, including 40 mg genistein and 28 mg daidzein), whereas the placebo group took 60 g of casein (an animal protein) without isoflavones. Treatment efficacy was assessed using the Kupperman index of menopausal symptoms, and patient diaries. The soy group experienced beneficial results within 4 weeks, and maximum benefits at 12 weeks. Gastrointestinal complaints were the main side effect in both groups. A total of 25 women dropped out of the study, 11 in the soy group and 14 in the placebo group. The researchers noted that these withdrawals were due not only to side effects but also to difficulties with ingesting glasses of "sticky powder." They believe that future, longer-term studies on the health-enhancing effects of soy must employ more "user-friendly" dosage forms to enhance patient compliance.[8]

SPECIFIC STUDIES

Menopause: Clinical Study (1998)

An Italian double-blind study involving 104 postmenopausal women found that daily consumption of 60 g of soy protein led to a 45 percent reduction in moderate to severe hot flashes over a 12-week period. In contrast, those taking placebo experienced a 30 percent reduction in hot flashes. During the study, women were randomly divided into two treatment groups. One group took 60 g

Cholesterol: Meta-analysis (1995)

A meta-analysis of 29 placebo-controlled studies showed that people who consumed 31 to 47 g of isolated soy protein or textured soy protein daily had a statistically significant decrease in total blood cholesterol levels (9 percent), LDL cholesterol (13 percent), and triglycerides (11 percent). People who started the trial with cholesterol levels higher than 335 mg/dl at baseline had the largest drops in total cholesterol and LDL levels, with reductions up to 20 percent.

Researchers concluded that replacing animal protein with soy protein can have a significant effect on high cholesterol levels. They also noted a 2.4 percent increase in healthful HDL cholesterol, though this change was not statistically significant. In most of the studies, people in both the soy and control groups consumed similar amounts of total fat and saturated fat.[7]

Breast Cancer: Case-Control Study (1997)

A case-control study conducted in Australia suggested that the risk of breast cancer is substantially less among women who have a high intake of isoflavones. Researchers compared 144 women with newly diagnosed early-stage breast cancer with 144 women without breast cancer who were matched for age and area of residence. Results were measured by means of questionnaires and urine samples, which were tested for levels of the isoflavones daidzein, genistein, and equol, as well as the lignans enterodiol, enterolactone, and matairesinol. The researchers tabulated the risk factors after adjusting for age at first menstruation, number of pregnancies, alcohol intake, and total fat intake. Most of the isoflavones listed previously, including those found in soy, were associated with a reduced risk of breast cancer. However, intake of the isoflavone equol (formed during metabolism of the soy isoflavone daidzein) and the lignan enterolactone (found primarily in flaxseed) was

linked to the greatest reduction of risk. Due to difficulties with the genistein assay, researchers were unfortunately unable to measure the association between this important isoflavone and breast cancer risk reduction.[14]

HOW IT WORKS

Most of the current research on soy has focused on the isoflavone consitutents genistein and daidzein. However, it is more likely that a whole range of constituents work together to produce soy's many health benefits. According to Stephen Barnes, Ph.D., a top soy researcher, "Although the isoflavones are one of the most promising of these agents, the role of interactions between the components of the soy bean are largely unexplored."[15]

Effects on Heart Health

Researchers haven't determined exactly how soy helps lower cholesterol, but they now believe that several components work together, including protein, isoflavones, and other potentially important constituents.[16] Attempts at focusing on isolated constituents have not provided a satisfactory explanation for soy's cholesterol-lowering ability. For example, in several studies with monkeys, researchers attempted to show that removal of the isoflavones from soy would eliminate its benefits on blood cholesterol levels.

However, the studies were flawed by the use of an alcohol extraction method to remove the isoflavones, a process that also eliminates other potential cholesterol-lowering constituents, including sterols and saponins.[17]

Because several plant constituents may be involved, it is likely that soy lowers blood cholesterol levels in several different ways. According to *in vitro* studies, genistein's antioxidant properties help prevent the harmful oxidation of LDL cholesterol, a significant factor in the development of atherosclerosis.[18] Some researchers also believe that genistein works by up-regulating (stimulating the activity of) LDL receptors so that the body eliminates more LDL cholesterol.[19] This theory is supported by a study of 12 people with severely elevated cholesterol levels. Researchers found that consumption of soy protein over a 4-week period led to an eightfold increase in the participants' ability to break down LDL cholesterol, compared with those who ate a low-fat animal protein diet. In this case, the protein component of soy was credited with the cholesterol-lowering benefits, rather than isoflavones.[20]

Another plausible theory is that soy isoflavones lower levels of lipoprotein(a) [Lp(a)], a cholesterol-carrying particle in the blood that is structurally similar to LDL cholesterol. Lp(a) is a more recently discovered risk factor for heart disease, and one that does not respond to standard dietary, lifestyle, or pharmacological approaches.

The only treatment that has been found to lower Lp(a) is estrogen therapy, an approach that carries serious health risks of its own. Researchers propose that isoflavones lower Lp(a) levels more safely than synthetic estrogen because of their structural similarity and ability to bind to estrogen receptors in the body. Further investigations are needed in this area.[17] *In vitro* evidence also suggests that the isoflavone genistein prevents the development of atherosclerotic plaque in the arteries by preventing the formation of abnormal blood clots (thrombi). Further studies are now needed to determine the therapeutic effects in humans.[21] In addition, some research suggests that soy protein lowers cholesterol by increasing blood levels of the hormone thyroxine.[22] Soy intake may also affect levels of insulin, glucagon and, in some cases, thyroid-stimulating hormone. These hormones are all known to be involved in cholesterol metabolism.[16]

Effects During Menopause

In China and Singapore, only 14 percent of women experience hot flashes during menopause, compared with 70 to 80 percent in North America and Europe.[23] Menopausal women in Asia also experience fewer related problems, such as cardiovascular disease and osteoporosis. Scientists now believe that these cultural differences may be explained, at least in part, by differences in soy intake. When estrogen levels are low, research shows that the soy isoflavones genistein and daidzein bind to estrogen receptors in the body. It is likely that this accounts for many of soy's effects on menopause-related problems.[24] In a recent laboratory study, researchers tested 150 herbs and found that soy was one of the top seven estrogen receptor-binding plants, along with red clover, licorice, hops, thyme, turmeric, and verbena.[25]

Currently, there is no evidence to suggest that soy's isoflavone content increases the risk of developing estrogen-dependent cancers. Researchers believe that isoflavones are safer than synthetic hormone replacement therapy (HRT) because they are 1,000 times weaker in action than estrogen.[25] Studies show that isoflavones bind to estrogen receptors but do not fully stimulate their nuclei, suggesting that their action is both milder and safer.[26]

Cancer Prevention

Although evidence for soy's anticancer effects is limited to epidemiological (population) and laboratory studies, the research is promising. In Asian countries, the risk of developing cancer is much lower than in Western nations. Migration studies consistently show that when Asian people move to the United States and adopt a standard American diet, they lose their protection against many forms of cancer. As a result, researchers do not believe that genetics account for the cultural differences. Although many dietary habits may play a role, including lower fat consumption, researchers believe that high intake of soy is one of the most important factors.[24]

In vitro (test tube) studies indicate that soy foods work through several mechanisms to protect against cancer. Several studies show that genistein, one of soy's major constituents, has strong antioxidant properties. This could give soy the ability to fight cancer by neutralizing free radicals, unstable molecules that damage DNA, the body's genetic material.[27,28] There is evidence that genistein directly interferes with a tumor's ability to grow by blocking the formation of new blood vessels (angiogenesis), thereby interfering with the supply of oxygen and nutrients to the tumor.[29] Genistein may also prevent the growth of tumors by stimulating apoptosis, a process that causes diseased cells to die.[30] Additional research suggests that genistein inhibits enzyme systems known as protein tyrosine kinases and DNA topoisomerases which are associated with cancer growth.[30,31]

Researchers are currently experimenting with combinations of genistein and standard anticancer drugs in an effort to reduce drug toxicity. In one laboratory experiment, genistein helped prevent cancer cell growth in three human breast cancer cell lines, and demonstrated even greater effects in combination with the drug Adriamycin (doxorubicin).[12] A second study showed that genistein and the drug tiazofurin caused a 5.9-fold decrease in cancer cell growth (proliferation) and a similar increase in the percentage of differentiating cells, a measure of the cells' ability to act like "normal" cells. By comparison, when genistein was used separately it produced only a 1.1-fold increase in the percentage of differentiating cells, and tiazofurin alone produced a 2.8-fold increase.[13] The results of these preliminary studies suggest that genistein may serve as an adjunct treatment against cancer.

BREAST CANCER

Asian women who consume a traditional diet have a four- to sixfold lower risk of developing breast cancer than Western women. Moreover, when breast cancer does occur, the tumors tend to be less serious and more responsive to treatment. Many dietary factors may be responsible for this, including a high intake of soy foods. This theory is supported by results from animal models of breast cancer and human cell culture studies, showing that genistein has anticarcinogenic activity.[24]

In spite of evidence from epidemiological and laboratory studies, researchers haven't determined exactly how soy helps protect against breast cancer. Some scientists have proposed that soy isoflavones act as estrogen antagonists, protecting against more harmful forms of estrogen by competing with them at receptor sites. This would give soy an action similar to that of Tamoxifen, a drug that fights breast cancer by interfering with estrogen binding at receptor sites. However, current evidence suggests that this may not be the way soy works.[24]

It is likely that genistein and other constituents from soy protect against breast cancer in different ways, depending on when they are administered. For example, consumption of soy foods before puberty accelerates the maturation rate of the mammary glands, according to recent research by Coral Lamartiniere, Ph.D. and colleagues. This is desirable because the breasts are more susceptible to carcinogens in the earlier stages of maturation. More specifically, genistein stimulated the terminal end buds (which are more susceptible to cancer) to mature into lobules (which are less susceptible), a process known as gland differentiation. Although this study was conducted in mice, the maturation of breast tissue is similar in human females.[32] As outlined previously, soy may work to protect against breast cancer in several different ways during other stages of the life cycle.

PROSTATE CANCER

Recent evidence suggests that soy plays a major role in protecting Asian men against prostate cancer. According to the American Cancer Society, Japanese men have one-fourth the rate of death from prostate cancer of American men. A 20-year study of 8,000 men of Japanese ancestry living in Hawaii showed that low intake of tofu (once or less per week) increased the likelihood of developing prostate cancer threefold compared with those who ate tofu more regularly. Many dietary factors were measured in this study, but researchers concluded that tofu intake was the most protective factor.[33]

Despite a low rate of prostate cancer, Asian and American men have a similar incidence of latent cancerous lesions. This has led researchers to believe that soy protects against prostate cancer during the promotional phase, when cancer growth is stimulated.[15,34] Although several constituents may be involved, the isoflavones genistein and daidzein appear to be especially important. Studies show that isoflavones help prevent the formation of a type of testosterone called dihydrotestosterone (DHT), which has been linked to benign prostate enlargement and prostate cancer.[33,35] As outlined above, soy may help protect against prostate cancer in several additional ways.

COLON CANCER

Population studies in Japan link high soy intake to a much lower rate of colon cancer. Phytosterols in soy may play a key protective role because they pass through the small intestine unabsorbed, exerting their anticancer effects in the colon.[36] In laboratory experiments, saponins from soy reduced the incidence of aberrant crypt foci, an important indicator of colon cancer. Researchers believe that saponins exert their effects during the initiation phase of cancer development, working through several mechanisms. These include preventing cholesterol oxidation in the colon, reducing the formation of secondary bile products, scavenging free radicals, and stimulating overall immune

function. Like phytosterols, saponins are broken down by friendly bacteria (acidophilus and others) in the large intestine.[37]

Osteoporosis and Bone Health

Lower levels of estrogen increase a woman's risk of developing osteoporosis during and after menopause. While synthetic estrogen is often prescribed to lower this risk, estrogen therapy is associated with serious dangers of its own, including an increased risk of breast and endometrial cancers. According to population studies, the rate of hip fracture in Hong Kong is one-third that of the United States, a fact that researchers attribute mainly to a high intake of soy foods.[17]

Although research is still preliminary, several animal studies suggest that soy may help prevent bone loss caused by estrogen deficiency. One study in animals with experimentally induced menopause showed that soy protein was effective in preventing bone loss in the fourth lumbar vertebra and somewhat effective in the right femur.[11] In a more recent study, the same research team tested the ability of soy to *reverse* bone loss caused by estrogen deficiency. Although soy was somewhat effective in reversing femoral bone-density loss, the overall results of the study were disappointing. Researchers concluded that it is easier to prevent osteoporosis than to reverse it. However, they also noted that the soy product used in this study was more than one year old, so low potency may have affected the results.[38]

Two studies attributed soy's effects on bone health to isoflavones, including a clinical study in postmenopausal women. This study found that a diet of soy protein with a high concentration of isoflavones significantly improved bone mineral density and content in the lumbar spine, compared with a soy diet lower in isoflavones and a diet of non-fat dry milk without isoflavones.[10,39]

Soy's effects on bone health may also be due to its protein content. Currently, over-consumption of animal protein is thought to be a major contributing factor to the high rate of osteoporosis in Western countries. Researchers found that consumption of soy protein leads to a lower rate of calcium excretion than protein from animal sources. Soy protein may be more beneficial because it is lower in sulfur amino acids than animal protein.[11] It is also theorized that soy protein supports bone health by stimulating the production of growth hormone, which in turn stimulates bone formation.[38]

MAJOR CONSTITUENTS

Isoflavones (genistein and daidzein), saponins, phytosterols, protein

SAFETY

Soybeans have a long history of use as a food and are generally recognized as safe (GRAS) by the U.S. Food and Drug Administration.

- **Side effects:** The most common side effects reported in clinical studies were bloating, nausea, and constipation. These complaints were attributed to the form of soy used in many of these studies (soy protein powder), which was difficult to metabolize. Although some people have soy allergies, most of those who consume soy foods such as tempeh and tofu experience no side effects.
- **Contraindications:** Do not regularly eat raw soybeans, soy flour, or protein powder made from raw, unroasted, or unfermented beans, because they can damage the pancreas over time (see Safety Issues with Raw Soybeans).[40,41]
- **Drug interactions:** None known.

Safety Issues with Raw Soybeans

For years, soy skeptics have been discussing two potentially harmful components in soybeans that may interfere with protein digestion and mineral absorption. Raw soybeans contain trypsin inhibitors, compounds that interfere with the metabolism of protein by the pancreatic enzyme trypsin. This can potentially damage the pancreas over time. They also contain high levels of phytates, which bind with minerals such as iron and zinc and prevent their absorption by the body. In 1998, the FDA declared that these problems are not an issue for any soy product that has been subjected to heat through cooking.[42] This includes nearly all soy foods, with the exception of products like un-toasted soy flour. These questionable sub-stances are almost completely eliminated from traditional soy foods like tempeh and miso during the fermentation process.

What's more, some researchers are now finding that the small amounts of trypsin in-hibitors left behind after cooking may even have protective effects against cancer and heart disease.[43–45] Likewise, low levels of phytates can act as powerful antioxidants by binding harmful levels of unbound iron in the intestines.[46] A study conducted by the U.S. Department of Agriculture found no difference in levels of zinc and iron absorp-tion in families eating beef extended with soy protein compared with those eating plain beef.[40]

DOSAGE

The following estimated dosages come from clinical studies. See table 1 for the amounts of isoflavones and soy protein found in vari-ous soy foods.

- **Cholesterol regulation:** 25 g or more of soy protein a day
- **Menopause:** 50 to 75 mg isoflavones a day
- **Osteoporosis prevention:** 55 to 90 mg isoflavones a day

STANDARDIZATION

Many soy foods now contain standardized levels of isoflavones and/or soy protein in each serving. Check the labels on soymilk, tofu, tempeh, and other prepared soy prod-ucts for this information.

Table 1
Isoflavone and Protein Content of Common Soy Foods*

SOY FOOD	ISOFLAVONES (MG)	PROTEIN (G)
Tempeh (¹/₂ cup)	60	18
Miso (¹/₃ cup)	—	12
Firm tofu (¹/₂ cup)	38	14
Soymilk (1 cup)	20	9
Roasted soynuts (¹/₂ cup)	167	—
Toasted soy flour (¹/₂ cup)	88	16
Soy protein concentrate (4 oz)	—	58
Soy protein isolate (4 oz)	—	80

*Dashes signify that no information was available.

Note: Keep in mind that a healthy bal-ance of friendly bacteria (acidophilus and others) in the digestive tract is important for proper absorption of soy products. Re-searchers have found that bacteria in the in-testines turn the dietary isoflavone daidzein into a useable form called equol.[47] Fer-mented soy products like tempeh and miso also contribute to healthy intestinal flora balance.[40,41]

REFERENCES

1. Brasher P. Soy may soar on health labels. *Daily Camera,* October 27, 1999.

2. Coward L, Barnes NC, Setchell KDR, et al. Genistein, daidzein, and their ß-glycoside conjugates: antitumor isoflavones in soybean foods from American and Asian diets. *Journal of Agricultural Food Chemistry* 1993; 41: 1961–1967.

3. Fukutake M, Takahashi M, Ishida K, et al. Quantification of genistein and genistin in soybeans and soybean products. *Food and Chemical Toxicology* 1996; 34: 457–461.

4. Messina M. Modern applications for an ancient bean: soybeans and the prevention and treatment of chronic disease. *Journal of Nutrition* 1995; 125: 567S–569S.

5. Anon. Archer Daniels Midland tells US farmers to segregate GE Crops. *Natural Business* October 1999; 3.

6. Anon. Media informs public with reports on GMOs. *Whole Foods* October 1999; 31–32.

7. Anderson JW, Johnstone BM, Cook-Newell ME. Meta-analysis of the effects of soy protein intake on serum lipids. *The New England Journal of Medicine* 1995; 333: 276–282.

8. Albertazzi P, Pansini F, Bonaccorsi G, et al. The effect of dietary soy supplementation on hot flushes. *Obstetrics and Gynecology* 1998; 91: 6–11.

9. Clarkson TB, Anthony MS, Williams JK, et al. The potential of soybean phytoestrogens for postmenopausal hormone replacement therapy. *Proceedings of the Society for Experimental Biology and Medicine* 1998; 217: 365–368.

10. Rotter SM, Baum JA, Teng H, et al. Soy protein and isoflavones: their effects on blood lipids and bone density in postmenopausal women. *American Journal of Clinical Nutrition* 1998; 68(suppl):1375S–1379S.

11. Arjmandi BH, Alekel I, Hollis BW, et al. Dietary soybean protein prevents bone loss in an ovariectomized rat model of osteoporosis. *Journal of Nutrition* 1996; 126: 161–167.

12. Monti E, Sinha BK. Antiproliferative effect of genistein and adriamycin against estrogen-dependent and -independent human breast carcinoma cell lines. *Anticancer Research* 1994; 14: 1221–1226.

13. Li W, Weber G. Synergistic action of tiazofurin and genistein on growth inhibition and differentiation of K-562 human leukemic cells. *Life Sciences* 1998; 63(22): 1975–1981.

14. Ingram D, Sanders K, Kolybaba M, et al. Case-control study of phyto-estrogens and breast cancer. *The Lancet* 1997; 350: 990–994.

15. Barnes S. Evolution of the health benefits of soy isoflavones. *Proceedings of the Society for Experimental Biology and Medicine* 1998; 217: 386–392.

16. Potter SM. Overview of proposed mechanisms for the hypocholesterolemic effect of soy. *Journal of Nutrition* 1995; 125: 606S–611S.

17. Tham DM, Gardner CD, Haskell WL. Clinical review 1997: potential health benefits of dietary phytoestrogens: a review of the clinical, epidemiological, and mechanistic evidence. *Journal of Clinical Endocrinology and Metabolism* 1998; 83: 2223–2235.

18. Anderson JW, Diwadkar VA, Bridges SR. Selective effects of different antioxidants on oxidation of lipoproteins from rats. *Society for Experimental Biology and Medicine* 1998; 218: 376–381.

19. Sirtori CR, Lovati MR, Manzoni C, et al. Soy and cholesterol reduction: clinical experience. *Journal of Nutrition* 1995; 125: 598S–605S.

20. Lovati MR, Manzoni C, Canavesi A, et al. Soybean protein diet increases low density lipoprotein receptor activity in mononuclear cells from hypercholesterolemic patients. *Journal of Clinical Investigation* 1987; 80: 1498–1502.

21. Wilcox JN, Blumenthal BF. Thrombotic mechanisms in atherosclerosis: potential impact of soy proteins. *Journal of Nutrition* 1995; 125: 631S–638S.

22. Forsythe WA. Soy protein, thyroid regulation and cholesterol metabolism. *Journal of Nutrition* 1995; 125: 619S–623S.

23. Knight DC, Eden JA. A review of the clinical effects of phytoestrogens. *Obstetrics and Gynecology* 1996; 87(5): 897–904.

24. Zava DT, Duwe G. Estrogenic and antiproliferative properties of genistein and other flavonoids in human breast cancer cells *in vitro*. *Nutrition and Cancer* 1997; 27(1): 31–40.

25. Zava DT, Dollbaum CM, Blen M. Estrogen and progestin bioactivity of foods, herbs, and spices. *Proceedings of the Society for Experimental Biology and Medicine* 1998; 217 (3): 369–378.

26. Cassidy A, Bingham S. Biological effects of isoflavones in young women: importance of the chemical composition of soyabean products. *British Journal of Nutrition* 1995; 74: 587–601.

27. Peterson G, Barnes S. Genistein and biochanin A inhibit the growth of human prostate cancer cells but not epidermal growth factor receptor tyrosine autophosphorylation. *Prostate* 1993; 22: 335–345.

28. Wei H. Isoflavones scavenge reactive oxygen species and protect DNA from oxidative DNA damage. *Proceedings of the American Association for Cancer Research* 1994; 35: 619.

29. Fotsis T, Pepper M, Adlercreutz H, et al. Genistein, a dietary-ingested isoflavonoid, inhibits cell proliferation and in vitro angiogenesis. *Journal of Nutrition* 1995; 125:790S–797S.

30. Yanagihara K, Ito A, Toge T, et al. Antiproliferative effect of isoflavones on human cancer cell lines established from the gastrointestinal tract. *Cancer Research* 1993; 53: 5815–5821.

31. Peterson G, Barnes S. Genistein inhibition of the growth of human breast cancer cells: independence from estrogen receptors and the multi-drug resistance gene. *Biochemical Biophysical Research Communications* 1991; 179(1): 661–667.

32. Lamartiniere CA, Murrill WB, Manzolillo PA, et al. Genistein alters the ontogeny of mammary gland development and protects against chemically-induced mammary

cancer in rats. *Proceedings of the Society for Experimental Biology and Medicine* 1998; 217(3): 358–364.

33. Holt S. Prostatic health: part 1, the optimal diet. *Alternative and Complementary Therapies* September/October 1996; 302–305.

34. Adlercreutz H, Markkanen H, Watanabe S. Plasma concentrations of phyto-estrogens in Japanese men. *The Lancet* 1993; 342: 1209–1210.

35. Bland JS. Diet and prostate problems. *Alternative Therapies* 1995; 1(4): 75–76.

36. Friedrich JA. Protective and regulatory benefits of soy: clinical perspectives. *Alternative and Complementary Therapies* February 1997: 53–58.

37. Koratkar R, Rao AV. Effect of soya bean saponins on azoxymethane-induced pre-neoplastic lesions in the colon of mice. *Nutrition and Cancer* 1997; 27(2): 206–209.

38. Arjmandi BH, Getlinger MJ, Goya NV, et al. Role of soy protein with normal or reduced isoflavone content in reversing bone loss induced by ovarian hormone deficiency in rats. *American Journal of Clinical Nutrition* 1998; 68(suppl6): 1358S–1363S.

39. Goyal N, Getlinger MJ, Sun P, et al. Effect of soy protein, with and without isoflavonoids, on bone in ovariectomized rats. *Journal of Bone Mineral Research* 1995; 10 (suppl 1): S453 (abstract).

40. Liener IE. Possible adverse effects of soybean anticarcinogens. *Journal of Nutrition* 1995; 125: 744S–750S.

41. Fallon SW, Enig MG. How safe is soy? *New Life* May 1996; 35–39.

42. Federal Register. Food labeling health claims: soy protein and coronary heart disease (Docket No. 98P-0683). November 10, 1998; 63(217): 62977–63015.

43. Messina M, Messina V. *The Simple Soybean and Your Health.* Garden City Park, NY: Avery, 1994.

44. Lo GS, Goldberg AP, Lim A, et al. Soy fiber improves lipid and carbohydrate metabolism in primary hyperlipidemic subjects. *Atherosclerosis* 1986; 62: 239–248.

45. Kennedy AR. The evidence for soybean products as cancer preventive agents. *Journal of Nutrition* 1995 (suppl); 733S–743S.

46. Graf E, Eaton JW. Suppression of colonic cancer by dietary phytic acid. *Nutrition and Cancer* 1993; 19(1): 11–19.

47. Lampe JW, Karr SC, Hutchins AM, et al. Urinary equol excretion with a soy challenge: influence of habitual diet. *Proceedings of the Society for Experimental Biology and Medicine* 1998; 217(3): 335–339.

St. John's Wort

HYPERICUM PERFORATUM
CLUSIACEAE
(SYNONYMS HYPERICACEAE
AND GUTTIFERAE)

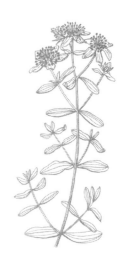

State of Knowledge: Five-Star Rating System

Clinical (human) research	✳✳✳✳
Laboratory research	✳✳✳✳
History of use/traditional use	✳✳✳✳
Safety record	✳✳✳✳
International acceptance	✳✳✳✳

PART USED: *Flower, leaf*

PRIMARY USES

Internal (extract)

- *Depression*
- *Anxiety related to depression*
- *Insomnia and fatigue related to depression*

External (oil infusion)

- *Wounds (traditional)*
- *Bruises (traditional)*
- *First-degree burns (traditional)*

St. John's wort rocketed to fame in the United States when the media picked up on the wealth of European clinical research confirming its effectiveness in the treatment of depression. The news came as no surprise to herbalists, who have long used St. John's wort not only for depression but also for the treatment of wounds, burns, injured nerves, sciatica, inflammations, ulcers, anxiety, and other ailments. Today, St. John's wort is one of the most frequently prescribed treatments for mild to moderate depression in Germany and has become one of the top ten best-selling dietary supplements in the United States. It is also the subject of continuing research by such prestigious organizations as the National Institutes of Health.

All of this attention is well deserved. Few herbs have been examined with the rigorous scientific scrutiny that St. John's wort has undergone. More than 25 high-quality, double-blind, controlled clinical trials on the use of St. John's wort in mild to moderate depression have been conducted since 1979. Comparative studies have shown St. John's wort to be more effective than placebo and just as effective as certain prescription antidepressants, but with a much lower rate of side effects. St. John's wort's exemplary safety record contributes greatly to the herb's popularity. Although often helpful in relieving symptoms, prescription anti-depressant medications can cause a variety of troublesome side effects, including problems with memory and concentration, drowsiness, lethargy, confusion, dry mouth, and weight gain.

Current estimates hold that as many as 3 to 5 percent of the world's population—at least 100 million people—suffer from depression.[1] Herbalists and other practitioners remind us that treatment for depression should address emotional factors, lifestyle issues, and constitutional differences among individuals, not just chemical imbalances. But it is clear that for many, St. John's wort can be a welcome alternative to standard prescription medications for the safe treatment of mild to moderate depression. Research is now underway on the potential of this medicinal herb for treating even serious depression.

HISTORY

St. John's wort has been esteemed as a medicine for centuries, and ancient Europeans believed it had magical protective powers against disease and evil. Even before it was recognized for melancholy, the herb was thought effective against demonic possession. It is quite possible that people who seemed "possessed" were actually suffering from mental illness that could be treated with St. John's wort. Ancient herbalists from Hippocrates to Dioscorides valued St. John's wort not only for the treatment of "melancholia" and other emotional disorders, but also for burns, wounds (particularly those involving nerve injuries), neuralgia or nerve pain, inflammations, ulcers, and more. After its introduction to America by early European settlers, the herb became firmly established as a vulnerary (wound-healing) and antidepressant herb among American herbalists, including the Eclectic physicians, a group of American doctors who practiced in the late nineteenth and early twentieth centuries.

The origin of the name "St. John's wort" remains a matter of speculation. Some believe the name refers to the fact that the plant blooms in midsummer, around the time of St. John's Day (June 24). Another theory holds that the reddish color produced when the buds and flowers are crushed was considered a symbol for the blood of John the Baptist.

International Status

St. John's wort is listed as an approved herb in the *German Commission E Monographs,* indicated for internal use in the treatment of depressive moods, anxiety and/or nervous unrest (extract), and for external use in the treatment of wounds, myalgia (muscle pain), and first-degree burns (oil preparation).[2] It is also approved in the United Kingdom and in France for topical application.

Botany

St. John's wort's bright yellow flowers are a familiar roadside sight in many parts of North America during its midsummer blooming season. When mature, the plant stands 1 to 3 feet tall, with branching, two-edged stems and numerous flowers. The edges of the small oval leaves (and to a lesser degree, the flowers) are perforated with many tiny dots, which give the plant its species name, *perforatum.*

The fresh flowers and unopened buds contain the highest concentrations of the constituent *hypericin,* the marker compound to which most St. John's wort extracts are standardized. If you crush a fresh flower bud, you'll notice that the hypericin in the "juice" leaves a purple stain on your fingers. Hypericin is the compound that gives good-quality St. John's wort tinctures and oil infusions their characteristic deep red color.

Native to Europe and Asia, St. John's wort is now naturalized in many parts of the world, including North and South America, Africa, and Australia. The healthiest wild populations of St. John's wort reportedly grow within 200 miles of the seacoast. In the United States, St. John's wort flourishes in northern California and southern Oregon. Under the right growing conditions, it can be quite invasive. Consequently, in spite of its value as a medicinal herb, St. John's wort is considered a noxious weed in certain circles. Ranchers regard the plant as a pest species because it can be toxic to livestock grazing on large quantities of it. In 1946, beetles were released as a biological control in an attempt to control further spread of the plant. This eradication program has vastly reduced plant populations in some areas of former abundance.

Benefits

- Alleviates psychological symptoms of mild to moderate depression, including despondency, poor concentration, and inability to perform daily tasks
- Eases physical (somatic) symptoms of mild to moderate depression, such as fatigue
- Relieves the anxiety and insomnia that often accompany depression

- May help people with masked (hidden) depression and seasonal affective disorder (SAD)
- Fewer side effects than prescription antidepressant drugs

SCIENTIFIC SUPPORT

Since the early 1980s, more than 25 double-blind European clinical studies involving more than 2,000 people have confirmed the benefits of St. John's wort in the treatment of mild to moderate depression. Standardized St. John's wort extract proved to be not only better than placebo, but also as effective as the antidepressant drugs to which it was compared—with far fewer side effects. St. John's wort may be helpful for people with masked depression, a condition in which a person does not realize that he or she is depressed but instead complains of physical (somatic) problems, such as fatigue or aches and pains.[3] The herb may also help people with seasonal affective disorder (SAD), a common form of depression believed to be caused by lack of exposure to light during fall and winter.[4]

To evaluate the effectiveness of the test preparations, most of the St. John's wort trials used a standard assessment tool for depression called the Hamilton Depression Rating Scale (HAMD), which measures improvements in symptoms such as depressive mood, insomnia, fatigue, anxiety, listless-ness, inability to perform daily tasks, anxiety, and somatic (physical) symptoms of depression, including fatigue.

Nearly all of the clinical research on St. John's wort has been conducted in people with mild or moderate depression, but researchers have begun to investigate the effects of the herb in people with severe depression. A German study that compared the effects of St. John's wort with those of the synthetic tricyclic antidepressant drug imipramine in people with severe depression showed that the two test substances were comparable in effectiveness for patients with severe depression (see Specific Studies). Because the patients were severely depressed, the investigators used dosages of St. John's wort and imipramine that were twice as high as those used in earlier trials.[5] The results of this study are promising, but more research is needed before St. John's wort can be recommended for people with severe depression.

In laboratory experiments, compounds isolated from St. John's wort demonstrated potent activity against a variety of viruses, including influenza, herpes simplex, Epstein-Barr, and retroviruses such as human immunodeficiency virus (HIV). Encouraged by these results, some people with AIDS began taking St. John's wort and reported benefits such as a more positive outlook, more energy, and less fatigue. However, it appears that these benefits were related to antidepressant effects rather than to a direct antiviral activity.[6]

SPECIFIC STUDIES

Mild to Moderate Depression: Meta-analysis (1996)

An analysis of 23 randomized European clinical investigations involving a total of 1,757 patients concluded that standardized St. John's wort extract was significantly more effective than placebo and just as effective as standard antidepressant medications in the treatment of mild or moderate depression. Fifteen of these studies were placebo controlled, and six compared St. John's wort extract with conventional drug treatments for depression, including maprotiline, imipramine, bromazepam, and amitriptyline. (The other two studies compared a combination product containing St. John's wort and valerian with synthetic antidepressants.) In the comparative trials, 35.9 percent of those taking conventional medications reported adverse effects, compared with 19.8 percent of those taking St. John's wort extract. Most of the studies utilized the Hamilton Depression Rating Scale to measure efficacy.[7]

Severe Depression: Clinical Study (1997)

This German study was the first to compare St. John's wort with a standard antidepressant medication in people with severe depression. Results of the controlled, randomized 6-week trial showed that standardized St. John's wort extract produced benefits comparable to those of the tricyclic antidepressant drug imipramine, but with far fewer side effects. The 209 participants in the trial were randomly divided into two groups: one group received treatment with 600 mg St. John's wort extract three times a day, and the other took 50 mg imipramine three times a day. The 1,800-mg daily dose of St. John's wort extract used in the study and the 150-mg dose of imipramine were both twice as high as doses used in earlier trials that compared the two substances. Over the 6-week treatment period, the study groups experienced a comparable improvement in depression symptoms, according to HAMD scores. These results seem promising, but the authors admitted that, "a definite proof of efficacy would . . . only have been possible if both treatment regimens had been tested against placebo." Side effects were reported by 41 percent of those in the imipramine group, compared with 23 percent taking St. John's wort.[5]

Mild to Moderate Depression: Clinical Study (1997)

Standardized St. John's wort extract at a total daily dose of 900 mg was as helpful as the sedating tricyclic antidepressant drug amitriptyline (25 mg three times daily) in relieving symptoms in 165 people with mild to moderate depression. According to results of the randomized controlled study, there was no statistically significant difference in effectiveness between the two study groups, although the amitriptyline group demonstrated a tendency toward a better response rate. However, there was a significant difference between the groups with regard to adverse effects. Sixty-four percent of participants taking amitriptyline reported side effects, compared with 37 percent in the St. John's wort group.[8]

Seasonal Affective Disorder: Clinical Study (1994)

This small controlled single-blind study suggested that treatment with standardized St. John's wort extract shows promise for relieving symptoms of seasonal affective disorder. SAD is a common form of depression associated with seasonal changes and is believed to be caused by reduced levels of light in winter months. Light therapy, a relatively new treatment for this type of depression, has demonstrated favorable results in a number of controlled clinical trials, but some people find it too time-consuming. In this study, 20 people with SAD were randomized to receive 4 weeks of treatment with standardized St. John's wort extract (300 mg three times a day) in combination with 2 hours of daily treatment with either bright light (3,000 lux) or dim light (less than 300 lux). According to the HAMD, both treatment groups experienced significant improvement in SAD symptoms, such as fatigue, despondency, and bad temper, and statistical analysis showed that there was

no significant difference between the two treatment groups. The researchers concluded that St. John's wort does have antidepressant effects in people with SAD, and that the herb might be even more effective if combined with light therapy. Further trials with greater numbers of participants are needed to confirm these results.[4]

HOW IT WORKS

Although it is clear that St. John's wort works, it is still not clear exactly *how* it works. Based on limited evidence from laboratory experiments, researchers at first believed that St. John's wort inhibits a substance called monoamine oxidase (MAO), which regulates levels of neurotransmitters in the brain. Subsequent research indicated that this was not the case and the theory fell out of favor, allaying fears that *Hypericum* could cause the same kind of serious side effects as prescription antidepressant drugs called monoamine oxidase inhibitors (MAOIs). Several other theories are currently under investigation. One proposes that St. John's wort raises levels of a neurotransmitter called serotonin, the way Prozac and similar antidepressant drugs do.[9] Others suggest that *Hypericum* lowers levels of the stress hormone cortisol or affects receptor sites for gamma-aminobutyric acid (GABA), a neurotransmitter.

Also yet to be determined is which constituents are the "active ingredients" responsible for St. John's wort's antidepressant action. Current candidates under investigation include hypericin, hyperforin, and pseudohypericin. For a time, many researchers regarded hypericin as the most active compound; consequently, hypericin became the marker compound to which most St. John's wort extracts are standardized. Most recently, however, research interest has focused on the constituent hyperforin. In one laboratory study, hyperforin inhibited reuptake of serotonin, dopamine, noradrenaline, GABA, and L-glutamate.[10]

The theory that hyperforin is the constituent responsible for St. John's wort's antidepressant effectiveness was put to the test in a study of 147 people with mild or moderate depression. For the double-blind, placebo-controlled trial, participants were randomized into three groups. One group received treatment with a St. John's wort extract containing 0.5 percent hyperforin (300 mg three times a day), one took a St. John's wort extract with a 5 percent hyperforin content (300 mg three times a day), and one group took placebo. According to statisical analysis of HAMD scores, the 5 percent hyperforin extract was significantly superior to placebo in relieving symptoms of depression, while results with the 0.5 percent hyperforin extract were comparable to those seen with placebo. The investigators concluded that results with the 5 percent extract were comparable with those seen with St. John's wort extracts standardized to 0.3 percent hypericin, and that overall, the

5 percent hyperforin extract was an effective antidepressant treatment.[11] These results are supported by animal studies using a 4.5 percent hyperforin extract.[10,12] Hyperforin is naturally present in St. John's wort in larger amounts than hypericin. However, neither hyperforin nor hypericin have been shown to be effective antidepressants by themselves.

Clearly, research on St. John's wort's mechanism of action remains inconclusive. As is the case with many herbs, it is likely that a variety of different plant compounds working together account for the herb's antidepressant effects. Some researchers speculate that there is a synergistic action among a number of different St. John's wort constituents, including hypericin, hyperforin, and flavonoid compounds.[10,13]

MAJOR CONSTITUENTS

Hypericin, hyperforin, pseudohypericin, flavonoids, xanthones, essential oil

SAFETY

St. John's wort is well tolerated by most people, and there are no reports of major side effects with recommended doses. Side effects are rare, and those that do occur are generally mild.

• **Side effects:** In clinical trials, only a few people experienced minor side effects, such as mild stomach upset. A drug-monitoring study that evaluated the safety and effectiveness of St. John's wort in 3,250 people documented a side effect rate of only 2.4 percent. The most common complaints were gastrointestinal irritations, allergic reactions, tiredness, and restlessness.[14]

In livestock, St. John's wort has been known to cause photosensitivity, an allergic skin reaction that occurs with exposure to sunlight. Photosensitivity does not appear to be a big problem for humans, but it may be wise to be cautious about sun exposure while taking St. John's wort, especially if you are fair-skinned.[15] Phototoxicity may be more likely if recommended dosage is exceeded.

• **Contraindications:** Currently, St. John's wort is recommended for use by people with mild to moderate depression, not severe depression.

• **Drug interactions:** There have been no reports of interactions between St. John's wort and drugs. However, if you are currently taking a prescription antidepressant medication, do not discontinue or change your dosage without the advice of your doctor. St. John's wort should not be taken in combination with prescription antidepressant medications or alcohol.

DOSAGE

St. John's wort is considered suitable for the treatment of mild to moderate depression, not severe depression that interferes with the ability to function in daily life. The dosage used in most clinical trials was 300 mg three times a day (a total daily dose of 900 mg) of extract containing 0.3 percent hypericin. Two to three weeks of regular use may be needed before antidepressant effects are seen.

• **Standardized extract:** 300 mg three times a day (a total daily dose of 900 mg)
• **Tincture:** 20 to 30 drops three times a day
• **Powdered extract:** 300 mg three times a day

STANDARDIZATION

St. John's wort extracts are typically standardized to 0.3 percent hypericin. The 900-mg daily dose contains 2.7 mg of hypericin. Some products are now standardized to 5 percent hyperforin.

REFERENCES

1. Lieberman S. Treating depression with St. John's wort. *Alternative and Complementary Therapies* June 1998; 163–168.
2. Blumenthal M, Busse W, Goldberg A, et al., eds. *The Complete German Commission E Monographs.* Austin, TX: The American Botanical Council; Boston: Integrative Medical Communications, 1998.

3. Hübner W-D, Lande S, Podzuweit H. Treatment of masked depressions with hypericum [in German]. *Nervenheilkunde* 1993; 12: 278–280.

4. Martinez B, Kasper S, Ruhrmann S, et al. Hypericum in the treatment of seasonal affective disorders. *Journal of Geriatric Psychiatry and Neurology* 1994; 7(suppl 1): S29–S33.

5. Vorbach EU, Arnoldt KH, Hübner W-D. Efficacy and tolerability of St. John's wort extract LI 160 versus imipramine in patients with severe depressive episodes according to ICD-10. *Pharmacopsychiatry* 1997; 30(suppl): 81–85.

6. Bergner P. Hypericum and AIDS. *Medical Herbalism* 1990; 2(1): 1–6.

7. Linde K, Ramirez G, Mulrow CD, et al. St. John's wort for depression—an overview and meta-analysis of randomized clinical trials. *British Medical Journal* 1996; 313: 253–258.

8. Wheatley D. LI 160, an extract of St. John's wort, versus amitriptyline in mildly to moderately depressed outpatients—a controlled 6-week trial. *Pharmacopsychiatry* 1997; 30(suppl): 77–80.

9. Müller WEG, Rossol R. Effects of *Hypericum* extract on the expression of serotonin receptors. *Journal of Geriatric Psychiatry and Neurology* 1994; 7(suppl 1): S63–S64.

10. Chatterjee SS, Bhattacharya SK, Wonnemann N, et al. Hyperforin as a possible antidepressant component of *Hypericum* extracts. *Life Sciences* 1998; 63(6): 499–510.

11. Laakmann G, Schüle C, Baghai T, et al. St. John's wort in mild to moderate depression: the relevance of hyperforin for the clinical efficacy. *Pharmacopsychiatry* 1998; 31(suppl): 54–59.

12. Bhattacharya SK, Chakrabarti A, Chatterjee SS. Activity profiles of two hyperforin-containing *Hypericum* extracts in behavioral models. *Pharmacopsychiatry* 1998; 31(suppl): 22–29.

13. Reuter HD. Chemistry and biology of *Hypericum perforatum* (St. John's wort). In: Lawson LD, Bauer R, eds. *Phytomedicines of Europe.* Washington, DC: American Chemical Society, 1998.

14. Woelk H, Burkard G, Grünwald J. Benefits and risks of the *Hypericum* extract LI 160: drug monitoring study with 3,250 patients. *Journal of Geriatric Psychiatry and Neurology* 1994; 7(suppl 1): S34–S38.

15. McGuffin M, Hobbs C, Upton R, et al., eds. *American Herbal Products Association Botanical Safety Handbook.* Boca Raton, FL: CRC Press, 1997.

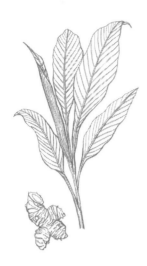

Turmeric

CURCUMA LONGA
ZINGIBERACEAE

State of Knowledge: Five-Star Rating System

Clinical (human) research	✶✶
Laboratory research	✶✶✶
History of use/traditional use	✶✶✶✶
Safety record	✶✶✶✶
International acceptance	✶✶✶

PART USED: *Rhizome*
PRIMARY USES

- *Inflammatory disorders, including arthritis*
- *Cancer protection (experimental)*
- *Antioxidant*
- *Liver and heart health*

Long before people understood how antioxidants worked to prevent disease, ancient people promoted good health by spicing food with golden-yellow turmeric. As a mainstay remedy in traditional Indian Ayurvedic medicine and other Asian healing systems, turmeric has been used through the ages in the treatment of arthritis and other inflammatory conditions.

Scientists have now identified potent antioxidant compounds in turmeric that account not only for many of its medicinal virtues, but also for its traditional use as a food preservative in hot tropical countries.

Although clinical research on turmeric is still in preliminary stages, studies conducted to date have generated excitement among scientists and health practitioners. Among the numerous scientifically documented actions that turmeric and its constituent curcumin possess are anti-inflammatory, antioxidant, anticancer, liver-protective, choleretic (bile-stimulating), antiplatelet, and antiviral. Current research is investigating the clinical potential of curcumin in the prevention and treatment of cancer, AIDS, elevated cholesterol, ulcers, gallbladder and liver disease, and inflammatory disorders such as arthritis.

Turmeric caught the attention of Western scientists in the 1970s, when research shed new light on the medicinal value of turmeric compounds called *curcuminoids*. This important class of antioxidant and anti-inflammatory constituents also gives turmeric its brilliant yellow-orange color. Much of the research on turmeric has centered on one particular curcuminoid known as *curcumin*. As an antioxidant, curcumin is estimated to be 30 times as potent as zingerone, an antioxidant compound in ginger.[1]

Turmeric is a major ingredient of curry blends, which are mixtures of spices that may also contain ginger, cloves, fenugreek, and other healthful herbs. In the United States today, the main use of turmeric is as a coloring agent for bright yellow prepared mustards.

flammations, sprains, painful joints, wounds, and various skin problems. In traditional Chinese medicine, turmeric has been used to treat inflammation, dysmenorrhea (painful menstruation), liver disorders, and wounds. Turmeric was also known to ancient Western healers such as the Greek herbalist Dioscorides, who mentioned it in his writings in the first century.

An important dye plant, turmeric produces a brilliant yellow-gold hue that has been used to color foods, paper, wood, cosmetics, and fabrics—even the golden robes worn by Thai Buddhist monks.

INTERNATIONAL STATUS

In Europe, turmeric is listed as an approved herb in the *German Commission E Monographs,* indicated for the treatment of dyspeptic conditions (indigestion).[2]

HISTORY

Turmeric's long and colorful history encompasses centuries of use as a spice, food preservative, medicine, and dye in many Asian cultures. Among other uses, turmeric is employed in the Ayurvedic healing tradition in the treatment of liver disease, urinary tract problems, and indigestion. It is applied externally in salves and poultices to treat in-

BOTANY

A member of the ginger family (Zingiberaceae), *Curcuma longa* is a perennial plant that is widely cultivated in tropical and subtropical regions of south and southeast Asia. Turmeric is believed to have originated in southern India, and to this day, India is still the largest producer of turmeric for the world market. Other important turmeric-growing nations include China, Indonesia, Malaysia, and Jamaica. After harvest, the fleshy yellow turmeric rhizomes are boiled, dried, and polished before further processing.

BENEFITS

- Acts as an anti-inflammatory agent
- Inhibits oxidation of blood fats (serum lipid peroxides)
- Increases bile production (choleretic)
- Lowers cholesterol
- Inhibits platelet aggregation
- Protects the liver against injury from toxins (experimental)
- Inhibits replication of human immunodeficiency virus (experimental)

SCIENTIFIC SUPPORT

Most of the limited clinical research on turmeric and curcumin has been performed in India. Some of the most interesting of these studies have investigated turmeric as an anti-inflammatory agent, providing scientific validation for this important Ayurvedic use of the plant. In other studies, turmeric has demonstrated impressive cancer-protective effects[3-9] as well as an ability to lower cholesterol and levels of blood lipid peroxides in healthy volunteers.[10,11]

In clinical and laboratory studies evaluating its effects against inflammation, curcumin appeared to be as effective as the nonsteroidal anti-inflammatory drugs (NSAIDs) against which it was tested.[12,13] These powerful synthetic drugs are a standard treatment for reducing the pain, stiffness, and inflammation of arthritis, but can cause a variety of serious side effects, including gastrointestinal ulceration and hemorrhage and kidney damage. In two studies, curcumin was tested against phenylbutazone, a particularly powerful NSAID that can cause side effects such as intestinal ulceration, anemia and other blood problems, rashes, fluid retention, and liver problems. Turmeric, on the other hand, has a long history of safe use as a food, and its constituent curcumin has caused no adverse effects in clinical trials.

Curcumin may have antimutagenic properties, meaning that it can help prevent genetic mutations that can lead to cancer. In laboratory experiments, both turmeric and curcumin have demonstrated impressive anticancer effects at all stages of cancer development. In numerous studies, curcumin reduced the number and size of tumors in animals with experimentally induced cancers, including cancers of the skin, colon, and stomach.[4-9]

Turmeric and curcumin have also shown promise in clinical studies involving people with cancer and precancerous conditions. In one 18-month study of 62 people with ulcerating oral or skin cancers (squamous cell carcinomas) that did not respond to conventional therapies, topical treatment with 9.5 percent curcumin ointment (for skin cancer) or an alcohol extract of turmeric (for oral cancer) was effective for many patients in reducing smell, itching, and exudate (oozing). A small number of patients experienced reductions in lesion size and pain.[14]

Laboratory studies indicate that turmeric can increase bile solubility and output,[15] suggesting the herb has potential value for preventing and treating gallstones and for lowering cholesterol. Experimental evidence indicates that turmeric's antioxidant activity may help protect against the formation of cataracts.[16] In other studies, curcumin protected the liver against powerful toxins.[17,18] Curcumin also interfered with the replication of the human immunodeficiency virus (HIV) in laboratory tests.[19]

In addition, in a recent laboratory study of 150 herbs, turmeric ranked among the seven herbs with the highest estrogen receptor–binding activity, and among the six with the highest progesterone-binding activity, suggesting that turmeric may have effects on hormone levels. (The other six highest estrogen-binding herbs were soy, licorice, red clover, thyme, hops, and verbena; the other five highest progesterone-binding herbs were oregano, verbena, thyme, red clover, and damiana.)[20]

Specific Studies

Postoperative Inflammation: Clinical Study (1986)

In this double-blind, placebo-controlled trial, both curcumin and the nonsteroidal anti-inflammatory drug phenylbutazone produced a significantly greater anti-inflammatory response than placebo after 6 days of treatment in people with postoperative inflammation. The study involved 45 men with edema (swelling) and tenderness of the spermatic cord following surgical correction of a hernia or hydrocele (an accumulation of fluid in the scrotum or spermatic cord). Five of the original participants developed wound infections and were excluded from the trial, so results from only 40 were available for assessment. Of these, 13 men received treatment with curcumin (450 mg three times a day), 14 with phenylbutazone (100 mg three times a day), and 13 with placebo. All of the men also took the antibiotic ampicillin during the course of the study. Curcumin decreased the intensity of all four measures of inflammation evaluated: pain at surgical site, tenderness at site, spermatic cord edema, and cord tenderness. Phenylbutazone, on the other hand, reduced only three of the four measures of inflammation. Reduction in total intensity scores by the end of the 6-day period was 84.2 percent for curcumin, 86 percent for phenylbutazone, and 61.8 percent for placebo.[12]

Arthritis:
Clinical Study (1980)

In this small, short-term, double-blind study in 18 people with rheumatoid arthritis, significant improvements were noted in morning stiffness, joint swelling, and walking ability after 2 weeks of treatment with either curcumin (1,200 mg per day) or the synthetic drug phenylbutazone (300 mg per day). The investigators saw improvement with both study medications, although the patients in the study felt that there was more significant improvement with phenylbutazone.[13]

Cholesterol and Lipid
Peroxides: Clinical Study (1992)

Results of this small study point out the potential value of curcumin as a form of protection against heart disease. After 7 days of treatment with curcumin at a daily dose of 500 mg, the 10 healthy volunteers demonstrated significant reductions in levels of serum lipid peroxides (33 percent) and total serum cholesterol (11.65 percent). A significant increase in levels of beneficial high-density lipoprotein (HDL) cholesterol was also observed (29 percent). The investigators suggested that because of its antioxidant activity, curcumin may be of value in the prevention of atherosclerosis (hardening and narrowing of the arteries).[11]

Cancer-Preventive Effects:
Biomonitoring Study (1992)

Tobacco smoke is a major source of mutagens and carcinogens, and cigarette smokers are known to excrete high levels of tobacco-derived mutagens in their urine. In this small controlled 30-day study, 16 chronic smokers who took 1.5 grams of turmeric a day had significant reductions in excretion of urinary mutagens compared with baseline levels. A control group of 6 nonsmokers who did not take turmeric showed no changes in levels of urinary mutagens. The investigators concluded that "dietary turmeric is an effective antimutagen and that it may be useful in chemoprevention" of cancer.[3]

HOW IT WORKS

Current research suggests that the antioxidant curcuminoids (including curcumin) are the major contributors to turmeric's health-protective benefits. Numerous studies, including human trials, have shown that turmeric and curcumin act as free radical scavengers, preventing the formation of oxidants in the body. Turmeric also appears to enhance the activity of the body's own antioxidant system.

Antioxidant Effects

Oxidants cause cell and organ damage that has been implicated in many serious health conditions, including cancer, heart disease, inflammatory disorders, and age-related decline. Turmeric protects against the formation of a variety of different oxidants, including lipid peroxides (oxidized blood fats). Lipid peroxides are associated with the development of heart disease such as atherosclerosis, a hardening and narrowing of the arteries that is largely due to the buildup of plaque deposits in the blood vessels.

Antiplatelet Effects

Another way that turmeric may help protect against disease is by inhibiting platelet aggregation, that is, the tendency of blood platelets to stick together and "thicken" the blood. Some platelet aggregation is essential for blood clotting and other body functions. However, too much platelet aggregation is implicated in the development of a number of diseases, including heart disease, asthma, and inflammatory disorders. Studies suggest that turmeric and curcumin inhibit platelet aggregation by interfering with the synthesis of thromboxanes, which encourage platelet aggregation, while at the same time increasing prostacyclin, which acts in the opposite manner.

Anti-Inflammatory Action

It is still unclear exactly how turmeric works to reduce inflammation, but the herb's antiplatelet and antioxidant proper-

ties are thought to play at least a partial role. Other theories under investigation include inhibition of leukotriene synthesis and effects on adrenal corticosteroids. Researchers believe that curcumin and the volatile oil component of turmeric are both responsible for its anti-inflammatory effects.

In addition, like capsaicin from cayenne, curcumin has been shown to deplete nerve endings of substance P, the neurotransmitter responsible for transmitting pain messages.

MAJOR CONSTITUENTS

Curcuminoids (including curcumin), volatile oil (primarily turmerone, atlantone, and zingiberone)

SAFETY

Turmeric has been safely used as a food for thousands of years. As a supplement, it is generally considered safe when used as directed. No toxicity has been observed in toxicology studies, and no adverse effects have been reported in clinical studies.

Any safety concerns for turmeric are based on the therapeutic use of large quantities, not on consumption of moderate amounts as a spice.[21]

- **Side effects:** None known.[21]
- **Contraindications:** Turmeric should not be taken in therapeutic doses

during pregnancy, because laboratory tests suggest it may stimulate uterine contractions.[21] In addition, because it increases the output of bile, turmeric should not be taken by people with bile duct obstructions. If you have gallstones, consult your health-care practitioner before taking turmeric.[2]

• **Drug interactions:** None known.[2,21]

DOSAGE

For reducing inflammation, some sources recommend a therapeutic dosage of 400 to 600 mg curcumin three times a day. To ingest an equivalent amount of curcumin in the form of whole turmeric would necessitate the consumption of 8,000 to 60,000 mg of turmeric three times a day (8 to 60 g).[22] For health maintenance and antioxidant effects, appropriate dosages of standardized turmeric extract or whole turmeric are much lower than this.

• **Standardized turmeric extract:** One 450-mg capsule three times a day
• **Whole-plant turmeric:** Up to 2 g a day (2,000 mg)
• **Curcumin:** 400 to 600 mg three times a day (for therapeutic effects)

STANDARDIZATION

Turmeric extracts are typically standardized to 95 percent curcuminoids.

REFERENCES

1. Reddy ACP, Lokesh BR. Studies on spice principles as antioxidants in the inhibition of lipid peroxidation of rat liver microsomes. *Molecular and Cellular Biochemistry* 1992; 111: 117–124.

2. Blumenthal M, Busse W, Goldberg A, et al., eds. *The Complete German Commission E Monographs.* Austin, TX: The American Botanical Council; Boston: Integrative Medical Communications, 1998.

3. Polasa K, Raghuram TC, Krishna TP, et al. Effect of turmeric on urinary mutagens in smokers. *Mutagenesis* 1992; 2: 107–109.

4. Limtrakul P, Lipigorngoson S, Namwong O, et al. Inhibitory effect of dietary curcumin on skin carcinogenesis in mice. *Cancer Letters* 1997; 116: 197–203.

5. Deshpande SS, Ingle AD, Maru GB. Inhibitory effects of curcumin-free aqueous turmeric extract on benzo[a]pyrene-induced forestomach papillomas in mice. *Cancer Letters* 1997; 118: 79–85.

6. Rao CV, Rivenson A, Simi B, et al. Chemoprevention of colon cancer by dietary curcumin. *Annals of the New York Academy of Sciences* 1995; 768: 201–204.

7. Huang M-T, Deschner EE, Newmark HL, et al. Effect of dietary curcumin and ascorbyl palmitate on azoxymethanol-induced colonic epithelial cell proliferation and focal areas of dysplasia. *Cancer Letters* 1992; 64: 117–121.

8. Huang M-T, Robertson FM, Lysz T, et al. Inhibitory effects of curcumin on carcinogensis in mouse epidermis. In: Huang MT, Ho CT, Lee CY, eds. *Phenolic Compounds in*

Food and Their Effects on Health II. Washington, DC: American Chemical Society, 1992: 338–349.

9. Nagabhushan M, Bhide SV. Curcumin as an inhibitor of cancer. *Journal of the American College of Nutrition* 1989; 8(5): 450. Abstract 96.

10. Ramirez-Boscá A, Soler A, Gutierrez MAC, et al. Antioxidant *Curcuma* extracts decrease the blood lipid peroxide levels of human subjects. *Age* 1995; 18: 167–169.

11. Soni KB, Kuttan R. Effect of oral curcumin administration on serum peroxides and cholesterol levels in human volunteers. *Indian Journal of Physiology and Pharmacology* 1992; 36(4): 273–275.

12. Satoskar RR, Shah SJ, Shenoy SG. Evaluation of anti-inflammatory property of curcumin (diferuloyl methane) in patients with postoperative inflammation. *International Journal of Clinical Pharmacology, Therapy and Toxicology* 1986; 24(12): 651–654.

13. Deodhar SD, Sethi R, Srimal RC. Preliminary study on antirheumatic activity of curcumin (diferuloyl methane). *Indian Journal of Medical Research* 1980; 71: 632–634.

14. Kuttan R, Sudheeran PC, Josph CD. Turmeric and curcumin as topical agents in cancer therapy. *Tumori* 1987; 73: 29–31.

15. Ammon HPT, Wahl MA. Pharmacology of *Curcuma longa. Planta Medica* 1991; 57: 1–6.

16. Awasthi S, Srivatava SK, Piper JT, et al. Curcumin protects against 4-hydroxy-2-trans-nonenal-induced cataract formation in rat lenses. *American Journal of Clinical Nutrition* 1996; 64: 761–766.

17. Reddy ACP, Lokesh BR. Effect of curcumin and eugenol on iron-induced hepatic toxicity in rats. *Toxicology* 1996; 107: 39–45.

18. Kiso Y, Suzuki Y, Watanabe N, et al. Antihepatoxic principles of *Curcuma longa* rhizomes. *Planta Medica* 1983; 49: 185–187.

19. Mazumder A, Raghavan K, Weinstein J, et al. Inhibition of human immunodeficiency virus type-1 integrase by curcumin. *Biochemical Pharmacology* 1995; 49(8): 1165–1170.

20. Zava DT, Dollbaum CM, Blen M. Estrogen and progestin bioactivity of foods, herbs, and spices. *Proceedings of the Society for Experimental Biology and Medicine* 1998; 217(3): 369–378.

21. McGuffin M, Hobbs C, Upton R, et al., eds. *American Herbal Products Association Botanical Safety Handbook.* Boca Raton, FL: CRC Press, 1997.

22. Murray M. *The Healing Power of Herbs.* Rocklin, CA: Prima Publishing, 1995.

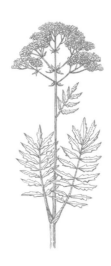

Valerian

VALERIANA OFFICINALIS
VALERIANACEAE

State of Knowledge: Five-Star Rating System

Clinical (human) research	✶✶
Laboratory research	✶✶
History of use/traditional use	✶✶✶
Safety record	✶✶✶
International acceptance	✶✶✶

PART USED: *Rhizome, root*
PRIMARY USES

- *Insomnia*
- *Mild anxiety or restlessness*
- *Muscle spasms and cramping (traditional)*
- *Menstrual cramps (traditional)*
- *Intestinal cramping/colic (traditional)*

Valerian's popularity as a sedative herb seems to be increasing along with the stresses of modern life. For at least 500 years, valerian has been among the most popular remedies in the United States and Europe, where it is now approved by Germany's Commission E for restlessness and sleeping disorders. Today, according to the National Institutes of Health, as many as one-third of American adults have trouble getting a good night's sleep. The majority of adults get less sleep than they actually need, and more than 60 percent of the American population functions with a chronic sleep deficit. Most people who suffer from sleep disturbances report being under some kind of emotional stress, and an estimated nine million Americans turn to potentially addictive pharmaceutical sleep aids each year in an effort to cope.

What's wrong with conventional sleeping pills? Our most common sleep aids are sedative drugs called benzodiazepines, which include Valium, Xanax, and Dalmane.

Research shows that this type of drug is addictive and actually worsens abnormal sleep patterns over time by interfering with rapid eye movement (REM) sleep. Side effects often include dizziness, impaired coordination, headaches, blurred vision, nausea, and even more serious negative effects on memory, behavior, and mood. People who are withdrawing from these drugs after long-term use often experience nightmares as REM sleep reverts to normal.

Fortunately, scientific evidence indicates that valerian can offer many sleepless Americans a safer, nonaddictive alternative for a refreshing night's sleep. The plant gets its name from the Latin word for "well-being" and is often used in combination with other calming herbs such as hops *(Humulus lupulus)*, passionflower *(Passiflora incarnata)*, lemon balm *(Melissa officinalis)*, chamomile *(Matricaria recutita)*, or skullcap *(Scutellaria lateriflora)*. If you are currently taking sedative drugs and want to switch to valerian, consult an herbally aware physician for advice on making a smooth transition. Many practitioners are actually prescribing valerian to ease withdrawal symptoms from sedative drugs. Keep in mind that valerian seems to be most effective when taken daily, rather than just taken as needed.

HISTORY

The ancient Greeks and Romans used valerian for digestive disorders, menstrual cramps, flatulence, nausea, urinary tract problems, and epilepsy. Ironically, there is only one early mention of valerian's sleep-inducing properties, by the physician Galen in A.D. 2. By the late sixteenth century, growing numbers of Europeans were reaching for valerian tinctures to help ease anxiety, insomnia, and nervous digestive disturbances. As late as the nineteenth century, the plant was also the chosen treatment for hysteria and vapors, two "female nervous conditions."

In 1620, the English colonists brought valerian roots to North America, along with their most precious belongings. The plant eventually became part of the Eclectic physicians' repertoire for nervous system conditions and muscle or bronchial spasms. The Eclectics were a group of prominent American physicians who practiced during the early twentieth century, primarily using herbal remedies. Valerian was an official remedy in *The United States Pharmacopoeia* from 1820 until 1936 and was featured in the *National Formulary* from 1888 to 1946. During the First World War, it was an important treatment for "shellshock" in soldiers and civilians. Until the rise of synthetic sedative drugs in the 1940s, the plant was included in standard medical textbooks in England and the United States. Today, valerian is an approved over-the-counter medicine in Germany, Belgium, France, Switzerland, and Italy. It is also recognized by the World Health Organization (WHO) as a mild hypotensive (blood pressure–lowering) herb.

Once known as the *herbe aux chats* (herb of cats), valerian has a long history of appeal for felines. Many cats find the signature dirty-sock smell euphoric and have been known to scratch at the labels on apothecary jars of valerian. In the eighteenth century, a prominent physician suggested that cats be employed to judge valerian quality! (So far, not a single herb company has followed his advice.) Legend also has it that it was valerian, not a magic flute, that the Pied Piper used to lure the rats out of Hamelin. It is interesting to note that fresh valerian root does not have the objectionable scent. As the root dries, it changes chemically, producing isovaleric acid, the plant compound responsible for the distinctive smell.

INTERNATIONAL STATUS

Valerian is approved in Germany, the United Kingdom, Belgium, and France for the treatment of nervous tension and stress, restlessness, disturbed sleep patterns, and anxiety states.

BOTANY

Originally from Europe and parts of northern Asia, *Valeriana officinalis* was carried to North America on the *Mayflower* and eventually escaped cultivation, spreading beyond its original range. Over time, the plant became naturalized from Nova Scotia to Pennsylvania, and from Ohio to Minnesota and Quebec. Sixteen naturalized *Valeriana* species grow in North America. About 200 other species are distributed around the globe.

Valerian is a moisture-loving perennial, commonly found along riverbanks, in woodlands, and in damp meadows. The stems reach heights of 2 to 5 feet, and the small, fragrant pink or white flowers bloom from June through September. Valerian's roots and rhizomes are harvested in the spring or autumn and dried at very low temperatures in order to preserve the volatile oils. The plant is raised commercially in Europe and the United States. It grows relatively easily as a garden plant in a variety of climates, spreading quickly on its many runners—just be sure to protect it from the neighborhood cats!

BENEFITS

- Decreases sleep latency (the length of time it takes to get to sleep) and the number of nighttime awakenings
- Improves overall sleep quality
- May improve well-being by decreasing nervousness and anxiety
- Does not cause side effects that are common with sedative drugs, including addiction and morning "hangovers"

SCIENTIFIC SUPPORT

Clinical research shows that valerian improves overall sleep quality, shortening the length of time it takes to fall asleep and helping people sleep more soundly. Overall, the herb seems to help poor sleepers the most, having little effect in people who already enjoy a peaceful slumber.[1] In one double-blind study on sleep disorders, 44 percent of the test group reported "perfect" sleep and 89 percent noted significant improvement after taking valerian, in comparison with placebo.[2] A large multicenter study has also demonstrated valerian's effectiveness in children with sleeping problems related to nervousness.[3] Overall, the positive results of five placebo-controlled trials and those of several large multicenter studies in more than 11,000 people offer convincing scientific evidence of valerian's value.

Several clinical studies suggest that valerian may be a useful alternative to antidepressant and antianxiety drugs in the treatment of mild depression, nervousness, and anxiety. Researchers compared a valerian and St. John's wort combination with the standard antidepressant drug amitriptylin in two randomized double-blind trials with neurotic, mildly depressed individuals. One study found the valerian/St. John's wort product comparable in efficacy to the antidepressant, while the other found it superior to standard treatment. The herbal therapy was associated with fewer side effects.[4,5] In another study of 182 people, those who took an herbal combination product containing valerian experienced more significant relief from anxiety symptoms than the placebo group. The herbal blend tested was a popular French product containing valerian and passionflower (Passiflora incarnata), in addition to smaller amounts of hawthorn (Crataegus spp.), black horehound (Ballota spp.), guarana (Paullinia cupana), and kola nut (Cola nitida). All of the participants in the study had been diagnosed with adjustment disorder with anxious mood, a condition that is normally treated with benzodiazepine drugs.[6] These three studies fit nicely into current trends in the field of psychology, which are aimed at reducing the side effects and dependence potential of standard treatments for mood disorders.

SPECIFIC STUDIES

Insomnia: Clinical Study (1996)

In a randomized, double-blind, placebo-controlled study of 121 people with insomnia, participants taking valerian reported significantly better sleep quality, psychological well-being, and dream recall, along with less daytime fatigue, than those receiving placebo. The dosage of valerian root extract was 2 tablets (300 mg each) 1 hour before bedtime. By the end of the 4-week study, the valerian group showed a statistically significant improvement on a self-evaluation sleep questionnaire (Gortelmeyer SF-B) and the State of Being Scale according to von Zerssen (Bf-S), compared with placebo. According to the Clinical Global Impression Scale (CGI) the researchers used to evaluate results, the change was "dramatically better" or "much better" in 56 percent of people in the valerian group at day 14, compared with only 26 percent in the placebo group. No side effects were reported, and overall tolerability was rated by the doctors as "very good" in 92 percent of participants.[7]

Nervous Conditions/Insomnia: Clinical Study (1984)

Participants taking valerian experienced statistically significant improvements in anxiety, depression, difficulty falling asleep, and sleeping through the night compared with placebo in a randomized double-blind study of 78 elderly people suffering from sleep disturbances and nervous conditions. During the 2-week study, the subjects took either standardized valerian (2 tablets three times daily) or placebo. No psychotropic drugs were allowed during the course of the study. The results were based on a subjective set of symptoms (the von Zerssen scales of subjective well-being) reported by the participants and on NOSIE, an objective behavioral rating scale that was processed by a nurse. Within 7 days, the participants taking valerian extract showed improvements that were statistically significant on both scales of measurement. Improvements in falling asleep and sleeping through the night were statistically significant in the valerian group within 14 days of treatment, compared with placebo. No side effects were reported with valerian treatment.[8]

Depression: Clinical Study (1988)

A combination formula containing valerian and St. John's wort was just as effective as the antidepressant drug amitriptyline in treating symptoms of depression—with far fewer side effects. The multicenter, randomized, double-blind study involved 130 depressed people who took either 1 capsule of the herbal formula three times daily or 1 (25 mg) capsule of amitriptyline three times daily over a 6-week period. After 4 days of treatment, the dosage for both therapies was increased to 2 capsules three times daily, for 9 participants in the herb group and 5 in the antidepressant group. During the study, 80 percent of the herb group and 88 percent of the drug group experienced a minimum 50 percent reduction in depressive symptoms, as measured by the Hamilton Depression Rating Scale. Attending physicians rated the improvement in both groups as equivalent, according to the Clinical Global Impressions Scale. There were no significant side effects in the valerian/St. John's wort group. However, five patients in the drug group required a dosage reduction due to unpleasant side effects, including dizziness, dryness of the mouth, heart palpitations, and day-time fatigue.[4]

How It Works

Researchers haven't determined exactly how valerian produces its relaxing effects. However, in 1989, a groundbreaking *in vitro* study offered one convincing piece of the puzzle. This study suggested that valerian and its constituents promote relaxation by binding to benzodiazepine receptors in the brain. In the experiment, valerian displaced fluorodiazepam (a standard sedative drug) from an isolated benzodiazepine receptor.[9] This mode of action is similar to that of sedative drugs such as Valium, though valerian's binding activity is milder. In a more recent study involving 23 women with sleeping disorders, valerian produced electroencephalogram (EEG) readings similar to diazepam (Valium), but had fewer effects on alpha waves, which are associated with wakefulness. This may help explain why benzodiazepine drugs provide more immediate relief, while valerian is more effective and safer in the long term.[10]

In a pharmacological study, researchers found relatively high levels of gamma-aminobutyric acid (GABA), a neurotransmitter that directly blocks the arousal of brain centers, in valerian extract. However, scientists aren't certain how relevant this finding is, since GABA does not readily cross the blood-brain barrier. This makes it doubtful that the plant extract binds to GABA receptor sites in the brain, although it is possible that the GABA present in valerian acts on the nervous system in other ways.[11] Valerian also contains high concentrations of glutamine, an amino acid that *is* capable of crossing the blood-brain barrier. Glutamine is metabolized into GABA by GABA-ergic neurons in the brain. Researchers are currently evaluating the relevance of this finding in studies using live animals.[11]

Several other theories have been proposed to explain valerian's mode of action. Some researchers believe that two valerian constituents (valerenolic acid and acetylvalerenolic acid) inhibit the breakdown of GABA in the brain, thereby prolonging a state of relaxation.[12] Others have speculated that the valerian constituent hydroxypinoresinal inhibits the uptake of a neurotransmitter called serotonin (5-HT), an action similar to that of Prozac and related antidepressant drugs.[13]

Valerian's active ingredients are still unidentified. In the early 1990s, laboratory evidence began to refute the idea that volatile oils were responsible for the plant's effects at benzodiazepine receptors.[14] Valerian's sedative effects may be due to volatile oils, valepotriates, and unidentified water-soluble constituents.

MAJOR CONSTITUENTS

Volatile oils, valepotriates (including valtrate), valerenic acid

SAFETY

Valerian is considered safe for consumption when used appropriately.[15]

• **Side effects:** A few people experience mild stomach upset with valerian use. A very small percentage of people are actually stimulated by the plant. This may be due to differences in the method of preparation or dosage, or whether the extract was prepared from fresh or dried plant material. It is most likely a matter of individual (idiosyncratic) reactions, the same factor that makes synthetic sleep aids and other drugs ineffective for some people. Extracts made from fresh plants are generally considered to be the highest quality.[16] Traditional Chinese medicine holds that valerian's warming energy is inappropriate for extroverted, "yang"-type people who become further heated by the plant and therefore energized.[17]

• **Contraindications:** Do not take valerian before driving or operating machinery.[15]

• **Drug interactions:** Valerian may potentiate the effects of alcohol and other sedative drugs.

DOSAGE

Valerian can be used as a tea, tablet, capsule, or tincture. If you are using valerian for sleep, take the following dose 1 hour before bed. The dose can be divided in half for daytime anxiety, and can be used in combination with other calming herbs such as skullcap, lemon balm, or chamomile. Valerian may take 2 to 4 weeks to improve mood and sleep patterns in some individuals.

Note: When making valerian tea, be sure to keep the pot covered to prevent the therapeutic volatile oils from escaping. If you are a bath lover, you can brew a very strong pot of valerian tea, strain it, and add it to the warm bath water. (Just be careful not to fall asleep in the tub!)

• **Standardized extract:** 300 to 400 mg a day
• **Capsules/tablets:** 300 to 500 mg a day
• **Tincture:** $1/2$ to 1 teaspoon a day
• **Tea:** 1 to 2 cups a day

STANDARDIZATION

There is little agreement as to which is the most appropriate constituent for standardization. Some valerian extracts are standardized to 0.8 to 1 percent valerenic acid, some to 1 to 1.5 percent valtrate, and others to 0.5 percent essential oil.

REFERENCES

1. Leathwood PD, Chauffard F, Heck E, et al. Aqueous extract of valerian root (*Valeriana officinalis* L.) improves sleep quality in man. *Pharmacology, Biochemistry & Behavior* 1982; 17: 65–71.

2. Lindahl O, Lindwall L. Double blind study of a valerian preparation. *Pharmacology, Biochemistry & Behavior* 1989; 32: 1065–1066.

3. Seifert T. Therapeutic effects of valerian in nervous disorders: a field study. *Therapeutikon* 1988; 2: 94–98.

4. Kniebel R, Burchard JM. The treatment of depressive moods in medical practice [in German]. *Zeitschrift Allgemeiner Medizin* 1988; 64: 689–696.

5. Steger W. A randomized, double-blind study to compare the effectiveness of a plant-based combination of metabolic substances to a synthetic antidepressant in depressive states [in German]. *Zeitschrift Allgemeiner Medizin* 1985; 61: 914–918.

6. Bourin M, Bougerol T, Guitton B, et al. A combination of plant extracts in the treatment of outpatients with adjustment disorder with anxious mood: controlled study versus placebo. *Fundamental Clinical Pharmacology* 1997; 11: 127–132.

7. Vorbach EU, Görtelmeyer R, Brüning J. Therapy for insomnia: efficacy and tolerability of a valerian preparation [in German]. *Psychopharmakotherapie* 1996; 3 (3): 109–115.

8. Kamm-Kohl AV, Jansen W, Brockmann P. Modern valerian therapy of nervous disorders in elderly patients [in German]. *Medwelt* 1984; 35: 1450–1454.

9. Holzl J, Godau P. Receptor binding studies with *Valeriana officinalis* on the benzodiazepine receptor. *Planta Medica* 1989; 55: 642.

10. Schulz V, Hübner WD, Ploch M. Clinical trials with phyto-psychopharmacological agents. *Phytomedicine* 1997; 4 (4): 379–387.

11. Santos MS, Ferreira F, Faro C, et al. The amount of GABA present in aqueous extracts of valerian is sufficient to account for (H)GABA release in synaptosomes. *Planta Medica* 1994; 60: 475–476.

12. Riedel E, Hansel R, Ehrke G. Inhibition of aminobutyric acid catabolism by valerenic acid derivatives [in German]. *Planta Medica* 1982; 46: 219–220.

13. Wong AHC, Smith M, Boon HS, et al. Herbal remedies in psychiatric practice. *Archives of General Psychiatry* 1998; 55: 1033–1044.

14. Mennini T, Bernasconi P, Bombardelli E, et al. In vitro study on the interaction of extracts and pure compounds from *Valeriana officinalis* roots with GABA,

benzodiazepine and barbiturate receptors in rat brain. *Fitoterapia* 1993; 64: 291–300.

15. McGuffin M, Hobbs C, Upton R, Goldberg A, eds. *American Herbal Products Association Botanical Safety Handbook.* Boca Raton and New York: CRC Press LLC, 1997.

16. Foster S, Tyler V. *Tyler's Honest Herbal,* 4th ed. New York and London: Haworth Herbal Press, 1999: 377–379.

17. Tierra M. *Planetary Herbology.* Santa Fe, NM: Lotus Press 1988: 353.

Vitex (Chasteberry)

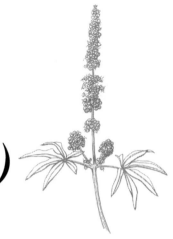

VITEX AGNUS-CASTUS
VERBENACEAE

State of Knowledge: Five-Star Rating System

Clinical (human) research	✶✶✶
Laboratory research	✶✶✶
History of use / traditional use	✶✶✶✶✶
Safety record	✶✶✶✶
International acceptance	✶✶✶✶

PART USED: *Berry*

PRIMARY USES

- *Female reproductive system health*
- *Premenstrual syndrome (PMS)*
- *Heavy or frequent menstrual cycles*
- *Absence of menstruation (amenorrhea)*
- *Certain types of infertility*
- *Milk production in nursing women (lactation)*
- *Menopause (traditional)*

As one of the oldest medicinal plants, vitex attests to the fact that women have a long history of dealing with menstrual cramps, imperfect cycles, and other women's health issues. As early as the fourth century B.C., Hippocrates recommended vitex berries steeped in red wine to help support female reproductive health. Today, clinical studies are revealing that vitex may be useful in treating PMS and other menstrual problems, as well as uterine fibroids, breast tenderness, low milk flow in nursing women, and even infertility.

Although studies demonstrate that vitex has the ability to affect and regulate hormone levels, the plant does not actually contain hormones. Like many herbs, vitex works more indirectly than drug therapies, in this case by acting on the pituitary gland to help the body regain its own natural hormonal balance.

HISTORY

As the common name "chasteberry" suggests, vitex has a historical reputation for "repressing the ardors of Venus." This use appears to be based more in ritual and wishful thinking than scientific fact. Rooted in Greek mythology, the association with chastity was later adopted by the Christian church. Even today, the colorful symbolism continues in Italy, where vitex flowers are strewn at the feet of novice monks and nuns. The other common name for vitex, "monk's pepper," refers to the tradition of sprinkling the ground herb on food to quell the passion and to literally spice up monastery life!

In the Mediterranean, vitex has been used for treating gynecological problems for more than 2,500 years. During the late 1800s, American physicians discovered the medicinal value of the plant and began prescribing it to women with menstrual disorders and low milk production during nursing. By 1950, German researchers were actively conducting scientific studies to find out how vitex works.

INTERNATIONAL STATUS

Vitex is approved for the treatment of irregular menstrual cycles, premenstrual prob-

lems, and mastodynia (breast tenderness) by Germany's Commission E.

BOTANY

Vitex is a water-loving shrub that grows along stream beds and riverbanks throughout the southeastern United States. Native to the Mediterranean and western Asia, the plant can now be found throughout Europe, where it is also raised commercially. Predominantly a woman's herb, vitex has elegant finger-shaped leaves, spikes of pretty violet flowers, and dark purple, aromatic berries the size of peppercorns. As monks discovered centuries ago, vitex berries smell and taste something like freshly ground pepper.

BENEFITS

- Helps resolve PMS symptoms, irregular cycles, and heavy or frequent periods by increasing progesterone levels and decreasing prolactin levels
- Often helps in cases of infertility caused by hormonal imbalances
- Increases the flow of milk in breastfeeding women
- May help during menopause, especially when there is a mixture of PMS and menopause symptoms

SCIENTIFIC SUPPORT

In the past 40 years, research has focused mainly on the use of vitex in PMS and other menstrual difficulties. Other large-scale, uncontrolled studies have reported favorable results in treating uterine fibroids, breast pain, and infertility caused by deficient progesterone levels. Several clinical studies have also confirmed the age-old use of vitex for increasing the flow of milk in nursing mothers. In a large study, 353 new mothers with poor milk production experienced significant improvement with vitex after 7 days, compared with 102 women taking vitamin B_1 and 362 taking placebo.[1] Researchers also report that vitex has demonstrated beneficial effects on hormonally induced acne.[2] Although no studies have been conducted in menopausal women, vitex is often recommended by European health-care practitioners for "the change of life."

SPECIFIC STUDIES

Premenstrual Syndrome: Clinical Study (1997)

Vitex was superior to pyridoxine (vitamin B_6) in relieving symptoms of PMS in a randomized, double-blind, controlled study of 127 women. Subjects received either one capsule containing 3.5 to 4.2 mg dried vitex extract plus one placebo capsule, or two 100-mg capsules of pyridoxine for three

menstrual cycles. Compared with the pyridoxine group, those taking vitex had a greater reduction in typical PMS symptoms, including breast tenderness, edema (swelling), tension, headache, constipation, and depression, according to the Premenstrual Tension Syndrome scale. Overall, 77 percent of the vitex group reported improvement, compared with 61 percent of those taking pyridoxine.

Eighty percent of supervising physicians felt that both treatments provided "adequate" efficacy. However, 25 percent rated vitex treatment as "excellent" according to the Clinical Global Impression scale, compared with only 12 percent who gave that rating to pyridoxine. Minor side effects, including headache, gastrointestinal and lower abdominal complaints, and skin problems, were reported by 5 women in the pyridoxine group and 12 in the vitex group. Although women wishing to conceive were excluded at the beginning of the study, 5 participants in the vitex group became pregnant during the course of the trial.[3]

Premenstrual Syndrome and Menstrual Disorders: Clinical Study (1994)

In an uncontrolled study of women experiencing menstrual disorders or PMS, symptoms resolved completely in 29 percent of subjects and improved significantly in an additional 52 percent after treatment with vitex. The 551 women in the study took 40 drops of standardized vitex extract daily for periods of time ranging from 1 week to 19 months. The average length of treatment was four menstrual cycles. Within the first 4 weeks, 32 percent of participants demonstrated improvement. The majority of subjects (84 percent) showed improvement by the end of the third cycle. There were minor side effects in just 5 percent of the women. Researchers also noted that 42 percent of 33 women with infertility problems became pregnant while taking vitex.[4]

Breast Pain: Clinical Study (1997)

Women taking vitex experienced a statistically significant reduction in breast pain compared with placebo, in a randomized, double-blind study of 104 subjects. All of the women in the trial had suffered from breast pain for at least three menstrual cycles and approximately half demonstrated borderline normal or elevated levels of prolactin prior to treatment. Participants took vitex as a liquid extract (30 drops of vitex two times daily plus 1 placebo tablet) or as a tablet (1 Vitex tablet plus 30 drops of placebo two times daily). The control group took 30 drops of placebo two times daily plus an additional placebo tablet.

By the second treatment cycle, the two vitex groups demonstrated statistically significant reductions in breast pain compared with the placebo group. Effectiveness was measured using the Visual Linear Analog Pain Scale. By the end of the 3-month study, those taking vitex also reported improvement in other premenstrual problems, including abdominal complaints, edema, headaches, and psychological symptoms. Levels of the hormone prolactin fell significantly and estrogen (estradiol) levels declined slightly in the vitex group, compared to those taking placebo. Researchers noted that the average prolactin decrease in this study was similar to that seen in a study of women who were given the drug bromocriptine for breast pain. Levels of progesterone, follicle-stimulating hormone, and luteinizing hormone remained unchanged. Mild side effects such as stomach upset and nausea were reported in a small percentage of women, but they occurred just as frequently in the placebo group.[5]

Menstrual Disorders: Clinical Study (1990)

Nearly 90 percent of women taking vitex experienced complete or significant improvement in menstrual disorders such as PMS during a large-scale study of 1,571 women. Prior to the study, all of the women had inadequate ovarian function due to low progesterone and elevated estrogen levels. The women underwent treatment for an average of 4.5 months, taking 40 drops of standardized vitex extract daily. The efficacy of treatment was rated as "very good," "good," or "satisfactory" in 90 percent of subjects, according to physicians' reports. There were minor side effects in just 2 percent of participants.[2]

HOW IT WORKS

Vitex works indirectly to modify the body's balance of progesterone and estrogen, rather than having a direct hormonal effect. Pharmacological investigations show that it acts on the hypothalamus and pituitary gland, which are responsible for regulating the body's hormones. Specifically, vitex stimulates the pituitary to increase the production of luteinizing hormone (LH), resulting in higher levels of progesterone during the second phase of a woman's menstrual cycle (the luteal phase). When there is a progesterone deficiency, estrogen continues to dominate the luteal phase of the cycle, contributing to a variety of female problems such as heavy periods and PMS.[6] Clinical studies have shown an increase in progesterone levels during vitex therapy.[7]

In clinical trials, vitex also lowered levels of a third hormone, prolactin.[5,7] In excess, prolactin can create breast tenderness, disturbances in the menstrual cycle, and even infertility. Prolactin levels are further increased during stress of any kind. In one large clinical study, low progesterone levels and high prolactin levels were diagnosed as the cause of infertility in 62 percent of 753 women.[8] Vitex decreases prolactin levels by binding directly to dopamine receptors in the pituitary gland, according to in vitro and animal research. So far, scientists have identified three dopaminergic compounds in vitex that prevent the release of prolactin.[9]

MAJOR CONSTITUENTS

Flavonoids, iridoids (agnuside and aucubin)

SAFETY

Clinical studies have shown that vitex is reasonably safe, even when taken for extensive periods of time.

- **Side effects:** Side effects are rare but can include minor skin irritations.[10,11] Stomach upset, nausea, headaches, and other minor complaints were reported by 2 to 5 percent of women in clinical studies.
- **Contraindications:** Vitex may counteract the effectiveness of birth control pills. Although generally not recommended during pregnancy, vitex has been used to prevent miscarriage in the first trimester for women with progesterone insufficiency.[10]

- **Drug interactions:** Do not combine vitex with dopamine-receptor antagonists.[11]

DOSAGE

Vitex can be taken as a tincture, capsule, tablet, or tea. Although many women notice results within two menstrual cycles, it can take more time to resolve long-standing health issues. For permanent results, health practitioners often recommend taking vitex for 6 months to 1 year. During the first month of treatment, the length of the cycle may temporarily shorten or lengthen before stabilizing.

- **Standardized extract:** The dosage used in clinical studies was 40 drops of standardized vitex extract taken once a day.
- **Capsules/tablets:** One 650-mg capsule/tablet up to three times a day.[12]
- **Tincture:** 40 drops up to three times a day.
- **Tea:** 1 cup two to three times a day.

STANDARDIZATION

Typical standardization for vitex is to 0.6 percent agnuside.

REFERENCES

1. Mohr H. Clinical investigations of means to increase lactation [in German]. *Deutsche Medizinische Wochenschrift* 1954; 79(41): 1513–1516.
2. Feldmann HU, Albrecht M, Lamertz M, et al. The treatment of corpus luteum insufficiency and premenstrual syndrome experience in a multicentre study under practice conditions. *Gyne* 1990; 42: 1–5.
3. Lauritzen CH, Reuter HD, Repges R, et al. Treatment of premenstrual tension syndrome with *Vitex agnus castus*: controlled, double-blind study versus pyridoxine. *Phytomedicine* 1997; 4(3): 183–189.
4. Peters-Welte C, Diessen M, Albrecht K. Menstrual abnormalities and PMS: *Vitex agnus-castus* in a study of application [in German]. *Gynakologie* 1994; 7: 49–52.
5. Wuttke W, Splitt G, Gorkow C, et al. Treatment of cyclical mastalgia with a medication containing *Agnus castus*: results of a randomised, placebo-controlled, double-blind study [in German] *Geburtshilfe und Frauenheilkunde* 1997; 57: 569–574.
6. Brown DJ. Vitex agnus castus: clinical mongraph. *Quarterly Review of Natural Medicine*, Summer 1994; 111–120.
7. Milewicz A, Gejdel E, Sworen H, et al. *Vitex agnus-castus* extract in the treatment of luteal phase defects due to latent hyperprolactinaemia: results of a randomized placebo-controlled double blind study [in German]. *Arzneimittel-Forschung* 1993; 43 (2): 752–756.

8. Winterhoff H. *Vitex agnus-castus* (chaste tree): pharmacological and clinical data. In: Lawson L and Bauer R, eds. *Phytomedicines of Europe: Chemistry and Biological Activity.* Washington DC: American Chemical Society, 1998.

9. Wuttke W, Gorkow CH, Jarry H. Dopaminergic compounds in *Vitex agnus castus* [In German]. In: Loew D, ed. *Phytopharmaka: Forschung und Klinische Anwendung.* Darmstadt: Steinkopff, 1995.

10. McGuffin M, Hobbs C, Upton R, et al., eds. *American Herbal Products Association Botanical Safety Handbook.* Boca Raton, FL: CRC Press, 1997.

11. Blumenthal M, Busse W, Goldberg A, et al., eds. *The Complete German Commission E Monographs.* Austin, TX: The American Botanical Council; Boston: Integrative Medical Communications, 1998.

12. Foster S. *101 Medicinal Herbs.* Loveland, CO: Interweave Press, 1998.

Part III

Appendixes

APPENDIX A

Recommended Reading List

For book purchases, check the Herb Research Foundation's website bookstore at http://www.herbs.org or contact the American Botanical Council at (800) 373-7105 or http://www.herbalgram.org.

GENERAL HERB REFERENCES

Brown DJ. *Herbal Prescriptions for Better Health: Your Everyday Guide to Prevention, Treatment, and Care.* Rocklin, CA: Prima Publishing, 1996.

Foster S. *Herbs for Your Health: A Handy Pocket Guide For Knowing and Using 50 Common Herbs.* Loveland, CO: Interweave Press, 1996.

Foster S. *101 Medicinal Herbs: An Illustrated Guide.* Loveland, CO: Interweave Press, 1999.

Foster S, Tyler V. *Tyler's Honest Herbal: A Sensible Guide to the Use of Herbs and Related Remedies,* 4th ed. New York and London: The Haworth Herbal Press, 1999.

Gladstar R. *Herbs for Longevity and Well-Being.* Pownal, VT: Storey Books, 1999.

Gladstar R. *Herbs for the Home Medicine Chest.* Pownal, VT: Storey Books, 1999.

Hobbs C. *Foundations of Health: The Liver and Digestive Herbal.* Capitola, CA: Botanica Press, 1992.

Hobbs C. *Handbook for Herbal Healing: A Concise Guide to Herbal Products.* Capitola, CA: Botanica Press, 1994.

Hobbs C. *Herbal Remedies for Dummies.* Foster City, CA: IDG Books Worldwide, 1998.

Hobbs C. *Natural Liver Therapy: Herbs and Other Natural Remedies for a Healthy Liver.* Capitola, CA: Botanica Press, 1993.

Hobbs C. *Stress and Natural Healing.* Loveland, CO: Interweave Press, 1997.

Hoffmann D. *The Complete Illustrated Holistic Herbal: A Safe and Practical Guide to Making and Using Herbal Remedies.* Boston: Element Books, 1996.

Hoffmann D. *The Herbal Handbook: A User's Guide to Medical Herbalism.* Rochester, VT: Healing Arts Press, 1988.

McIntyre A. *Herbs for Common Ailments: How to Use Familiar Herbs to Treat More Than 100 Health Problems.* New York: Fireside Books, 1992.

Murray M. *Natural Alternatives to Over the Counter and Prescription Drugs.* New York: William Morrow, 1994.

Murray M. *The Healing Power of Herbs: The Enlightened Person's Guide to the Wonders of Medicinal Plants.* Rocklin, CA: Prima Publishing, 1995.

Murray M, Pizzorno J. *Encyclopedia of Natural Medicine,* 2nd ed. Rocklin, CA: Prima Publishing, 1998.

Ody P. *Healing with Herbs: Simple Treatments for More Than 100 Common Ailments.* Pownal, VT: Storey Books, 1999.

Ody P. *Herbs for First Aid,* 2nd ed. Los Angeles: Keat's Publishing, 1999.

Pederson M. *Nutritional Herbology: A Reference Guide to Herbs*. Winona Lake, IN: Wendell Whitman, 1994.

Robbers JE, Tyler V. *Tyler's Herbs of Choice: The Therapeutic Use of Phytomedicinals*. New York and London: The Haworth Herbal Press, 1999.

Tierra M. *The Way of Herbs,* 4th ed. New York: Pocket Books, 1998.

Weil A. *Natural Health, Natural Medicine: A Comprehensive Manual for Wellness and Self Care*. Boston: Houghton Mifflin, 1990.

Willard T. *Wild Rose Scientific Herbal*. Alberta, Canada: Wild Rose College of Natural Healing, 1991.

TECHNICAL REFERENCES

Bisset NG, ed. *Herbal Drugs and Phytopharmaceuticals*. Boca Raton, FL: CRC Press, 1994.

Bruneton J. *Pharmacognosy, Phytochemistry, Medicinal Plants*. Paris: Lavoisier, 1995.

Chadha YR, ed. *The Wealth of India: A Dictionary of Indian Raw Materials and Industrial Products*. New Delhi: Publications and Information Directorate, CSIR, 1976.

De Smet PAGM. *Adverse Effects of Herbal Drugs*. 2 vols. New York: Springer-Verlag, 1993.

Duke J. *Handbook of Medicinal Herbs*. Boca Raton, FL: CRC Press, 1988.

Duke J. *Handbook of Phytochemical Constituents of GRAS Herbs and Other Economic Plants*. Boca Raton, FL: CRC Press, 1992.

Evans WC. *Trease and Evans' Pharmacognosy,* 13th ed. Philadelphia: Bailliere Tindall (Curtis Center), 1989.

Felter HW. *King's American Dispensatory*. Vol. 1 and 2. Portland, OR: Eclectic Medical Publications, 1983.

Goodman LS, Gilman A, Rall T, et al., eds. *Goodman and Gilman's The Pharmacological Basis of Therapeutics,* 8th ed. New York: McGraw Hill, 1990.

Hoffmann D. *The Information Sourcebook of Herbal Medicine*. Freedom, CA: The Crossing Press, 1994.

Lawson LD, Bauer R, eds. *Phytomedicines of Europe: Chemistry and Biological Activity*. Washington, DC: American Chemical Society, 1998.

Leung A, Foster S. *Encyclopedia of Common Natural Ingredients Used in Food, Drugs, and Cosmetics,* 2nd ed. New York: John Wiley and Sons, 1996.

Lewis WH. *Medical Botany, Plants Affecting Man's Health*. New York: Wiley and Sons, 1977.

Mabberly DJ. *The Plant Book*. New York: Press Syndicate of University of Cambridge, 1987.

Moerman D. *Medicinal Plants of Native America*. Vol. 1 and 2. Ann Arbor: Regent of the University of Michigan, Museum of Anthropology, 1986.

Reynolds J, ed. *Martindale: The Extra Pharmacopoeia,* 30th ed. London: The Pharmaceutical Press, 1993.

Tyler V. *Pharmacognosy,* 8th ed. Philadelphia: Lea and Febiger, 1981.

Upton R, ed. *American Herbal Pharmacopoeia Monographs*. (See appendix E for more information.)

Wagner H, Bladt S. *Plant Drug Analysis,* 2nd ed. Berlin and Heidelberg: Springer-Verlag, 1996.

Wagner H, Farnsworth NR. *Economic and Medicinal Plant Research*. San Diego: Academic Press, 1991.

REFERENCE GUIDES FOR PRACTITIONERS

Blumenthal M, Busse WR, Goldberg A, et al., eds. *The Complete German Commission E Monographs*. Austin, TX: American Botanical Council; Boston: Integrative Medicine Communications, 1998.

Bradley PR, ed. *British Herbal Compendium*. Vol 1. Dorset: British Herbal Medicine Association, 1992.

Bradley PR, ed. *British Herbal Pharmacopoeia*. Vol 1. Dorset: British Herbal Medicine Association, 1990.

McGuffin M, Hobbs C, Upton R, et al., eds. *American Herbal Products Association Botanical Safety Handbook*. Boca Raton, FL: CRC Press, 1997.

Miller LG, Murray WJ, eds. *Herbal Medicinals: A Clinician's Guide*. New York: Pharmaceutical Products Press, 1998.

Murray M, Werbach M. *Botanical Influences on Illness*. Tarzana, CA: Third Line Press, 1994.

Pierce A. *The American Pharmaceutical Association Practical Guide to Natural Medicine*. New York: William Morrow, 1999.

Pizzorno J. *A Textbook of Natural Medicine*. Vol. 1 and 2. Seattle: John Bastyr College Publications, 1993.

Schulz V. *Rational Phytotherapy: A Physician's Guide to Herbal Medicine,* 3rd ed. New York: Springer-Verlag, 1998.

Walker LP. *The Alternative Pharmacy*. Paramus, NJ: Prentice Hall, 1998.

Weiss RF. *Herbal Medicine*. Beaconsfield, England: Beaconsfield Publishers, 1988.

Werbach M. *Nutritional Influences on Illness*. New Canaan, CT: Keats Publishing, 1988.

Werbach M. *Nutritional Influences on Mental Illness*. Tarzana, CA: Third Line Press, 1991.

Willard T. *Textbook of Advanced Herbology*. Alberta, Canada: Wild Rose College of Natural Healing, 1992.

Willard T. *Textbook of Modern Herbology,* 2nd ed. Alberta, Canada: Wild Rose College of Natural Healing, 1993.

FIELD GUIDES

Angier B. *Field Guide to Edible Wild Plants*. Harrisburg, PA: Stackpole Books, 1974.

Angier B. *Field Guide to Medicinal Wild Plants*. Harrisburg, PA: Stackpole Books, 1978.

Foster S, Peterson RT, Duke J. *Field Guide to Medicinal Plants. Eastern and Central North America*. Boston: Houghton Mifflin, 1998.

Krochmal A. *A Field Guide to Medicinal Plants*. New York: New York Times Books, 1984.

Moore M. *Medicinal Plants of the Desert and Canyon West*. Santa Fe, NM: Museum of New Mexico Press, 1989.

Moore M. *Medicinal Plants of the Mountain West*. Santa Fe, NM: Museum of New Mexico Press, 1979.

Moore M. *Medicinal Plants of the Pacific West*. Santa Fe, NM: Red Crane Books, 1993.

Tilford G. *The EcoHerbalist's Fieldbook: Wildcrafting in the Mountain West*. Coner, MT: Mountain Weed Publishing, 1993.

Willard T. *Edible and Medicinal Plants of the Rocky Mountains and Neighbouring Territories*. Alberta, Canada: Wild Rose College of Natural Healing, 1992.

Women's Health

Crawford AM. *Herbal Menopause Book: Herbs, Nutrition, and Other Natural Therapies*, 2nd ed. Freedom, CA: The Crossing Press, 1997.

Crawford AM. *Herbal Remedies for Women: Discover Nature's Wonderful Secrets Just for Women!* Rocklin, CA: Prima Publishing, 1997.

Gladstar R. *Herbal Healing for Women: Simple Home Remedies for Women of All Ages*. New York: Fireside Books, 1993.

Hobbs C, Keville K. *Women's Herbs, Women's Health*. Loveland, CO: Interweave Press, 1998.

Hudson T. *Women's Encyclopedia of Natural Medicine*. Los Angeles: Keats Publishing, 1999.

McIntyre A. *The Complete Woman's Herbal: A Manual of Healing Herbs and Nutrition for Personal Well-Being and Family Care*. New York: Henry Holt, 1995.

Northrup C. *Women's Bodies, Women's Wisdom: Creating Physical and Emotional Health and Healing*. New York: Bantam Books, 1994.

Soule D. *A Woman's Book of Herbs: The Healing Power of Natural Remedies*. Secaucus, NJ: Citadel Press, 1998.

Weed S. *Breast Cancer? Breast Health! The Wise Woman Way*. Woodstock, NY: Ash Tree Publishing, 1996.

Weed S. *Healing Wise: A Wise Woman Herbal*. Woodstock, NY: Ash Tree Publishing, 1989.

Weed S. *Menopausal Years: The Wise Woman Way—Alternative Approaches for Women*. Woodstock, NY: Ash Tree Publishing, 1992.

Weed S. *Wise Woman Herbal for the Childbearing Years*. Woodstock, NY: Ash Tree Publishing, 1986.

Herbs for Children

Bove M. *Encyclopedia of Natural Healing for Infants and Children*. Los Angeles: Keat's Publishing, 1996.

Gladstar R. *Herbal Remedies For Children's Health*. Pownal, VT: Storey Books, 1999.

White LB, Mavor S. *Kids, Herbs, Health: Practical Solutions for Your Child's Health, from Birth to Puberty*. Loveland, CO: Interweave Press, 1998.

Zand J, Walton R, Rountree B. *Smart Medicine for a Healthier Child: A Practical A-to-Z Reference to Natural and Conventional Treatments for Infants and Children*. Garden City Park, NY: Avery Publishing Group, 1994.

Traditional Chinese Medicine

Beinfeld H, Korngold E. *Between Heaven and Earth: A Guide to Chinese Medicine*. New York: Ballantine Books, 1991.

Bensky D, Gamble A. *Chinese Herbal Medicine: Materia Medica*. Seattle: Eastland Press, 1993.

Kaptchuk T. *The Web That Has No Weaver: Understanding Chinese Medicine*. New York: St. Martin's Press, 1984.

Leung AY. *Chinese Herbal Remedies*. New York: Universe Books, 1984.

Tierra L. *The Herbs of Life*. Freedom, CA: Crossing Press, 1992.

AYURVEDIC MEDICINE

Chopra D. *Creating Health: How to Wake Up the Body's Intelligence*. New York: Houghton Mifflin, 1991.

Chopra D. *Perfect Digestion: The Key to Balanced Living*. New York: Three Rivers Press, 1995.

Chopra D. *Restful Sleep: The Complete Mind/Body Program for Overcoming Insomnia*. New York: Three Rivers Press, 1994.

Frawley D. *Ayurvedic Healing*. Sandy, UT: Passage Press, 1992.

Kapoor LD. *A Handbook of Ayurvedic Medicinal Plants*. Boca Raton, FL: CRC Press, 1990.

Lad V. *The Yoga of Herbs*. Santa Fe, NM: Lotus Press, 1990.

Svoboda RE. *Ayurveda: Life, Health, and Longevity*. New York: Penguin Press, 1992.

Tirtha SS. *The Ayurvedic Encyclopedia: Natural Secrets to Healing, Prevention, and Longevity*. Bayville, NY: Ayurveda Holistic Center Press, 1998.

CULTIVATING HERBS

Duke JA, duCellier JL. *CRC Handbook of Alternative Cash Crops*. Boca Raton, FL: CRC Press, 1993.

Foster S. *Herbal Bounty! The Gentle Art of Herb Culture*. Layton, UT: Gibbs M. Smith, 1984.

Hartung T. *Growing 101 Herbs that Heal: Gardening Techniques, Recipes, and Remedies*. Pownal, VT: Storey Books, 2000.

McIntyre A. *The Medicinal Garden: How to Grow and Use Your Own Medicinal Herbs*. New York: Henry Holt, 1997.

Miller RA. *The Potential of Herbs As a Cash Crop*. Berkeley, CA: Ten Speed Press, 1992.

Shores S. *Growing and Selling Fresh-Cut Herbs*. Pownal, VT: Storey Books, 1999.

Sturdivant L, Blakley T. *Medicinal Herbs in the Garden, Field, and Marketplace*. Friday Harbor, WA: San Juan Naturals, 1999.

HERBAL MEDICINE-MAKING

Hobbs C. *Handmade Medicines: Simple Recipes for Herbal Health*. Loveland, CO: Interweave Press, 1998.

St. Claire D. *The Herbal Medicine Cabinet*. Berkeley, CA: Celestial Arts, 1997.

SINGLE HERBS

Bergner P. *The Healing Power of Garlic: The Enlightened Person's Guide to Nature's Most Versatile Plant*. Rocklin, CA: Prima Publishing, 1996.

Bergner P. *The Healing Power of Ginseng & the Tonic Herbs: The Enlightened Person's Guide*. Rocklin, CA: Prima Publishing, 1996.

Foster S. *Echinacea: Nature's Immune Enhancer*. Rochester, VT: Healing Arts Press, 1991.

Fulder S. *The Book of Ginseng*. Rochester, VT: Healing Arts Press, 1993.

Hobbs C. *Echinacea: The Immune Herb*, 3rd ed. Capitola, CA: Botanica Press, 1992.

Hobbs C. *Ginkgo, Elixir of Youth*. Capitola, CA: Botanica Press, 1991.

Hobbs C. *Medicinal Mushrooms: An Exploration of Tradition, Healing, and Culture.* Santa Cruz, CA: Botanica Press, 1995.

Hobbs C. *Milk Thistle: The Liver Herb*, 2nd ed. Capitola, CA: Botanica Press, 1992.

Hobbs C. *Reishi Mushroom.* Seattle: Sylvan Press, 1995.

Hobbs C. *Valerian: The Relaxing and Sleep Herb.* Capitola, CA: Botanica Press, 1993.

Hobbs C. *Vitex: The Women's Herb.* Capitola, CA: Botanica Press, 1993.

Koch HP, Lawson LD, eds. *Garlic: The Science and Therapeutic Application of* Allium sativum *L. and Related Species,* 2nd ed. Baltimore: Williams and Wilkins, 1996.

Lau B. *Garlic and You: The Modern Medicine.* Vancouver, Canada: Apple Publishing, 1997.

Schulick P. *Ginger: Common Spice and Wonder Drug,* 2nd ed. Brattleboro, VT: Herbal Free Press Ltd, 1994.

AROMATHERAPY

Buckle J. *Clinical Aromatherapy in Nursing.* San Diego: Singular Publishing Group, 1997.

England A. *Aromatherapy for Mother and Baby: Natural Healing with Essential Oils during Pregnancy and Early Motherhood.* Rochester, VT: Healing Arts Press, 1994.

Keville K, Green M. *Aromatherapy: A Complete Guide to the Healing Art.* Freedom, CA: The Crossing Press, 1995.

Lavabre M. *Aromatherapy Workbook.* Rochester, VT: Healing Arts Press, 1990.

Lawless J. *The Illustrated Encyclopedia of Essential Oils.* Rockport, MA: Element Books, 1995.

Schnaubelt K. *Advanced Aromatherapy: The Science of Essential Oil Therapy.* Rochester, VT: Healing Arts Press, 1998.

Schnaubelt K. *Medical Aromatherapy: Healing with Essential Oils.* Berkeley, CA: North Atlantic Books, 1999.

Tisserand R, Balacs T. *Essential Oil Safety: A Guide for Health Care Professionals.* New York: Churchill Livingstone, 1995.

NATURAL HEALTH CARE FOR PETS

de Bairacli Levy J. *The Complete Herbal Handbook for Farm and Stable.* Boston: Faber and Faber, 1991.

de Bairacli Levy J. *The Complete Herbal Handbook for the Dog and Cat.* Boston: Faber and Faber, 1991.

Pitcairn R. *Natural Health for Dogs and Cats.* Emmaus, PA: Rodale Press, 1982.

Stein D. *Natural Healing for Dogs and Cats.* Freedom, CA: Crossing Press, 1993.

Stein D. *The Natural Remedy Book for Dogs and Cats.* Freedom, CA: Crossing Press, 1994.

OTHER TOPICS

DeLuca D. *Botanica Erotica: Arousing Body, Mind, and Spirit.* Rochester, VT: Healing Arts Press, 1998.

Gladstar R. *Herbal Remedies for Men's Health.* Pownal, VT: Storey Books, 1999.

Gladstar R. *Herbs for Natural Beauty.* Pownal, VT: Storey Books, 1999.

Gladstar R. *Herbs for Reducing Stress and Anxiety.* Pownal, VT: Storey Books, 1999.

Hoffmann D. *An Elder's Herbal: Natural Techniques for Health and Vitality.* Rochester, VT: Healing Arts Press, 1993.

Hoffmann D. *An Herbal Guide to Stress Relief.* Rochester, VT: Healing Arts Press, 1991.

APPENDIX B

Recommended Periodicals

GENERAL

The Business of Herbs
439 Ponderosa Way
Jémez Springs, NM 87025-8025

The Canadian Journal of Herbalism
11 Winthrop Place
Stoney Creek, Ontario, Canada L8G 3M3

The Herb Companion
Interweave Press, Inc.
201 East 4th Street
Loveland, CO 80537
Phone: (970) 669-7672;
(800) 272-2193

The Herb Quarterly
Long Mountain Press
PO Box 548
Boiling Springs, PA 17007
Phone: (717) 245-2764

Herbs for Health
Interweave Press, Inc.
201 East 4th Street
Loveland, CO 80537
Phone: (970) 669-7672;
(800) 272-2193
(Also available with Herb Research
Foundation membership)

Robyn's Recommended Reading
6101 Shadow Circle Drive
Bozeman, MT 59715
Phone: (406) 585-8006
E-Mail: rrr@wtp.net
Website: http://www.wtp.net/~rrr

TECHNICAL

Alternative Agriculture News
9200 Edmonston Road, Suite 117
Greenbelt, MD 20770
Phone: (301) 441-8777

American Journal of Alternative Agriculture
9200 Edmonston Road, Suite 117
Greenbelt, MD 20770
Phone: (301) 441-8777

Economic Botany
PO Box 1897
Lawrence, KS 66044-8897
Phone: (800) 627-0629

HerbalGram
PO Box 144345
Austin, TX 78714-4345
Phone: (512) 926-4900
(Also available with Herb Research
Foundation membership)

The Herb, Spice, and Medicinal Plant Digest
Department of Plant and Soil Sciences
Stockbridge Hall,
University of Massachusetts
Amherst, MA 01003
Phone: (413) 545-2349

Journal of Ethnopharmacology
Elsevier Science
PO Box 945
New York, NY 10159-0945
Phone: (212) 633-3730;
(888) 4ES-INFO

Journal of Natural Products
American Chemical Society
PO Box 3337
Columbus, OH 43210
Phone: (614) 447-3776;
(800) 333-9511

Pharmaceutical Biology
Swets & Zeitlinger
PO Box 825
2160 SZ Lisse
The Netherlands

Phytomedicine
Stockton Press
The Subscription Dept.
Houndmills, Basingstoke
Hants RG 21 6XS
United Kingdom
Phone: (800) 747-3187

FOR PRACTITIONERS

Alternative and Complementary Therapies
Mary Ann Liebert, Inc.
2 Madison Avenue
Larchmont, NY 10538
Phone: (914) 834-3100

Alternative Therapies in Health and Medicine
Innovision Communications
101 Columbia
Aliso Viejo, CA 92656
Phone: (800) 899-1712

Australian Journal of Medical Herbalism
PO Box 61 Broadway
Australia 2007

International Journal of Integrative Medicine
PO Box 12496
Green Bay, WI 54307-2496
Phone: (920) 434-8884

Medical Herbalism
PO Box 20512
Boulder, CO 80308
Phone: (303) 541-9552
Website: www.medherb.com

Nutrition Science News
1301 Spruce Street
Boulder, CO 80302
Phone: (303) 939-8440

Quarterly Review of Natural Medicine
Natural Products Research Consultants, Inc.
600 First Avenue, Suite 205
Seattle, WA 98104
Phone: (206) 623-2520

APPENDIX C

Library Resources

Initial literature search sources should include local university libraries that are linked through the ILL (Inter-Library Loan) program, which provides copies of articles from other institutions. Many libraries also have technical research services that can access online databases such as MEDLINE (National Library of Medicine). Private research firms also perform this service. Libraries can provide citations and abstracts of articles, and also full-text document retrieval. For more ideas, see *The Information Sourcebook of Herbal Medicine* by David Hoffmann (Freedom, CA: Crossing Press, 1994).

Herb Research Foundation

1007 Pearl Street, Suite 200
Boulder, CO 80302
Phone: (303) 449-2265
Website: http://www.herbs.org

HRF is a specialty library with more than 200,000 articles on file about the clinical research pharmacology, toxicology, chemistry, horticulture, analysis, and history of herbs used in food and for health care. The HRF research department provides custom botanical research, abstracts of scientific articles on herbs, full-text documents, and online research services.

Lloyd Library

917 Plum Street
Cincinnati, Ohio 45202
Phone: (513) 721-3707
Website: http://www.libraries.uc.edu/Lloyd

Possibly the world's most extensive collection of botanical reference material, the Lloyd Library is a private library containing approximately 200,000 volumes, 600 domestic and foreign journal titles, and many other publications. It has many rare and antique holdings as well as one of the largest collections of pharmacopoeias in the world. Open to the public, no charge, 8:30 A.M. to 4:00 P.M., Monday through Friday.

National Agricultural Library, USDA

10301 Baltimore Boulevard, Room 111
Beltsville, MD 20705
Reference: (301) 504-5479
Circulation Desk/Journals: (301) 504-5755

The National Agricultural Library provides extensive literature searches and bibliographies on various herb-related topics, offering current information to growers, medicinal herbalists, marketers, and others.

Internet Resources

Agricola

http://www.nalusda.gov/general_info/
agricola/agricola.html
Database of agricultural information on a wide
variety of plants, including herbs.

**Algy's Home Page—
Medicinal**

http://www.algy.com/herb/
Very comprehensive collection of herb information. Voted as being in the top five percent of
herb related websites.

American Botanical Council

http://www.herbalgram.org
Bookstore on site, book reviews; publisher of
HerbalGram, a quarterly journal co-produced
with the Herb Research Foundation.

American Herbalists Guild

http://www.healthy.com/herbalists
The official website of the American Herbalists
Guild, which represents professional herbalists
in the United States.

Ask Dr. Weil

http://www.drweil.com
This site, managed by TIME, Inc., provides a directory of health-care practitioners and information on health topics, including herbs.

**Center for Complementary and
Alternative Medicine**

http://www-camra.ucdavis.edu/
This site, maintained by the University of California at Davis, provides information on alternative therapies for the treatment of asthma and
allergies, with a focus on herbal medicine and
acupuncture.

**Columbia Medical School's
Database Links**

http://cpmcnet.columbia.edu/dept/
rosenthal/
Our friends at the Rosenthal Center at Columbia University have compiled an impressive
and useful list of the online databases in bio-
medicine *and* alternative and complementary
medicine.

**Garden Gate Glossary of
Botanical Names**

http://www.prairienet.org/ag/garden/botrts
.htm
More than 1,000 root words of botanical names
with their English meanings.

Health World

http://www.healthworld.com/
Part of an ambitious health Internet site offering
a wide range of information, including some
links to herb information resources.

Henriette's Herbal Homepage

http://metalab.unc.edu/herbmed/
This site is from the Webmaster of the Sunsite Herbal Collection at the University of North Carolina. It includes a very rich collection of links to other sites.

Herbal Hall

http://www.herb.com/herbal.htm
Contains lists of schools, herbalists, and online herbal information. Features Michael Moore's Herbal-Medical Dictionary.

HerbMed

http://www.amfoundation.org/herbmed.htm
An interactive herbal database providing hyperlinked access to scientific data underlying the use of herbs for health.

HerbNet

Sponsored by the Herb Growing and Marketing Network. Features *The Herbalist* newsletter, lists of courses, associations, and software. All this and music, too.

Herb Research Foundation

http://www.herbs.org
A comprehensive, award-winning site for herb information, featuring the latest science, political, business, and international news from the world of herbs. You can browse recommended links, view herbs in the photo gallery, order scientific papers, speak out on herbal topics, and ask herb questions online. Herb "green-papers" and research reviews highlight specific herbs and their medicinal uses.

Medical Herbalism

http://www.medherb.com
The electronic version of Paul Bergner's newsletter of the same name. Also includes a discussion board, bookstore, adverse events reporting site, and many other features.

Michael Moore's Home Page

http://www.rt66.com/hrbmoore/HOMEPAGE/
Features an excellent collection of medicinal plant images. Site is managed by the director of the Southwest School of Botanical Medicine.

National Institutes of Health Dietary Supplement Database

http://www.nal.usda.gov/fnic/IBIDS
Produced by NIH's Office of Dietary Supplements in conjunction with the U.S. Department of Agriculture's Food and Nutrition Information Center of the National Agricultural Library, this database contains bibliographic records and abstracts on vitamins, minerals, and herbal dietary supplements.

New York Botanical Garden

http://www.nybg.org
One of the United States' foremost botanical gardens, also accessible in virtual form.

Paracelsus

http://www.teleport.com/~ibis/paracib.html
This site provides valuable information about the integrated use of a wide range of therapeutic methods in health care. The information is updated frequently by teams of clinicians and researchers from many diverse fields.

Phytonet

http://www.ex.ac.uk/phytonet/
The home of the European Scientific Cooperative on Phytomedicine (ESCOP) provides a forum (in five languages) for reporting adverse reactions to herbal products.

Phytopharmacognosy

http://www.phytochemistry.freeserve.co.uk
Professional herb information, including the Internet mailing list by the same name, which carries on a rather overwhelming discussion (sometimes dozens of messages per day) concerning various botanical topics.

UK Herb Society Home Page

http://sunsite.unc.edu/herbmed/HerbSociety/
Information on select herbs, conservation, events, and herbal legislation in the United Kingdom.

University of Texas Center for Alternative Medicine Research

http://www.sph.uth.tmc.edu/utcam/
A site dedicated to investigating the effectiveness of complementary therapies used for cancer prevention and treatment. Includes background information and a review of the available scientific research, including references and annotated bibliographies. There is also a section that describes clinical studies being conducted at the Center.

USDA: Phytochemical and Ethnobotanical Databases

http://www.ars-grin.gov/duke
This site contains Dr. James Duke's searchable databases. You can search by plant, chemical, activity, or ethnobotany.

Herb Organizations and Associations

American Botanical Council
PO Box 144345
Austin, TX 78714-4345
Phone: (512) 926-4900
Website: http://www.herbalgram.org

This nonprofit herbal research and education organization provides public education about herbs and promotes the safe and effective use of medicinal plants. The ABC bookstore offers an extensive selection of technical and popular books on herbs and other plants. ABC is the co-publisher, along with the Herb Research Foundation, of the peer-reviewed journal *HerbalGram*.

American Herb Association
PO Box 1673
Nevada City, CA 95959
Phone: (916) 265-9552

Public education about herbs and herbal products. Includes nationwide network of current data and resources for members. Laboratory projects, herb garden, library, quarterly newsletter.

American Herbal Pharmacopoeia
PO Box 5159
Santa Cruz, CA 95063
Phone: (831) 461-6335

The AHP is a nonprofit education organization dedicated to producing comprehensive, peer-reviewed monographs on botanical medi-

cines. Each monograph provides complete quality control and therapeutic information, including a thorough review of the available clinical and pharmacological literature; macroscopic, microscopic, and chemical identification; substantiated analytical methods; dosages; complete safety profile; substantiated structure/function claims; historical use; and botany.

American Herbal Products Association
8484 Georgia Avenue, Suite 370
Silver Springs, MD 20910
Phone: (301) 588-1171
Website: AHPA@ix.netcom.com

Current information on legal and regulatory issues affecting herbal products. Services include promotion and research activities, compiled statistics, advertising, newsletter, and membership directory.

American Herbalists Guild
PO Box 70
Roosevelt, UT 84066
Phone: (435) 722-8434
Website: http://www.healthy.net/herbalists

Professional body of herbal practitioners, educators, students, and supporters. Professional members (practitioners) undergo a peer-reviewed acceptance process. Membership includes a quarterly newsletter, *The Herbalist*.

The AHG sponsors annual seminars in different parts of the United States and publishes a comprehensive directory of herbal education programs ($10).

Herb Research Foundation

1007 Pearl Street, Suite 200
Boulder, CO 80302
Phone: (303) 449-2265
Website: http://www.herbs.org

With a primary goal of public education, HRF is a nonprofit international education and research organization that collects and disseminates accurate and reliable scientific information about herbs. A valuable resource for consumers, researchers, manufacturers, reporters, and writers. Membership includes a choice of publications (*HerbalGram* or *Herbs For Health*) and discounts on HRF services, including custom botanical research, herb information packets, and the Natural Healthcare Hotline.

Herb Society of America

9019 Kirtland-Chardon Road
Kirtland, Ohio 44094
Phone: (440) 256-0514

An organization for those interested in the diverse uses of herbs (not necessarily medical), including botanical and horticultural research as well as culinary and economic uses. Herb Society of America holds an annual convention and publishes a bimonthly newsletter and membership directory.

International Herb Association

PO Box 206
Mechanicsburg, PA 17055-0206
Phone: (717) 697-1500

Large trade organization for growers, retailers, wildcrafters, wholesalers, researchers, and extension service personnel. Members receive a bimonthly newsletter, special seminars and workshops, and discounts on conference fees and trade show booths.

The Northeast Herb Association

PO Box 10
Newport, NY 13416
(315) 845-6060

Members receive a triannual newsletter and membership directory and are welcome to attend an annual meeting to share with other Northeast herbalists.

Office of Small Scale Agriculture

Cooperative State Research
Education and Extension Service/USDA,
Stop 2244
Washington, DC 20250-2244
Phone: (202) 401-1805

Specialty information for small-scale and specialty agricultural growers and marketers, including information pertaining to herbs. Numerous sources and resources.

Rocky Mountain Herbalist Coalition

PO Box 165
Lyons, CO 80540
Phone: (303) 823-9255

Emphasis on wildcrafting ethics and animal rights.

Society for Economic Botany

PO Box 1897
Lawrence, KS 66044-8897
Phone: (800) 627-0629

International society offering multidisciplinary and scientific research on economically useful plants, including herbs. Members receive *Economic Botany* (a quarterly journal) and *Plants and People* (a quarterly newsletter).

HERB CONSERVATION ORGANIZATIONS

Friends of Echinacea
6101 Shadow Circle Drive
Bozeman, MT 59715
Phone: (406) 585-8006
E-mail: rrr@wtp.net
Website: http://www.wtp.net/~rrr

National Center for the Preservation of Medicinal Herbs
33560 Beech Grove Road
Rutland, OH 45775
Phone and fax: (740) 742-4401
E-mail: tim.blakley@frontiercoop.com

United Plant Savers
PO Box 98
East Barre, VT 05649
Phone: (802) 479-9825
Website: http://www.plantsavers.org

Herb Education Programs

For a more comprehensive list, contact the American Herbalists Guild at the following address and request their directory of herbal education programs ($10).

American Herbalists Guild
PO Box 70
Roosevelt, UT 84066
Phone: (435) 722-8434
E-mail: ahgoffice@earthlink.net
Website: http://www.healthy.net/herbalists

ARIZONA

Southwest School of Botanical Medicine
PO Box 4565
Bisbee, AZ 85603
Phone: (505) 255-9215
Website: http://www.rt66.com/hrbmoore/HOMEPAGE/HomePage.html
Intensive training program, classes, workshops. Catalog available.

CALIFORNIA

Aromatherapy and Herbal Studies
219 Carl Street
San Francisco, CA 94117
Phone: (415) 564-6785
Fax: (415) 564-6799
Classes, workshops, correspondence course. Catalog available.

The California School of Herbal Studies
PO Box 39
Forestville, CA 95436
Phone: (707) 887-7457
Intensive program, classes, workshops. Catalog available.

EastWest School of Herbology
PO Box 712
Santa Cruz, CA 95061
Phone: (800) 717-5010
Fax: (408) 336-4548
Correspondence course, workshops. Catalog available.

Flower Essence Society
PO Box 459
Nevada City, CA 95959
Phone: (800) 736-9222
Fax: (530) 265-6467
Classes, workshops. Catalog available.

The Pacific Institute of Aromatherapy
PO Box 6723
San Rafael, CA 94903
Phone: (415) 479-9121
Fax: (415) 479-0119
Correspondence course, classes, workshops. Catalog available.

Pacific School of Herbal Medicine
PO Box 3151
Oakland, CA 94760
Phone: (510) 845-4028
Classes, workshops. Class listings available.

Therapeutic Herbalism
2068 Ludwig Avenue
Santa Rosa, CA 95407
Phone: (707) 525-9772
Correspondence course.

COLORADO

Rocky Mountain Center for Botanical Studies
PO Box 19254
Boulder, CO 80308-2254
Phone: (303) 442-6861
Intensive training program, classes, workshops. Catalog available.

School of Natural Medicine
PO Box 7369
Boulder, CO 80306-7369
Phone: (303) 443-4882
Fax: (303) 443-8276
E-mail: snm@purehealth.com
Website: http://www.purehealth.com
Correspondence course, classes, workshops. Catalog available.

GEORGIA

Living with Herbs Institute
931 Monroe Drive #102-343

Atlanta, GA 30308
Phone: (404) 607-8222
Classes, workshops. Catalog available.

MASSACHUSETTS

Blazing Star Herbal School
PO Box 6
Shelburne Falls, MA 01370
Phone: (413) 625-6875
Classes, workshops. Catalog available.

MONTANA

Rocky Mountain Herbal Institute
PO Box 579
Hot Springs, MT 59845
Phone: (406) 741-3811
E-mail: rmhi@rmhiherbal.org
Website: http://www.rmhiherbal.org
Chinese medicine. Classes, workshops, correspondence course. Catalog available.

Sweetgrass School of Herbalism
6101 Shadow Circle Drive
Bozeman, MT 59715
Phone: (406) 585-8006
Classes, workshops. Catalog available.

NEW JERSEY

Herbal Therapeutics
PO Box 553
Broadway, NJ 08808
Phone: (908) 835-0822

Fax: (908) 835-0824
E-mail: dwherbal@cencom.net
Intensive training program.

New Mexico

Ayurvedic Institute
PO Box 23445
Albuquerque, NM 87192-1445
Phone: (505) 291-9698
Fax: (505) 294-7572
Correspondence course, classes, workshops.
Catalog available.

National College of Phytotherapy
3030 Isleta SW
Albuquerque, NM 87105
Phone and fax: (505) 452-3468
Training program, classes. Catalog available.

New York

Ayurveda Holistic Center of New York
82-A Bayville Avenue
Bayville, NY 11709
Phone and fax: (516) 628-8200
Website: http://www.ayurvedahc.com
Correspondence course, classes, workshops.
Catalog available.

The New College for Wholistic Health Education and Research
6801 Jericho Turnpike
Syosset, NY 11791-4413
Phone: (516) 364-0808
Fax: (516) 364-0989
Website: http://www.nycollege.edu

Wise Woman Center
PO Box 64
Woodstock, NY 12498
Phone and fax: (914) 246-8081
Correspondence course, classes, workshops.
Catalog available.

Oregon

The Australasian College of Herbal Studies
PO Box 57
Lake Oswego, OR 97034
Phone: (503) 635-6652; (800) 487-8839
Fax: (503) 636-0607
Correspondence course, workshops.
Catalog available.

Utah

The School of Natural Healing
25 West 200 South, #16
Springville, UT 84663
Phone: (801) 489-4254
Fax: (801) 489-8341
Correspondence course, classes, workshops.
Catalog available.

Vermont

Sage Mountain Herbal Center and Native Plant Preserve
Education Department
PO Box 420
East Barre, VT 05649
Phone: (802) 479-9825
Correspondence course, classes, workshops.
Catalog available.

CANADA

Wild Rose College of Natural Healing

1228 Kensington Road, NW, #400
Calgary, Alberta
Canada T2N 4P9
Phone: (403) 270-0936
Fax: (403) 283-0799
Classes, correspondence course. Free catalog.

DEGREE PROGRAMS

Bastyr University

Admissions/Continuing Education
14500 Juanita Drive NE
Bothell, WA 98011
Phone: (425) 602-3070
Fax: (206) 823-6222
Degrees: ND and other degrees.

National College of Naturopathic Medicine

11231 SE Market Street
Portland, OR 97216
Phone: (503) 255-4860
Degree: ND

School of Phytotherapy

Bucksteep Manor, Bodle Street Green
Near Hailsham, East Sussex, UK, BN27 4RJ
Phone: 01323-833-812-4
Fax: 01323-833-869
E-mail: medherb@pavilion.co.uk
Degrees: BS in phytotherapy

Southwest College of Naturopathic Medicine and Health Sciences

2140 East Broadway Road
Tempe, AZ 85282
Phone: (602) 858-9100
Degrees: ND, MA in acupuncture

ETHNOBOTANY PROGRAMS

A comprehensive list of schools offering courses and programs in ethnobotany is available from the *Economic Botany* business office.

Economic Botany

PO Box 368
Lawrence, KS 66044
E-mail: tflaster@rmi.net
Website: http://www.econ.bot.org

Index

About the Herb Research Foundation

The Herb Research Foundation (HRF) is internationally recognized as one of the foremost sources of accurate scientific information in the field of botanical medicine. Founded by Rob McCaleb in 1983 as a nonprofit educational organization, HRF remains dedicated to promoting better world health through the responsible and informed use of herbs. With a focus on public education, HRF provides scientific information on the health benefits and safety of plants to the public, the media, health-care professionals, and legislators. We also advocate plant conservation and cultivation in the United States and abroad, and are actively involved in fostering sustainable botanical agribusiness projects in developing nations. HRF is guided by a professional advisory board composed of 19 of the world's leading medicinal plant experts, as well as a board of directors that helps establish HRF's overall direction.

When HRF was founded, there was no major repository of scientific literature about the use of herbs in health care. For years, we quietly built one of the world's best collections of modern, research-based documentation of the safety and effectiveness of herbs. In the early 1990s, the value of HRF's library resources became critically apparent. As the move for better regulation of herbs began and the U.S. Congress began debating the merits of the Dietary Supplement Health and Education Act (DSHEA), HRF provided—almost overnight—substantial and significant scientific documentation for the safety and efficacy of herbs. Legislators used this research to make informed decisions about supplement regulation. HRF's contribution was instrumental in the eventual passage of DSHEA—the most important and far-reaching piece of legislation passed to date on the regulation of dietary supplements.

As the growth of the American herb industry accelerated, HRF played a major role in helping to keep public opinion about herbs in perspective. At times when most of the publicity about herbs was unfairly negative, HRF provided the media with balanced, unbiased, positive information. Today, HRF reaches more than five million people a month through accurate information that we provide to the media, who call on us frequently for up-to-date herb facts and analysis of current issues.

Keeping our burgeoning library current is an ongoing process that involves working with professional bibliographers, scholars, herbalists, university libraries, botanical centers, inter-library loan services, herb industry members, online databases, and many other sources. To educate the public about herbs is our primary goal, and we are proud of our accomplishments in this area. As herbs are integrated into modern medical practice, HRF remains committed to staying on the forefront of this evolving field. Our work is made possible by our loyal members, whose support enables us to maintain our presence as a rational voice advocating the informed use of herbs.

How Is HRF Funded?

HRF is one of the world's leading specialty libraries of herb information, but unlike public or university libraries, we receive no government funding to help us maintain our collection or pay our overhead. Instead, we rely 100 percent on the support of our members and on our clients, who pay for our research services to fund the continued effort needed to keep our library collection current. Although we must charge for information services, the projects accomplished by our research department cost less than those provided by college libraries, despite the fact that those operations are subsidized by tax dollars.

If the work we do is important to you, please consider becoming an HRF member or making a contribution to one of our many ongoing projects. Please contact us at (303) 449-2265 to discuss membership, special project donations, or planned giving opportunities. HRF memberships and donations are tax deductible to the extent allowed by law.

How Does HRF Provide Herb Information?

Media Contact

Through our ongoing media outreach efforts, HRF staff members provide interviews, written materials, and fact-checking services for numerous media representatives every month. The major television networks, radio stations, magazines, newspapers, and wire services call us when they need facts. Although our name may not appear in every article, there's an excellent chance that HRF was contacted for fast and accurate information.

Publications

In cooperation with the American Botanical Council, HRF co-publishes the quarterly peer-reviewed journal *HerbalGram*, for which Rob McCaleb serves as technical editor. The HRF editorial department also manages the writing, editing, and peer-review process for the Research Reviews section of *HerbalGram*. Rob is also a member of the editorial boards of a number of other popular publications, including *Herbs for Health, Natural Health, Natural Foods Merchandiser,* and *Alternative Therapies in Health and Medicine.* He and other HRF staff members are regular contributors of articles and peer reviews for these and other publications. In addition, HRF publishes its own informative quarterly newsletter, *Herb Research News,* and a variety of other member-services publications, including *TechNotes* and *HerbWorld Update*.

Educational Presentations

HRF employees are frequently invited to make presentations on various herbal topics at conferences, workshops, continuing education courses, and symposia in the United States and around the world. Rob McCaleb is a regular presenter at annual medical continuing education courses sponsored by Columbia University, the University of Arizona, and Harvard Medical School, which are attended by growing numbers of health-care practitioners eager for research-based information on the health benefits and safety of herbs. HRF has also participated in numerous pharmacy education courses. The positive response from health-care practitioners has been strong and consistent. Scientifically validated information about herbs is currently one of the greatest needs of doctors and pharmacists in the rapidly changing world of integrated health care.

The Natural Healthcare Hotline

This unique, interactive telephone service was inspired by the growing public demand for up-to-date facts on the health benefits and safety of herbs. Today, the Hotline's information specialists answer dozens of questions daily from herb consumers, physicians, holistic health-care professionals, pharmacists, researchers, and many others for a nominal fee. Our staff is carefully trained to answer questions without diagnosing, prescribing, or recommending any particular brand or product. To reach the Natural Healthcare Hotline, call (303) 449-2265.

Herb Information Packets

HRF offers more than 180 information packets on single herbs, health conditions, and special herb-related topics. Each contains carefully chosen articles or discussions by experts on herbs and other supplements, and includes easy to understand review articles as well as more technical articles to appeal to a wide audience. This information answers the questions most commonly asked by the public and provides professionals with resources for further research.

Custom Botanical Research

The HRF research department provides current, in-depth botanical information for professional or personal use. Drawing on multiple online databases and a botanical library containing more than 200,000 scientific articles on thousands of herbs, HRF research professionals offer three basic research services: searches of multiple online databases, research by our professional staff in HRF's extensive botanical library, and document retrieval, through which HRF librarians track down and retrieve even hard-to-find articles. The HRF botanical library also contains a substantial collection of data on traditional and worldwide cultural uses of herbs, plus historical, horticultural, production, and marketing information.

Herb Abstracts

For serious researchers, we provide compilations of abstracts from major scientific literature on more than 400 plant genera. These reports include complete bibliographic citations and are arranged alphabetically by author.

Resource Lists

HRF provides resource lists on recommended reading; education programs; herb cultivation and sources of high-quality herbs, extracts or other ingredients; information on choosing herbal products and practitioners; and more.

Worldwide Website

Our award-winning website at www.herbs.org features top research and industry news, a question-and-answer forum, herbal *Greenpapers*, research reviews, online ordering of scientific papers, and other educational features.

OTHER HRF ACTIVITIES

Our strength in the areas of botanical research and education led the Foundation into other projects concerning the production, manufacturing, international trade, and regulation of herbal products. The use of herbs in health care is fostered and limited by a complex interaction of regulatory obstacles and controls, positive and negative press, the influence of legal and medical authorities, and public opinion.

THE REGULATORY ARENA

HRF has played a major role in shifting public opinion of herb use from one of ignorance and misconception to one of growing respectability. The Foundation has been called upon time after time by the U.S. Congress, the Food and Drug Administration, the Federal Trade Commission,

state health departments, the National Institutes of Health, and other agencies to provide expert testimony and documentation on the health benefits and safety of herbs. Rob McCaleb remains active in the regulatory field, having served from 1995 to 1997 on the Commission on Dietary Supplement Labels, and continues to provide testimony and information to the U.S. legislature on botanical regulatory matters.

HERB CONSERVATION AND DEVELOPMENT

Sustainable herb cultivation and conservation of wild medicinal plants are two other important areas of focus for HRF. We are deeply involved in international botanical agribusiness development, helping underprivileged farmers find a niche in the booming worldwide botanical market. These sustainable herb development projects change lives—boosting local economies with earth-friendly agriculture and providing communities with training, jobs, and better access to low-cost botanical medicine. They also provide a source of high-quality organic herbs for the worldwide market. To date, HRF's international development efforts have helped provide a much-needed source of training and income for hundreds of low-income African farming families.

Working in cooperation with the U.S. Department of Agriculture (USDA) and the U.S. Agency for International Development (USAID), HRF provides pre- and post-harvest technical assistance on herb growing and marketing. We also help farmers become proficient in the business aspects of botanical agriculture, from increasing crop quality and yield to finding buyers.

An additional goal of these projects is to protect and preserve native plants that are now endangered due to over collection. Exhaustion of the world's botanical resources threatens not only environmental well-being and diversity, but also the large portions of the world's population who rely on these plants as a part of their traditional medicinal systems. Identification and cultivation of endangered medicinal plants reduces the demand on wild plant populations and helps preserve traditional healing systems by ensuring a continued supply of native medicinal botanicals.

As is so often the case, price and cost dictate how a plant is produced. If it is cheaper to pick a plant from the wild, and if buyers do not insist on cultivated herbs, producers have no incentive to cultivate that plant. Sometimes though, farmers in a less-developed country can afford to compete with distributors of wild-harvested plants from developed countries. For this reason, HRF focuses on developing cultivated, sustainable herb supplies in various geographic and economic areas.

PLEASE JOIN HRF

We invite you to support us in our vital work and to share our vision of better world health through the informed use of herbs. HRF members include consumers, health-care professionals, media representatives, educators, researchers, and herb industry manufacturers from around the world. We all share a common vision: improved world health through the use of herbs, from the medicinal plants of the rain forest to the ones in your own backyard.

Members receive discounts on all HRF services, and more importantly, enable us to continue our essential work. Membership starts at just $35 a year, with many different membership options and categories. Your membership benefits include:

- Subscription to *HerbalGram* or *Herbs for Health* magazines (or both, for an additional $20)
- *Herb Research News*, HRF's informative quarterly newsletter
- A free herb information packet, containing up to 40 pages of practical information about herbs, when you join and each time you renew
- Discounts on custom botanical research and the Natural Healthcare Hotline service
- Additional services, publications, and discounts for higher level members

To join HRF or to receive more information about our services and work, please call, write, or email us:

Herb Research Foundation
1007 Pearl Street, Suite 200
Boulder, Colorado, USA 80302
Phone: (303) 449-2265
Fax: (303) 449-7849
E-mail: info@herbs.org
Website: www.herbs.org

About the Authors

Rob McCaleb is founder and president of the Herb Research Foundation. With more than 20 years of experience in botanical research, Rob has held the position of Research Director for Celestial Seasonings and has served on the Board of Directors of the American Herbal Products Association. He was appointed by President Clinton to the seven-member Commission on Dietary Supplement Labels, and has also served as an advisor to the U.S. Congress, the Office of Dietary Supplements, the Office of Alternative Medicine, and other federal and state agencies. Rob has educated hundreds of doctors and pharmacists through Harvard and Columbia Medical Schools and other continuing medical education programs. He lectures and writes widely on medicinal plants and serves on the editorial boards of a number of popular publications, including the peer-reviewed journal *HerbalGram*.

Evelyn Leigh is a medical writer and botanical specialist with more than 15 years experience writing for health-care professionals and the general public. She is senior writer and editor at the Herb Research Foundation, where she manages the production of HRF's quarterly newsletter, *Herb Research News*, as well as the writing and peer-review process for the Research Reviews section of the journal *HerbalGram*. She is an avid amateur botanist, and in her free time enjoys gardening, hiking, and writing poetry.

Krista Morien received her herbal training at the Rocky Mountain Center for Botanical Studies in Boulder, Colorado, and firsthand from the mountain plants surrounding her home. She has eight years of experience in the natural products field and has written professionally on a variety of health topics. When not at her computer, she enjoys hiking, traveling throughout the West, and writing haiku poetry.